Statistics Workbook for
Evidence-based Health Care

Statistics Workbook for
Evidence-based Health Care

Jennifer Peat
Consultant Biostatistician, Clinical Epidemiologist and Medical Writer
The Children's Hospital at Westmead
Sydney
Australia

Belinda Barton
Head, Children's Hospital Education Research Institute (CHERI)
The Children's Hospital at Westmead and Conjoint
Senior Lecturer
Discipline of Paediatrics and Child Health
Faculty of Medicine
University of Sydney
Sydney
Australia

Elizabeth Elliott
Professor of Paediatrics and Child Health, The University of Sydney
Consultant Paediatrician, The Children's Hospital at Westmead
Practitioner Fellow, National Health and Medical Research
Council of Australia and Director Centre for Evidence Based Paediatrics
Gastroenterology and Nutrition
Sydney
Australia

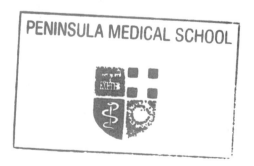
WILEY-BLACKWELL
A John Wiley & Sons, Ltd., Publication

BMJ|Books

This edition first published 2008

BMJ Books is an imprint of BMJ Publishing Group Limited, used under licence by Blackwell Publishing which was acquired by John Wiley & Sons in February 2007. Blackwell's publishing programme has been merged with Wiley's global Scientific, Technical and Medical business to form Wiley-Blackwell.

Registered office: John Wiley & Sons Ltd, The Atrium, Southern Gate, Chichester, West Sussex, PO19 8SQ, UK

Editorial offices: 9600 Garsington Road, Oxford, OX4 2DQ, UK
                       The Atrium, Southern Gate, Chichester, West Sussex, PO19 8SQ, UK
                       111 River Street, Hoboken, NJ 07030-5774, USA

For details of our global editorial offices, for customer services and for information about how to apply for permission to reuse the copyright material in this book please see our website at www.wiley.com/wiley-blackwell

Library of Congress Cataloging-in-Publication Data

Peat, Jennifer K.
Statistics workbook for evidence-based healthcare / Jennifer Peat, Belinda Barton and Elizabeth Elliot.
    p. cm.
   Includes bibliographical references and index.
   ISBN 978-1-4051-4644-9 (pbk. : alk. paper)
   1. Evidence-based medicine--Statistical methods. I. Barton, Belinda. II. Elliott, Elizabeth J. III. Title.
   R723.7.P428 2008
   610.72'7--dc22

                                                                              2008022220

ISBN: 978-1-4051-4644-9

A catalogue record for this book is available from the British Library.
Set in 9.5/12 pt Minion by Newgen Imaging Systems Pvt. Ltd, Chennai, India
Printed and bound in Singapore by COS Printers Pte Ltd

1   2008

Contents

Foreword

Before you read this book, you need to know some definitions. A 'statistic' is just a bit of numerical data. However, 'statistics' is not just a few of these data points put together. It is in fact, "the science and art of dealing with variation in data through collection, classification and analysis in such a way as to obtain reliable results."[1] What makes statistics unique is their ability to quantify uncertainty – to make uncertainty precise![2] Evidence-based health care denotes the integration of the best available evidence from clinical research with clinical expertise in the context of the patient's circumstances and preferences.

In order to practice evidence-based health care, a practitioner must be able to interpret reports of clinical research – and these reports are, of course, filled with statistics. In fact, these reports are filled with more and more statistics. In 1952, a reader of the journal *Pediatrics* who understood descriptive statistics such as means and standard deviations and just three inferential statistics (Student's *t*-test, chi-square and Pearson's *r*) could understand 97% of research articles; by 1982, this level of understanding only applied to 49% of the research articles in *Pediatrics*. By 2005, in order to interpret just 47% of the research in *Pediatrics*, a reader would need to be familiar with 10 of the most common types of statistical procedures.[3] But do not despair; this book will take the reader through all 10 of these procedures, and more.

The best way to learn to understand statistical concepts is to use them. This book is organised around active participation in the learning process. The authors have treated you (the reader) as a participant, not as an observer. The learning objectives for each chapter start with the words, "On completion of this unit, *participants* will be able to . . . ." In each unit, the objectives are clearly stated, the material discussed, and examples provided. The examples are not made up – they are real articles from the health science literature, replete with the complexities that real life presents. The authors also suggest further reading and test your understanding with questions that could also be used in group discussions.

Understanding statistics does not guarantee that you will practice evidence-based health care. However, it does make it considerably more likely that you will recognise the way in which statistics are used and can also at times, mislead. The book *How to Lie with Statistics* was first published over 50 years ago – and it is still very timely![4] Authors of scientific papers are human, after all, and they want to convince both their readers and themselves that their results are important. As readers of the literature, it is our job to critically assess study design, execution and analysis in order to determine whether the results of any given study can be applied to our patients. Therefore, this book also addresses statistics, the analysis, in the context of study design in a concise, easy to understand and learner-friendly format.

Let me suggest that you work through this book before you read another article!

Virginia A. Moyer MD, MPH

[1] Last JM. A dictionary of epidemiology. New York: Oxford University Press, 1983.

[2] Gonick L, Smith W. The cartoon guide to statistics. New York: Harper Collins, 1993.

[3] Hellems MA, Gurka MJ, Hayden GF. Statistical literacy for readers of pediatrics: a moving target. Pediatrics 2007;119:1083–1088.

[4] Huff D. How to Lie With Statistics. New York: W.W. Norton and Company, 1993.

Introduction

"If there were no individual variability, medicine would have been a science not an art." Sir William Osler, 1849–1919. Master physician, writer and inspiring teacher[1]

This book is designed to foster a better understanding of the medical statistics that are frequently used in the reporting of health care research and that underpin evidence-based practice. Learning how to use medical statistics is not a spectator sport and therefore this book is filled with practical hands-on exercises. Although this book is intended for group learning, it could be used equally well as a reference or text book in its own right.

We particularly focus on the interpretation of published results because critical appraisal has become an essential component of evidence-based health care.[2] Critical appraisal is now taught widely to clinicians to improve the evaluation and understanding of research and its translation into individual patient care and health care delivery. To inform these practices, it is crucial to distinguish the results that are believable from the results that are biased because incorrect statistical methods have been used. An understanding of medical statistics is an important part of understanding health care research and this informs provision of better patient care.[3] When critically appraising the literature to decide whether the evidence presented in a journal article is robust enough to warrant a change in clinical practice, or whether a new research study should be designed to collect better evidence, evaluation of the statistics methods that are used is essential.

In analysing research data, the choice of the most appropriate statistic depends on many factors – the study design, the sample size, the type of outcome measurements, the distribution of the measurements in the sample, the purpose of the study and much more. In this book, we draw on the related concepts of research design and medical statistics to help clinicians to incorporate statistical appraisal into evidence-based practice and to help researchers to interpret research results correctly. However, this book is not grounded in the field of clinical epidemiology and we do not explain either the strengths or weaknesses of different study designs or the various methods of participant selection, which are covered in detail in other texts.[4–6]

As clinicians or researchers, we should never lose track of the concept that science is a search for the truth. In this search, there is no place for bias as a result of inappropriate statistical methods or misinterpretation of summary results. The correct use of medical statistics is not only ethical because it leads to the correct interpretation of the data, but is imperative because so much information about how to do research well is now available. We hope that this book will help to bring researchers and clinicians one step closer towards being statistically savvy and critically astute in their reading of the research literature and their interpretation of research results.

References

1. O'Rourke MF. Editorial. William Osler: a model for the 21st century? Med J Aust 1999;171:577–579.
2. Moyer VA, Elliott EJ, *et al.* (eds.) Evidence based pediatrics and child health. BMJ Books 2004 (2nd Edition). London: BMJ Books.
3. Bland JM, Peacock J. Statistical questions in evidence-based medicine. New York: Oxford University Press, 2000.
4. Guyatt GH, Rennie D. Users' guide to the medical literature. Essentials of evidence-based practice. JAMA and Archives Journals, Chicago: AMA Press, 2002.
5. Sackett DL, Haynes RB, Guyatt GJ, Tugwell P. Clinical epidemiology. A basic science for clinical medicine. Boston: Little, Brown and Company, 1991.
6. Peat JK, Mellis CM, Williams K, Xuan W. Study design. Health science research. A handbook of quantitative methods. Crow's Nest, Australia: Allen and Unwin, 2001.

Overview

This book has been designed as either a group or individual learning workbook to promote the concepts of applying medical statistics in either a health care or research context. Each unit in this book contains:

- Specific learning objectives to clearly identify the learning goals.
- Basic information and formulas for key statistical concepts as they relate to evidence-based health care.
- Take home lists of key terms and concepts for easy identification of the fundamental concepts.
- Reprinted journal articles aimed at exposing the reader to a real example of the concepts as presented in the health care literature.

- Worked examples.
- Questions for readers to assess their understanding of concepts and calculations.
- A quick quiz to aid understanding and reinforce concepts.
- Critical appraisal checklists which are designed to assist the reader in evaluating reported research.

The back matter of the book also contains two valuable reader resources:

- A glossary for ready access to the definitions used.
- Answers to the set articles and the quiz in each unit.

UNIT 1

Hypothesis testing and estimation

Aims

To understand how the methods of hypothesis testing and estimation complement one another when deciding whether there are important differences in summary statistics between two or more study groups.

> **Learning objectives**
> On completion of this unit, participants will be able to:
> - understand and interpret P values;
> - describe the meaning of type I and II errors;
> - decide when to use a one-tailed or two-tailed test of significance;
> - estimate and interpret 95% confidence intervals.

Background

In health care research, significance tests are usually conducted to assess whether there is evidence for a real difference in the summary statistics of two or more study groups. The summary statistic may be, for example, the mean of the outcome measurement or a frequency rate. When comparing two or more groups, the probability that the difference between the groups has occurred by chance, which is expressed as a P value, is used to describe the statistical significance of the findings. However, P values convey only part of the information and therefore they should be accompanied by an estimation of the effect size, that is the size of the difference between the study groups that was found.[1] The estimation, which may be a statistic such as the size of the mean difference between two groups, allows readers to assess whether the observed difference is important enough to warrant a change in current health care practice or to warrant further research. Reporting the effect size enables readers to judge whether a statistically significant result is also a clinically important finding.

Hypothesis testing and *P* values

Most medical statistics are based on the concept of hypothesis testing and therefore an associated P value is usually reported. In hypothesis testing, a 'null hypothesis' is first specified, that is a hypothesis stating that there is no difference in the summary statistics of the study groups. In essence, the null hypothesis assumes that the groups that are being compared are drawn from the same population. An alternative hypothesis, which states that there is a difference between groups, can also be specified. The P value, that is, the probability that the difference between the groups would have occurred assuming the null hypothesis was 'true', is then calculated. A P value is obtained by first calculating a test statistic, such as a t-statistic or a chi-square value, which is then compared to a known distribution. The known distribution is used to determine the probability that the observed test statistic value (or a more extreme value) would occur, if the null hypothesis were true. In the following units in this book, the calculation and interpretation of the most commonly used test statistics will be explored.

A P value of less than 0.05, that is a probability of less than 1 chance in 20, is usually accepted as being statistically significant. If a P value is less than 0.05, we accept that it is unlikely that a difference between groups has occurred by chance if the null hypothesis was true. In this situation, we reject the null hypothesis and accept the alternative hypothesis, and therefore conclude that there is a statistically significant difference between the groups. On the other hand, if the P value is greater than or equal to 0.05 and therefore the probability with which the test statistic occurs is greater than 1 chance in 20, we accept that the difference between groups has occurred by chance. In this case, we accept the null hypothesis and conclude that there is no difference between the study groups beyond variations that can be attributed to sampling.

In accepting or rejecting a null hypothesis, it is important to remember that the P value only provides a probability value and does not provide absolute proof that the null hypothesis is true or false. A P value obtained from a test of significance should only be interpreted as a measure of the strength of evidence against the null hypothesis.[2] The smaller the P value, the stronger the evidence provided by the data that the null hypothesis can be rejected. Thus, P values of 0.01 or lower are conventionally regarded as being highly significant because they indicate that it is highly unlikely that the difference between groups has occurred by chance. Although the cut-off point between statistical significance and non-significance is generally accepted as a P value of less than 0.05, it is important to remember that P values of 0.07 and 0.04 indicate very similar strengths of evidence even though a P value of 0.07 is conventionally regarded as being non-significant and a P value of 0.04 as being statistically significant. To convey the strength of evidence rather than using pre-conceived arbitrary categories, actual P values should be reported, for example $P = 0.04$ rather than $P < 0.05$ and $P = 0.63$ rather than NS (not significant).

In measuring between-group effects, the absolute magnitude of the difference between the groups and the direction of the effect are not conveyed by the P value. Thus, when P values alone are reported, the results can only be interpreted as probability values that indicate statistical significance with no regard for the clinical importance of the result. A P value that is larger than 0.05 does not necessarily mean that the treatments or the groups that are being compared are similar, because the P value depends on both the size of difference between the groups and on the sample size.[3] By only using P values, it is not possible to answer questions of how confident we are, given the study results, that a treatment is beneficial or has no effect, or how much better we expect patients to become if they receive a new treatment.[4, 5] For this, we need an estimation of the size of the effect in addition to significance tests.

Estimation

In health care research, rather than enrolling an entire population in a study, which would usually be impractical, a sample of the population is usually selected and then statistics are used to make inferences about the entire population. When using estimation, a summary statistic is calculated that describes the effect size in the sample, together with a margin of precision around the statistic that depends on the size of the sample that was enrolled. Estimation allows us to make judgements on the certainty, or uncertainty, of summary statistics calculated from a sample, and therefore to make inferences about the population from which the sample was drawn.

When comparing two study groups, estimation involves calculating the actual size of the difference between the groups in addition to a P value. A limitation in the interpretation of P values is that they are heavily influenced by the sample size. Although P values provide a measure of the strength of evidence, they convey only a small part of the total information about the effectiveness of a treatment in clinical research or about differences between population samples in epidemiological studies. In a clinical study, the outcome of interest may be, for example, a difference in mean lung function measurements or a per cent reduction in

symptoms between groups receiving a new treatment compared to a standard treatment (control). These types of summary statistics indicate how much patients could expect their lung function to increase or their symptoms to improve if they received the new treatment compared to if they received the standard treatment. As such, the summary statistics quantify the actual effect of the new treatment in a way that complements the probability that the difference between groups arose by chance.

TAKE HOME LIST

- A P value indicates the strength of evidence against the null hypothesis.

- A P value of less than 0.05 indicates that there is a statistically significant difference between the study groups.

- Smaller P values provide stronger evidence that the null hypothesis is false.

- The actual P value, for example, $P = 0.04$ or $P = 0.56$, should be reported.

- A limitation of P values is that they only describe a probability and the statistical significance of a between-group difference.

- P values are strongly influenced by the sample size. The larger the sample size the more likely a difference between study groups will be statistically significant.

- Estimation provides an effect size between groups that complements the P value.

Confidence intervals

Confidence intervals are important in estimation in that they describe the precision around a summary statistic, such as a difference between study groups.[5] There is error in all estimates of effect because it is unlikely that the measured effect would be the same when a study is repeated in different random samples of the population. When different groups of people are sampled, variations in summary statistics occur simply because there is a large amount of inherent variation in human characteristics.

The confidence interval provides an estimated range of values that is likely to include the population value. The interpretation of a 95% confidence interval is that 95% of the confidence intervals calculated from many different samples would include the true value of the summary statistic that occurs in the population.[6] A simpler and perhaps more intuitive way to interpret a 95% confidence interval is that we can be roughly 95% certain, or confident, that the true value of the summary statistic in the population is within the 95% confidence interval calculated from a single study sample. Thus, confidence intervals provide an estimate of precision, or rather lack of precision, which can be attributed to sampling variation. In Unit 2, we explain how 95% confidence intervals for differences between study groups are calculated and show how these intervals can be used to make statistical inferences about differences between groups, sometimes without the need for computing a P value at all.

Confidence intervals are calculated from the standard error (SE), which is an estimate of the precision with which a summary statistic has been measured. The standard error can be used to calculate a 95% confidence interval as follows:

95% confidence interval = summary statistic ± (1.96 × SE)

In this calculation, the summary statistic may be a value such as a mean value, a percentage or an odds ratio and the SE is the standard error around the summary value. A critical value of 1.96, which is derived from the normal population distribution of the summary statistic, is used to compute 95% intervals when the group or sample size is larger than 50 participants. If the sample size is smaller than 50, a larger critical value than 1.96 that can be derived from a statistical table should be used.[6]

It is important to remember that a 95% confidence interval only applies to populations with the same characteristics as the population from which the data were sampled.[6] However, a 95% confidence interval provides important information over and above the P value. This is especially important when the P value is greater than 0.05 because a judgement about the clinical importance of the difference that has been measured can be made by assessing the width of the 95% confidence interval. As might be expected, the P values and confidence intervals from any study are closely related to one another. In most cases, if the value of the null hypothesis, for example a value equal to 0, falls within the 95% confidence interval then the P value will be greater than 0.05.[6]

When critically appraising the literature, it is important to calculate 95% confidence intervals if they are not reported. Although 95% confidence intervals for mean values are calculated from the standard error, which describes the precision around the mean value, the only descriptor of variance that is often reported is the standard deviation (SD), which describes the distribution of the spread or the variation of the actual data points. In describing the error and spread around a mean value, the terms standard error and standard deviation have important distinctions[7] and for this reason they are explained in more detail in Unit 6. To calculate 95% confidence intervals, the standard deviation around a mean value can easily be converted into a standard error as follows:

Standard error (SE) = SD/$\sqrt{n}$

where n is the sample size of the group from which the mean and the standard deviation were estimated.

As can be seen from the formula, the standard error is inversely related to the square root of the sample size. Thus, the standard error becomes smaller as the sample size increases. As the sample size becomes larger, the width of the 95% confidence interval for the same effect becomes smaller, indicating greater certainty in the precision of the result. On the other hand, as the sample size becomes smaller, the standard error becomes larger and thus the width of the 95% confidence interval becomes wider, indicating less certainty in the precision of the result. The above methods for estimating and calculating 95% confidence intervals apply to all summary statistics. The calculation of standard errors and the 95% confidence interval for proportions, for example incidence and prevalenvce rates, and for odds ratios are discussed in the following units.

Glossary	
Term	**Definition**
Null hypothesis	A hypothesis stating that there is no difference between the study groups.
P value	Probability that a difference between study groups would have occurred if the null hypothesis was true.
95% confidence interval	Range in which we can be approximately 95% certain that the true population value lies.

Type I and II errors

Confidence intervals clearly show the lack of precision around an estimate but, when only a P value is calculated, the degree of uncertainty about whether the null hypothesis should be accepted or rejected is easily overlooked. Obviously if a P value is very small, say less than 0.01, then the probability that the groups have been sampled from the same population is quite unlikely and we can be confident that there is a real difference. Similarly if the P value is large, say over 0.1, then we can be confident that there is no difference between the groups beyond sampling variation.

When testing between-group differences, the P value is closely related to the sample size. Thus, the larger the sample size, the smaller the P value will be for the same summary statistic, such as a mean difference between groups. The P value is smaller when the sample size is large because the summary statistic represents a more accurate estimate of the true value in the population from which the sample is drawn. Thus, the P value depends on both the size of the summary statistic and on the sample size. Therefore it is important to consider how the clinical importance of a difference (that is, the actual magnitude of the difference between groups) compares with the statistical significance (that is, the P value which is dependent on sample size). The decision about the size of difference between groups that is considered clinically important depends solely on expert knowledge and can only be made by health care practitioners and researchers with experience in the field.

When accepting or rejecting a null hypothesis it is possible that a type I or type II error has occurred. A 'type I error' occurs when the null hypothesis is incorrectly rejected. That is, it is concluded that there is a statistically significant difference between groups when no clinically important difference exists. The probability of a type I error occurring is reported as the P value. With a P value of 0.05, there is a chance of 5 in 100 or 1 in 20 that the significant results occurred by chance alone. So for every 20 statistical tests that are conducted, one test will be significant by chance alone. Type I errors frequently occur when data is repeatedly analysed, when there are multiple comparisons or multiple outcomes.

A 'type II error' occurs when the null hypothesis is incorrectly accepted. That is, it is concluded that there is no statistically significant difference between groups when a clinically important difference exists. The probability of avoiding a type II error is referred to as the power of the study, that is, the probability of correctly rejecting the null hypothesis. Type II errors typically occur when the sample size is too small for a clinically important difference to reach statistical significance. Because both type I and II errors are a product of the sample size, the risk of a type I error is reduced when the sample size becomes smaller but the risk of a type II error increases.

Although the occurrence of type I and II errors is usually related to the sample size, the consequences of these two types of errors are very different. For example, if a type I error occurs in a clinical trial then a new treatment will be incorrectly judged to be more effective than the control

over the control treatment even though many people who receive the new treatment will experience beneficial effects. Type I and II errors not only have clinical implications for interpretation of summary statistics but also have ethical implications. If the sample size is too small, the study may be unethical because too few participants are enrolled than are needed to test the study hypothesis, and therefore research

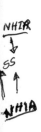

> ### TAKE HOME LIST
>
> - As the sample size increases, the width of the 95% confidence interval becomes smaller, indicating greater certainty in the precision of the result.
>
> - Summary statistics and their 95% confidence intervals should be reported, together with P values, to indicate the absolute size of the difference between the groups and the direction of effect.
>
> - Type I and II error rates are inversely related because both are influenced by sample size – when the risk of a type I error is reduced, the risk of a type II error is increased.

resources will also be wasted. If the sample size is too large, the study may be unethical because more participants are enrolled than are needed to test the study hypothesis and research resources will also be wasted. For these reasons, ethics committees often request that a statistician is consulted when a study is being designed to ensure that the probability of type I and II errors is minimised.

One-tailed and two-tailed tests of significance

The calculation of a P value is influenced by the expected direction of difference between study groups, which is generally specified as the alternative hypothesis. When the difference between two study groups is expected to occur in one direction only, for example when a group of people receiving one treatment could only show greater improvements than a group receiving another treatment, a one-tailed (or one-sided) test of significance is used. For one-tailed t-tests, the probability of the test statistic value or one more extreme occurring in only one direction, such as occurring in only the upper tail of the distribution, is calculated.

When the difference between two study groups is expected to occur in either direction, for example when a group of people receiving one treatment could show a larger or smaller improvement than a group receiving another treatment, a two-tailed (or two-sided) test of significance is used. For two-tailed tests, the probability of the test statistic occurring in either the upper or lower tail of the distribution is calculated. Since one-tailed tests involve calculating the probability using only one tail of the distribution of the test statistic, the P value is reduced by half so that it is more significant than when both tails are used in a two-sided test.

Glossary	
Term	**Definition**
Type I error	When the null hypothesis is incorrectly rejected. That is, a difference between groups is statistically significant although a clinically important difference does not exist.
Type II error	When the null hypothesis is incorrectly accepted. That is, a difference between groups is not statistically significant although a clinically important difference exists.

group treatment. If the new treatment is more expensive or has more severe side effects, recommendation of the new treatment will not confer benefit on average but will have an adverse impact on people to whom it is recommended. On the other hand, if a type II error occurs, the new treatment will be incorrectly judged to have no advantage

In most health care research studies, the use of one-tailed tests is rarely justified because we should expect that a result could be in either direction. It is most unusual for researchers to be certain about the direction of effect before the study is conducted and, if they were, the study would probably not need to be conducted at all.[7] For this reason, one-tailed statistics are rarely used. A search of the abstracts published in the *British Medical Journal* between 1994 and 2006 found only one study in thirteen years in which the results were described using a one-tailed significance test. If a one-tailed *P* value is reported, the *P* value can easily be converted into a two-tailed (or two-sided) value by doubling its numerical value.

In the vast majority of studies, two-tailed tests of significance are used unless there is a very good reason for not doing so.[9] In health care research, it is almost always important to allow for the possibility that extreme results could occur by chance and could occur equally often in either direction, which in clinical trials would mean towards a beneficial or towards an adverse effect. Two-tailed tests provide a more conservative result than one-tailed tests in that the *P* value is higher, that is, less significant. In this way, two-tailed tests reduce the chance that a between-group difference is declared statistically significant in error, and thus that a new treatment is incorrectly accepted as being more effective than an existing treatment. A conservative approach is essential because no health care practice should be modified on the basis of results that have arisen entirely by chance.

Reading and questions
Reprint
Berry G. Statistical significance and confidence intervals. Med J Aust 1986;144:618–619. (See p. 7.)

After reading Unit 1 and the reprint by Berry (1986) answer the following questions:

1 Can 95% confidence intervals be used to infer *P* values and vice versa?   *yes but not ver versa*
2 When might a significance test fail to detect a real effect?
   Type I   Small SS →
   error

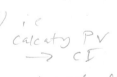

1) ic
calcaty PV
→ CI
whe cant calcu pv
but can have CI

3 When is the null hypothesis value outside the 95% confidence interval?
4 What type of error occurs when a difference between groups is not statistically significant but is large enough to be thought clinically important?   *Type II*
5 Who decides what size of difference between groups is clinically important?   *Medics*

Non sigtance P > 0.05

Worked example
Set article
Logroscino G, Kang, JH, Grodstein F. Prospective study of type 2 diabetes and cognitive decline in women aged 70–81 years. BMJ (Published 23 February 2004). (See p. 10.)

In the set article by Logroscino *et al.* (2004) the authors refer to Table 2 and state that "On every cognitive test, means baseline scores were lower for women with diabetes". Review this table and decide how this conclusion was reached.

- What statistical test was used?   *mean ;   scors*
- What do the authors mean by "lower"?   *by mean scores*
- Have the authors used hypothesis testing or estimation to reach this conclusion?   *NO*
- What is the size of the difference between groups and is it clinically important?   *little*
- Was there a type I or type II error?   *Type I ⓐ No pise A by chance*
- Would you reach the same conclusion?   *NO   Lack from line to Prefer score*

27/11/2018

Exercise

The standard deviation around each estimate in Table 2 from Logroscino *et al.* (2004) is easily converted first into an SE and then to a 95% confidence interval. In Table 1.1, calculate the SE and 95% confidence intervals for the participants with diabetes.

After completing the new estimations in Table 1.1 decide:
- What factors influence the 95% confidence intervals and in what way?
- Why are the confidence intervals so narrow?   *Larg Smpl √N*

Table 1.1 Mean and 95% CI cognitive scores at baseline in 1394 women with type 2 diabetes

	N	Mean	SD	SE	Lower 95% CI	Upper 95% CI
TICS (8–41 points)	1394	33.2	2.9	0.08	33.1	33.4
TICS 10 word list	1394	2.0	1.9	0.05	1.9	2.1
East Boston memory test – immediate recall	1394	9.3	1.8	0.05	9.2	9.4
East Boston memory test – delayed recall	1394	8.9	2.1	0.06 / 0.12	8.78 / 8.8	9.02

Table 1.2 Mean and 95% CI cognitive scores at baseline in 50 women with type 2 diabetes

	N	Mean	SD	SE	Lower 95% CI	Upper 95% CI
TICS (8–41 points)	50	33.2	2.9	0.41	32.4	34.0
TICS 10 word list	50	2.0	1.9			
East Boston memory test – immediate recall	50	9.3	1.8			
East Boston memory test – delayed recall	50	8.9	2.1			

Next calculate the SE and 95% confidence intervals if the sample comprised only 50 participants, rather than the enrolled number of 1394.

After completing the new estimations in Table 1.2 decide:

- What happens to the 95% confidence intervals when the sample size is smaller?
- Why does this happen?

Quick quiz

Tick the correct answer for each of the following questions.

1 A 95% confidence interval is:
(a) the range in which a mean value falls approximately 95% of the time;
(b) the range in which 95% of the study observations can be expected to lie;
(c) the range in which we are 95% certain that the true population value lies;
(d) the range calculated as the mean ± 1.96 standard deviations and which excludes 5% of the sample.

2 A type II error occurs when:
(a) a statistician makes an error in calculating a P value;
(b) an important difference between groups has a P value that is larger than 0.05;
(c) a clinically important effect is unlikely to have occurred by chance;
(d) a new treatment proves more effective than was thought when the sample size was calculated.

3 Two-tailed tests of significance are used because:
(a) that is what statisticians recommend as standard practice;
(b) statisticians are often unsure of what the study results will show;

(c) all studies have some degree of sampling variation that affects the results;
(d) a new treatment could turn out to be better or worse than the control treatment.

4 An estimation of the difference between study groups provides important information that is additional to a P value because:
(a) it conveys the size of the difference of effect between the groups;
(b) it provides a more reliable summary statistic;
(c) it conveys how well the new treatment works;
(d) it is an essential component of evidence-based practice.

References

1. Altman DG. Estimation or hypothesis testing? In: Practical statistics for medical research. London: Chapman & Hall, 1996; pp 174–175.
2. Bland JM. Principles of significance tests. In: An introduction to medical statistics. Oxford: Oxford University Press, 1996; p 136.
3. Freiman JA, Chalmers TC, Smith H, Keubler RR. The importance of the beta, the type II error and sample size in the design and interpretation of the randomised controlled trial. Survey of 71 "negative" trials. N Engl J Med 1978;299:690–694.
4. Shakespeare TP, Gebski VJ, Veness MJ, Simes J. Improving interpretation of clinical studies by use of confidence levels, clinical significance curves, and risk-benefit contours. Lancet 2001;357:1349–1353.
5. Gardner MJ, Altman DG. Confidence intervals rather than P values: estimation rather than hypothesis testing. BMJ (Clin Res Ed) 1986;292:746–750.
6. Bland JM, Peacock J. Interpreting statistics with confidence. TOG 2002;4:176–180.
7. Altman DG, Bland JM. Standard deviations and standard errors. BMJ 2005;331:903.
8. Altman DG. Two-sided or one-sided P values? In: Practical statistics for medical research. London: Chapman & Hall, 1996; pp 170–171.
9. Bland JM, Altman DG. One and two sided tests of significance. BMJ 1994;309:248.

Statistical significance and confidence intervals

Geoffrey Berry

Many papers in the Journal use statistical methods and one of the aims of the review process is to try to ensure that appropriate methods have been used. Often papers report results of comparative studies that are designed to answer questions such as whether one treatment is superior to another for a particular disease, or whether there is an association between some form of behaviour (for example, taking regular exercise or smoking) and the occurrence of some disease. Comparative studies are almost invariably carried out on a *sample* of individuals who are chosen from the *population* of individuals to whom it is intended to generalize the results. Data are collected on the sample in order to make inferences on the population. Valid inferences can only be drawn if the sample is chosen in such a way that it is representative of the population. Otherwise a bias could occur; epidemiological methods are designed to eliminate such biases.

Since the aim of a statistical analysis is to make inferences, it is paramount to express whatever inferences that can be drawn in the most informative way. There are several methods of statistical inference, but the two that are most commonly used are significance testing and confidence interval estimation. The former is well known and is featured by quoting *P* values. Many authors appear to be under the impression that a profusion of *P* values is necessary; regrettably this impression has been bolstered in the past by editors of biological journals. Significance testing has its place but, as mentioned by Healy in 1978,[1] "it is widely agreed among statisticians (if less so among the more naive users of statistics) that significance testing is not the be-all and end-all of the subject". In this leading article I would like to discuss the characteristics of both methods of inference, show that a confidence interval contains the result of a significance test, but not vice versa, and suggest that confidence intervals are the answers to the more interesting questions that data can be used to answer.

Any particular study is based on a particular sample; however, it is useful to imagine that the study is repeated with a different sample being selected each time. These hypothetical studies will give different results, because they contain different individuals, and individuals vary in any characteristic because of biological variability. The differences are termed *sampling variability*. It follows then that the results that are obtained from a particular sample

Associate Professor of Biostatistics, School of Public Health and Tropical Medicine The University of Sydney

can only be taken as an approximation to the actual situation in the whole population. Statistical methods are concerned with assessing the degree of approximation and what may be reasonably inferred, given that a different sample would have produced a different result.

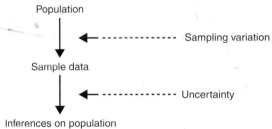

The methods are based on the assumption that it is a matter of chance which particular subjects are in the sample that is being studied, and the sampling variability is thus random variation which is determined by the laws of probability. Therefore, the inferences are expressed in terms of probability. The situation is illustrated below.

Taking a sample from the population involves sampling variation. As a consequence of this, inferences from the sample data back to the population involve uncertainty.

A statistical analysis may be thought of as asking questions of the data. In an investigation that compares two groups for the mean value of, for example, blood pressure or the prevalence of some disease, three questions may be posed: Is there a difference between the groups?; How large is the difference?; and How accurately is the size of the difference known?

As expressed, the first question expects the answer "yes" or "no"; although the answer cannot be given in precisely these terms, it is often reduced to two possibilities. The appropriate methodology is the *significance test*. The second question expects a numerical value to be the answer. This is an estimate and, as it is a single value, is referred to as a *point estimate*. In effect, the third question asks how reliable this point estimate is; the answer is a range of values which is referred to as an *interval estimate* or a *confidence interval*.

These questions represent two approaches to inference: hypothesis testing and estimation. Although at first sight they appear to be quite different, in concept they have much in common. Both make inferential statements about the value of a parameter. (A parameter is an unknown quantity which partly or wholly characterizes a population, for example, a mean or a measure of association.)

Originally published in *MJA* 1986; **144**: 618–19. Reproduced with permission.

The significance test is an appropriate technique when there is an a priori hypothesis to test. For the purpose of the statistical test this hypothesis is expressed in *null* form — such as when no difference exists between groups — and the test evaluates whether the data are consistent with the null hypothesis. If the data differ markedly from those which would be expected under the null hypothesis, to the extent that the probability of such an extreme result is low, then it is said that the result is statistically significant. Probability is measured on a continuum between 0 and 1, but in significance testing a probability is considered low if it is less than conventional values such as 0.05 (5%) or 0.01 (1%). A significant result is equated with the rejection of the null hypothesis or the claim of a real effect. By definition, when the null hypothesis is true, significant results will occur by chance with the same relative frequency as the significance probability. That is, real effects will be claimed when the null hypothesis is true; however, the probability of this error (type 1) is determined in the data analysis.

One disadvantage of a significance test is that it may fail to detect a real effect; that is, although the null hypothesis is false, the evidence is not strong enough to reject it. The probability of this error (type II) can be controlled at the design stage only, by appropriate selection of the sample size, and may be quite large. Thus, the trap of equating non-significance with no effect must be avoided; failure to reject the null hypothesis is not the same as accepting it.

In the approach of confidence interval estimation no particular hypothesis is considered; rather, the emphasis is on estimating those values of the parameter with which the data are consistent. These values form a range — the confidence interval. The range is calculated so that there is a high probability — conventionally 95% or 99% — that it contains the true value of the parameter.

A significance test is essentially a test of whether the data are consistent with a specified parameter value, and the confidence interval contains those parameter values with which the data are consistent. Therefore, a 5% significance test and a 95% confidence interval contain some information in common: significance implies that the null hypothesis value is outside the confidence interval; non-significance implies that the null hypothesis value is within the confidence interval. However, the confidence interval contains more information because it is equivalent to performing a significance test for all values of the parameter, not just a single value. A confidence interval enables a reader to see how large the effect may be, not simply whether it is different from zero.

The limitations of the interpretations that are provided by a significance test may now be considered.

The difference is significant. This means that there is a difference or, in other words, the size of the difference is not zero. We know no more than this. The difference may be large and of great importance or it may be small and of no practical importance. It is unsatisfactory that the test provides no way of distinguishing between these quite different possibilities.

The difference is not significant. This means that there is insufficient evidence to enable us to conclude that there is a difference. So the difference may well be zero. But this is not the same as saying that it is zero. The true difference may be quite large. Again, it is unsatisfactory that this possibility is not addressed.

The conclusions that may be drawn from a significance test are considered to be incomplete because it is rarely that one is interested solely in whether a null hypothesis is or is not true; indeed in many cases it may be recognized at the outset that the null hypothesis is unlikely to be true. Rather, the question is how large is the difference and is it possibly large enough to be important? The emphasis is on measuring rather than on testing. The addition of the concept of an important difference to that of a null hypothesis means that there are four possible interpretations to an analysis: (a) the difference is significant and large enough to be of practical importance; (b) the difference is significant but too small to be of practical importance; (c) the difference is not significant but may be large enough to be important; and (d) the difference is not significant and also not large enough to be of practical importance.

The size of difference that is considered to be large enough to be important is a matter for debate, and genuine differences of opinion may arise. It is a medical, not a statistical, question, although a medical statistician who is experienced in the subject area could contribute to setting a value. The fact that agreement on a unique value may be impossible in no way detracts from the argument. In fact, expressing the results as a confidence interval enables interpretations to be made for any particular value that is considered appropriate.

These possibilities are illustrated in the Figure where the confidence intervals are shown. The significant and

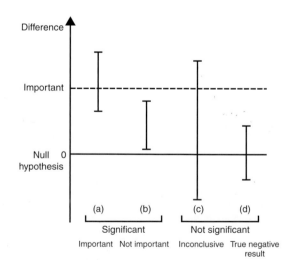

Figure Confidence intervals showing four possible conclusions in terms of statistical significance and practical importance.

Originally published in *MJA* 1986; **144**: 618–19. Reproduced with permission.

non-significant cases are distinguished by the confidence intervals that exclude or include zero respectively. The main point is that in each case the confidence interval gives the range of possible values for the true difference. Of particular concern is (c). Here there may be no true difference or there may be a large, important difference. In other words the study is completely inconclusive. Such a possibility is missed by the simple expression "not significant" with its lure of equating this falsely with "no effect". This situation will arise with a study that is carried out on too small a sample and this is why good study design demands attention to sample size to try to prevent the occurrence of an inconclusive result. Altman found that it was common for undue emphasis to be placed on "negative" findings from small studies,[2] while Freimen et al. noted that "negative" trials were often too small to constitute a fair test of therapies.[3] Similarly, a significance test will contrast (b) as significant and (d) as not significant but fails to recognize that they give essentially the same conclusion — that any difference is too small to be important.

As an example, consider some results which were obtained by Garraway et al. from a clinical trial for the management of acute stroke in the elderly.[4] Of 155 patients who were managed in a stroke unit, 78 were assessed as independent when they were discharged from the unit compared with 49 of 152 who were managed in a medical unit. The simplest analysis shows that the difference between the success rates of the two units is significant at the 1% level. Therefore, a genuine effect has been established. To appreciate the importance of this effect the advantage of the stroke unit may be measured by the difference between the two units in the percentage of subjects who were discharged as independent: 50.3% − 32.2% = 18.1%. This is the point estimate. The accuracy of this estimate is given by its standard error (5.5) and the 95% confidence limits (7.3% and 28.9%). Thus, the gain could be as large as 29% or as small as 7%.

Recently, Gardner and Altman have argued against the excessive use of hypothesis testing and urged a greater use of confidence intervals.[5] In an appendix to their paper they give methods to calculate confidence intervals for the commonly occurring two-sample comparisons.

In presenting the main results of a study it is good practice to provide confidence intervals rather than to restrict the analysis to significance tests. Only by so doing can authors give readers sufficient information for a proper conclusion to be drawn; otherwise readers have to rely upon the authors' own interpretation.[2] Therefore, intending authors are urged to express their main conclusions in confidence interval form (possibly with the addition of a significance test, although strictly that would provide no extra information). One of the aims of the Journal's statistical review process will be to ensure that where possible this is done.

References

1 Healy MJR. Is statistics a science? *J R Statist Soc A* 1978; 141: 385–393.
2 Altman DG. Statistics in medical journals. *Stat Med* 1982; 1: 59–71.
3 Freiman JA, Chalmers TC, Smith H Jr, Kuebler RR. The importance of beta, the type II error and sample size in the design and interpretation of the randomized control trial. *N Engl J Med* 1978; 299: 690–694.
4 Garraway WM, Akhtar AJ, Prescott RJ, Hockey L. Management of acute stroke in the elderly: preliminary results of a controlled trial. *Br Med J* 1980; 280: 1040–1043.
5 Gardner MJ, Altman DG. Confidence intervals rather than P values: estimation rather than hypothesis testing. *Br Med J* 1986; 292: 746–750.

Prospective study of type 2 diabetes and cognitive decline in women aged 70–81 years

Giancarlo Logroscino, Jae Hee Kang, Francine Grodstein

Abstract

Objective   To examine the association of type 2 diabetes with baseline cognitive function and cognitive decline over two years of follow up, focusing on women living in the community and on the effects of treatments for diabetes.

Design   Nurses' health study in the United States. Two cognitive interviews were carried out by telephone during 1995–2003.

Participants   18 999 women aged 70–81 years who had been registered nurses completed the baseline interview; to date, 16 596 participants have completed follow up interviews after two years.

Main outcome measures   Cognitive assessments included telephone interview of cognitive status, immediate and delayed recalls of the East Boston memory test, test of verbal fluency, delayed recall of 10 word list, and digit span backwards. Global scores were calculated by averaging the results of all tests with z scores.

Results   After multivariate adjustment, women with type 2 diabetes performed worse on all cognitive tests than women without diabetes at baseline. For example, women with diabetes were at 25–35% increased odds of poor baseline score (defined as bottom 10% of the distribution) compared with women without diabetes on the telephone interview of cognitive status and the global composite score (odds ratios 1.34, 95% confidence interval 1.14 to 1.57, and 1.26, 1.06 to 1.51, respectively). Odds of poor cognition were particularly high for women who had had diabetes for a long time (1.52, 1.15 to 1.99, and 1.49, 1.11 to 2.00, respectively, for ≥15 years' duration). In contrast, women with diabetes who were on oral hypoglycaemic agents performed similarly to women without diabetes (1.06 and 0.99), while women not using any medication had the greatest odds of poor performance (1.71, 1.28 to 2.281, and 1.45, 1.04 to 2.02) compared with women without diabetes. There was also a modest increase in odds of poor cognition among women using insulin treatment. All findings were similar when cognitive decline was examined over time.

Conclusions   Women with type 2 diabetes had increased odds of poor cognitive function and substantial cognitive decline. Use of oral hypoglycaemic therapy, however, may ameliorate risk.

Introduction

Several population based studies have shown that type 2 diabetes increases the risk of dementia.[1–5] Cognitive decline is an intermediate stage between normal ageing and dementia.[6] As dementia may be most effectively delayed in its initial stages, identifying diabetes as a modifiable risk factor for early cognitive decline could be of major public health importance. Estimates in the United States indicate that delaying onset of dementia by one year could lead to 800 000 fewer cases after 50 years.[7]

Though many investigations have examined diabetes in relation to early cognitive decline,[5,8–19] only one large prospective study has focused on women.[8] Type 2 diabetes disproportionately affects older women and is a stronger risk factor for cardiovascular disease in women than in men.[20] As cardiovascular disease is an independent risk factor for cognitive decline, we need to determine the impact of diabetes on cognition in women.[20] Moreover, few studies have evaluated the influence of different treatments for diabetes on the association between type 2 diabetes and cognition.

We assessed the associations between type 2 diabetes, different treatments for diabetes, and cognitive function in more than 16 000 women.

doi 10.1136/bmj.37977.495729.EE

Department of Epidemiology, Harvard School of Public Health, Boston, MA 02115, USA

Giancarlo Logroscino *associate professor of neuroepidemiology*

Channing Lab, Department of Medicine, Brigham and Women's Hospital, Harvard Medical School, Boston

Francine Grodstein *associate professor of medicine*
Jae Hee Kang *instructor of medicine*

Correspondence to: G Logroscino
(email: glogrosc@hsph.harvard.edu)

(*Accepted 27 November 2003*)

Originally published in *BMJ* 2004; **328**. Reproduced with permission.

Methods

The nurses' health study is a prospective cohort of 121 700 US female registered nurses, who were aged 30–55 years in 1976, when the study began. Participants' health information has been updated with biennial mailed questionnaires. Over 90% of the original cohort have been followed up to date.

From 1995–2001, participants aged 70 years and older who had not had a stroke were given baseline cognitive assessments by telephone. Overall, 93% completed the interview. Interviewers were blinded to participants' health status (including diabetes). For the baseline analyses of cognitive function, we included 18 999 women with complete information on education and without type 1 diabetes, gestational diabetes, or unconfirmed diabetes (see below).

The follow up cognitive assessment began about two years after the baseline interview. After the exclusion of the 3% who died, calls have been attempted for 98% to date. Of these, 92% (n = 16 596) completed the interview, 5% (n = 967) refused, 3% (n = 526) were unreachable. For analyses of cognitive decline, we included 16 596 participants who completed both assessments and excluded women in whom diabetes had been newly diagnosed between the baseline and second interviews.

Assessment of cognitive function

Our cognitive assessment has been previously described.[21] Briefly, we initially administered only the telephone interview for cognitive status (TICS) (n = 18 999)[22] but gradually added more tests: immediate (n = 18 295) and delayed recalls of the East Boston memory test (n = 18 268), test of verbal fluency (naming animals, n = 18 285), digit span backwards (n = 16 591), and delayed recall of a 10 word list (n = 16 582). To summarise performance, we calculated a global score averaging results of the six tests using z scores (16 563 women completed all six tests).

We have established high validity (r = 0.81 comparing the global score from our telephone interview to an in-person exam) and high reliability (r = 0.70 for two administrations of the TICS, 31 days apart)[21] for these telephone interviews in highly educated women.

Ascertainment of type 2 diabetes

We identified women who reported that diabetes had been diagnosed by a physician before the baseline cognitive interview. We then confirmed reports based on responses to a supplementary questionnaire including complications, diagnostic tests, and treatment; confirmations conformed to guidelines of the National Diabetes Data Group[23] until 1997, and revised criteria of the American Diabetes Association from 1998.[24] Validation studies found 98% concordance of our nurse participants' reports of type 2 diabetes with medical records.[25] We estimated duration of diabetes by subtracting date of diagnosis from date of baseline cognitive interview. We obtained information on recent drug treatment for diabetes from the biennial questionnaire before the baseline interview.

Statistical analyses

Baseline analyses—We examined the relation between type 2 diabetes and cognitive performance by comparing "poor scorers" to remaining women. "Poor scorers" on the TICS were those who scored <31 points (a pre-established cut off point[21]); on other tests, we defined poor scorers as those below the lowest 10th centile (≤ 7 for immediate recall and ≤ 6 for delayed recall on Boston memory test, ≤ 11 for verbal fluency test, ≤ 0 for delayed recall of the TICS 10 words list, and ≤ 3 for digit span backwards). Multivariate adjusted odds ratios of a poor score and 95% confidence intervals were calculated with logistic regression models. We also analysed scores continuously using multiple linear regression to obtain adjusted differences in mean score between women with and without diabetes.

Analyses of cognitive decline—We used logistic regression to calculate odds ratios of "substantial decline," defined as the worst 10% of the distribution of change from the baseline to the second interview (with cut off points for decline of ≥ 4 on the TICS, ≥ 6 on the category fluency test, and ≥ 3 on the other tests). We also used linear regression to estimate adjusted mean differences in decline by diabetes status.

Potential confounding factors—Data on potential confounders were identified from information provided as of the questionnaire immediately before the baseline cognitive assessment. All potential confounding variables were selected a priori based on risk factors for cognitive function in the existing literature (see tables 3 and 4). In analyses of cognitive decline, we adjusted for baseline performance.[26]

Results

At baseline interview 7.3% (n = 1394) of the women had type 2 diabetes, with a mean duration of 12 years since diagnosis. Of the 1248 women with diabetes who completed the most recent questionnaire, 901 reported recent medication for management of diabetes (294 (33%) insulin, 607 (67%) oral hypoglycaemic agents). As expected, women with diabetes had higher prevalence of several comorbid conditions (hypertension, high cholesterol, heart disease, obesity, depression) than women without diabetes (table 1), and used hormone therapy less and drank less alcohol. On every cognitive test, mean baseline scores were lower for women with diabetes (table 2).

We focused analyses on two measures of general cognitive function: the TICS and the global score (table 3). After we adjusted for potential confounding factors, women with diabetes were at 25–35% increased odds of poor baseline score compared with women without diabetes (odds ratio 1.34, 95% confidence interval 1.14 to 1.57, for TICS and 1.26, 1.06 to 1.51, for global score). Findings were consistent when we examined mean differences in scores; the mean score for women with diabetes was lower by −0.42 points, −0.58 to −0.27 points, on the TICS and by −0.09 units, −0.12 to −0.05 units, on the global score compared with women without diabetes. Associations became stronger with longer duration of diabetes. For those with diabetes for ≥ 15 years the odds

Table 1 Characteristics of women aged 70–81 years, according to type 2 diabetes. Figures are percentage of respondents unless stated otherwise*

	Without diabetes	With diabetes
No of participants	17 605	1394
Mean age (years)	74.2	74.2
Masters or doctorate degree	5.8	5.0
History of hypertension	53.2	78.1
History of hypercholesterolaemia	64.0	75.5
History of heart disease	5.2	15.2
Obesity (body mass index ≥30 kg/m²)	15.3	38.8
Self perceived low energy (<55 in SF-36 energy-fatigue index)	13.4	24.7
Self perceived depression (<52 in SF-36 mental health index)	2.6	5.0
Current antidepressant use	5.3	7.9
Current regular aspirin use	37.8	42.0
Current regular use of other non-steroidal inflammatory drugs	17.1	18.2
Current use of vitamin E	41.9	37.2
Current use of postmenopausal hormone	32.6	22.0
Mean (SD) age at menopause in years	48.3 (6.4)	47.7 (6.8)
Median physical activity in metabolic equivalents/week (25th–75th centile)	9.8 (3.2–21.9)	4.3 (1.0–14.0)
Current smoking	8.7	6.0
Median alcohol intake in g/day (25th–75th centile)	1.0 (0.0–6.4)	0.0 (0.0–0.9)

*Characteristics from questionnaire immediately before baseline cognitive test. Type 2 diabetes defined as diagnosis at any time before baseline cognitive test.

Table 2 Mean cognitive test scores at baseline in women aged 70–81, according to type 2 diabetes. Figures are means (SD)

Test (range of scores)	Without diabetes	With diabetes
TICS (8–41 points)	33.8 (2.8)	33.2 (2.9)
TICS 10 word list—delayed (0–10 points)	2.3 (2.0)	2.0 (1.9)
Global score (–4–2 standard units)	0.005 (0.6)	–0.1 (0.6)
East Boston memory test—immediate recall (0–12 points)	9.4 (1.7)	9.3 (1.8)
East Boston memory test—delayed (0–12 points)	9.0 (2.0)	8.9 (2.1)
Verbal fluency test (0–38 points)	16.9 (4.7)	16.3 (4.6)
Digit span backwards (0–12)	6.7 (2.4)	6.4 (2.4)

TICS = telephone interview of cognitive status.

of poor cognitive performance was 50% higher than for women without diabetes (1.52, 1.15 to 1.99, and 1.49, 1.11 to 2.00, respectively).

Odds of poor performance also seemed to differ across treatment groups (table 3). Compared with women without diabetes, we found high odds of poor performance for women with diabetes who did not report pharmaceutical treatment (1.71, 1.28 to 2.28, and 1.45, 1.04 to 2.02, respectively). Those taking insulin also had modestly increased odds of poor cognition (1.20, 0.85 to 1.70, and 1.38, 0.97 to 1.95, respectively). In the more powerful analyses of mean differences, the worst performance was among women using insulin (mean differences −0.40, 0.72 to −0.09, and −0.11, −0.18 to −0.03, respectively). In contrast, those taking oral medications had similar odds of poor cognitive performance as those without diabetes (odds ratios 1.06, 0.81 to 1.37, and 0.99, 0.74 to 1.33, respectively) and had the smallest mean difference in score (mean differences −0.35, −0.58 to −0.13, and −0.06, −0.11 to −0.01, respectively).

As cognitive impairment may be a cause rather than a consequence of not taking medications, we also examined use of medication at time of diagnosis (average of 12 years before cognitive assessment). However, results were similar: the odds ratios for poor score were 1.61, 1.19 to 2.16, and 1.43, 1.02 to 2.00, respectively, for women with diabetes who were not taking medication at diagnosis compared with women without diabetes.

In addition, as duration of diabetes, medication use, and level of control are correlated we conducted additional analyses to try to assess their independent effects. The results for duration of diabetes were largely similar after we adjusted for medication use, and results for medication use were largely unchanged after we included a term for duration in the model or stratified by duration of diabetes. For example, among women with diabetes, those not taking medication had a higher risk of poor cognitive performance on the TICS compared with those taking oral medication both in the group with duration of diabetes <10 years (1.73, 1.01 to 2.98) and

Table 3 Diabetes, duration of diabetes, and use of medication for diabetes in women aged 70–81 in relation to baseline cognitive function

	% of women	Odds ratio of poor cognitive performance (95% CI)		Mean difference in cognitive performance (95% CI)	
		TICS (n = 18 999)	Global score* (n = 16 563)	TICS (n = 18 999)	Global score* (n = 16 563)
Diagnosis					
No diabetes	92.7	1.00	1.00	0	0
Diabetes:					
Adjusted for age and education	7.3	1.44 (1.24 to 1.69)	1.37 (1.16 to 1.63)	−0.55 (−0.70 to −0.41)	−0.11 (−0.15 to −0.08)
Multivariate adjusted†	7.3	1.34 (1.14 to 1.57)	1.26 (1.06 to 1.51)	−0.42 (−0.58 to −0.27)	−0.09 (−0.12 to −0.05)
Duration of diabetes (years)					
No diabetes	92.7	1.00	1.00	0	0
Adjusted for age and education:					
≤4	1.5	1.35 (0.97 to 1.88)	1.53 (1.08 to 2.18)	−0.37 (−0.69 to −0.06)	−0.10 (−0.17 to −0.03)
5–9	2.1	1.16 (0.86 to 1.58)	0.91 (0.64 to 1.31)	−0.51 (−0.79 to −0.24)	−0.09 (−0.15 to −0.03)
10–14	1.6	1.59 (1.17 to 2.16)	1.44 (1.03 to 2.02)	−0.68 (−1.00 to −0.37)	−0.12 (−0.19 to −0.05)
≥15	2.1	1.69 (1.30 to 2.21)	1.68 (1.27 to 2.24)	−0.63 (−0.91 to −0.36)	−0.14 (−0.21 to −0.08)
P for trend		<0.0001	<0.0001	<0.0001	<0.0001
Multivariate adjusted†:					
≤4	1.5	1.27 (0.91 to 1.79)	1.48 (1.03 to 2.11)	−0.27 (−0.59 to 0.04)	−0.08 (−0.16 to −0.01)
5–9	2.1	1.10 (0.81 to 1.50)	0.86 (0.60 to 1.25)	−0.41 (−0.69 to −0.14)	−0.07 (−0.13 to −0.01)
10–14	1.6	1.48 (1.08 to 2.02)	1.31 (0.93 to 1.85)	−0.53 (−0.84 to −0.22)	−0.09 (−0.16 to −0.02)
≥15	2.1	1.52 (1.15 to 1.99)	1.49 (1.11 to 2.00)	−0.46 (−0.73 to −0.18)	−0.11 (−0.17 to −0.04)
P for trend		0.0002	0.007	<0.0001	<0.0001

Continued

Table 3 Continued

| | % of women | Odds ratio of poor cognitive performance (95% CI) | | Mean difference in cognitive performance (95% CI) | |
		TICS (n = 18 999)	Global score* (n = 16 563)	TICS (n = 18 999)	Global score* (n = 16 563)
Medication‡					
No diabetes	92.7	1.00	1.00	0	0
Adjusted for age and education:					
Insulin	1.5	1.27 (0.91 to 1.78)	1.48 (1.06 to 2.08)	−0.55 (−0.86 to −0.23)	−0.14 (−0.20 to −0.07)
Oral medication	3.2	1.05 (0.82 to 1.36)	0.99 (0.74 to 1.31)	−0.40 (−0.62 to −0.18)	−0.06 (−0.11 to −0.01)
No reported treatment	1.8	1.70 (1.28 to 2.26)	1.43 (1.03 to 1.98)	−0.42 (−0.71 to −0.13)	−0.09 (−0.16 to −0.02)
Multivariate adjusted†:					
Insulin	1.5	1.20 (0.85 to 1.70)	1.38 (0.97 to 1.95)	−0.40 (−0.72 to −0.09)	−0.11 (−0.18 to −0.03)
Oral medication	3.2	1.06 (0.81 to 1.37)	0.99 (0.74 to 1.33)	−0.35 (−0.58 to −0.13)	−0.06 (−0.11 to −0.01)
No reported treatment	1.8	1.71 (1.28 to 2.28)	1.45 (1.04 to 2.02)	−0.38 (−0.67 to −0.09)	−0.08 (−0.15 to −0.01)

TICS – telephone interview of cognitive status.

*Global score combines TICS, test of verbal fluency, delayed recall of TICS 10 word list, digit backwards test, immediate and delayed recalls of East Boston memory test.

†Adjusted for age at interview (years), highest attained education (registered nurse diploma, Bachelor's degree, Master's or Doctoral degree), history of high cholesterol (yes, no), history of high blood pressure (yes, no), use of vitamin E supplement (currently yes, no), age at menopause (<50, 50–52, ≥53 years), body mass index (<22, 22–24.9, 25–29.9, ≥30 kg/m²), cigarette smoking (current, past, never), antidepressant use (yes, no), alcohol intake (0, 1–4, 5–14, ≥15 g/day), use of aspirin (current use 1–5 times/week, use ≥6 times/week, no), use of other NSAID (current use, no), postmenopausal hormone use (currently yes, no), mental health index (0–52, 52–100), and energy-fatigue index (0–54, 55–100) from SF-36.

‡Data on medication use from questionnaire immediately before baseline cognitive assessment. Percentages do not total 100% as 0.8% who did not respond to medication question are not presented.

>10 years (1.90, 1.04 to 3.48). Furthermore, although we did not have detailed information on level of control (for example, data on haemoglobin A_{1c} concentration), all results were generally unchanged when we excluded data from women with metabolic complications (for instance, those with severely uncontrolled disease).

Finally, we restricted analyses to participants who did not report any difficulty with hearing (n = 12 099) to reduce confounding by hearing status. The results were similar when we compared women with and without diabetes (1.45, 1.18 to 1.78, and 1.37, 1.10 to 1.71, respectively).

Prospective analyses of decline

Although cognitive decline was measured over just a two year period, we observed a significantly increased odds of substantial decline on the TICS (1.26, 1.03 to 1.54) for women compared with women without type 2 diabetes (table 4). However, we observed little overall relation between diabetes and decline on the global score (1.11, 0.90 to 1.37). Similarly,

mean decline was greater among women with diabetes by −0.17 points (−0.33 to −0.01) on the TICS but was comparable in the two groups on the global score (mean difference in decline −0.01, −0.04 to 0.03). In addition, qualitative relations with longer duration diabetes and use of medication were generally similar to those observed with baseline cognitive function.

Discussion

In this large prospective study of women aged 70–81 years with type 2 diabetes who were living in the community we found that they had marginally worse baseline cognitive performance and greater cognitive decline than women without diabetes. Longer duration of diabetes resulted in larger associations. However, women who said they were on hypoglycaemic treatment seemed to have a similar likelihood of poor cognition as women without diabetes, while women not taking medication for diabetes or those taking insulin had worse performance.

A major strength of our study is the large sample size for assessing the relations between type 2 diabetes, duration, treatment, and cognition. Other strengths are the prospective assessment of diabetes and potential confounders over 25 years of follow up and the relative homogeneity of the sample in terms of education and access to health care, which should minimise confounding.

Limitations

Limitations should be considered. Firstly, as we relied on the women reporting their own diabetes status, we may have included some women with undiagnosed diabetes in the reference group, which could have led to underestimation of the true associations. However, undiagnosed diabetes was probably rare in these nurses. Among a random sample of those with no reported diabetes, plasma samples indicated just 2% had diagnostic signs of type 2 diabetes. Secondly, as in all studies of cognitive decline, there is regression to the mean on the repeat cognitive assessment. As women with type 2 diabetes had worse cognitive performance at baseline, regression to the mean would probably have attenuated the true magnitude of cognitive decline associated with diabetes.

In addition, there are important issues to consider in interpreting our findings regarding pharmaceutical treatment of diabetes. Participants who were not taking any treatment for diabetes probably included a heterogeneous group of women with untreated diabetes and diabetes controlled through

Table 4 Diabetes, duration of diabetes, use of medication for diabetes in women aged 70–81 in relation to cognitive decline over two years

	%	Odds ratio of substantial decline (95% CI)		Mean difference in cognitive decline (95% CI)	
		TICS (n = 16 596)	Global score* (n = 14 470)	TICS (n = 16 596)	Global score* (n = 14 470)
Diagnosis					
No diabetes	92.9	1.00	1.00	0	0
Diabetes:					
Adjusted for age and education	7.1	1.36 (1.12 to 1.65)	1.20 (0.97 to 1.47)	−0.29 (−0.44 to −0.13)	−0.03 (−0.06 to 0.00)
Multivariate adjusted†	7.1	1.26 (1.03 to 1.54)	1.10 (0.89 to 1.37)	−0.17 (−0.33 to −0.01)	−0.01 (−0.04 to 0.02)
Duration of diabetes (years)					
No diabetes	92.9	1.00	1.00	0	0
Adjusted for age and education:					
≤4	1.6	1.25 (0.83 to 1.88)	0.68 (0.40 to 1.17)	0.04 (−0.28 to 0.35)	0.05 (−0.01 to 0.12)
5–9	2.0	1.08 (0.74 to 1.59)	1.08 (0.73 to 1.59)	−0.10 (−0.38 to 0.18)	0.01 (−0.05 to 0.06)
10–14	1.6	1.35 (0.90 to 2.02)	1.53 (1.03 to 2.27)	−0.36 (−0.67 to −0.04)	−0.09 (−0.15 to −0.03)
≥15	1.9	1.77 (1.27 to 2.47)	1.51 (1.05 to 2.15)	−0.68 (−0.97 to −0.40)	−0.08 (−0.13 to −0.02)
P for trend		0.0004	0.005	<0.0001	0.001
Multivariate adjusted:					
≤4	1.6	1.15 (0.76 to 1.74)	0.65 (0.38 to 1.12)	0.14 (−0.18 to 0.46)	0.07 (0.01 to 0.13)
5–9	2.0	1.00 (0.68 to 1.47)	1.01 (0.68 to 1.49)	−0.01 (−0.29 to 0.27)	0.02 (−0.04 to 0.07)
10–14	1.6	1.26 (0.83 to 1.90)	1.40 (0.94 to 2.09)	−0.23 (−0.55 to 0.09)	−0.07 (−0.13 to 0.00)
≥15	1.9	1.64 (1.17 to 2.30)	1.35 (0.93 to 1.94)	−0.54 (−0.83 to −0.25)	−0.05 (−0.11 to 0.01)
P for trend		0.005	0.05	0.0004	0.05

Continued

Originally published in *BMJ* 2004; **328**. Reproduced with permission.

Table 4 Continued

	%	Odds ratio of substantial decline (95% CI)		Mean difference in cognitive decline (95% CI)	
		TICS (n = 16596)	Global score* (n = 14470)	TICS (n = 16596)	Global score* (n = 14470)
Medication‡					
No diabetes	92.9	1.00	1.00	0	0
Adjusted for age and education:					
Insulin	1.5	1.49 (0.99 to 2.25)	1.22 (0.79 to 1.89)	−0.59 (−0.92 to −0.26)	−0.08 (−0.15 to −0.01)
Oral medication	3.1	1.12 (0.82 to 1.51)	0.82 (0.58 to 1.14)	0.00 (−0.22 to 0.23)	0.02 (−0.03 to 0.06)
No reported treatment	1.8	1.35 (0.93 to 1.95)	1.67 (1.18 to 2.37)	−0.27 (−0.56 to −0.03)	−0.02 (−0.08 to 0.04)
Multivariate adjusted:					
Insulin	1.5	1.39 (0.91 to 2.10)	1.08 (0.69 to 1.68)	−0.44 (−0.77 to −0.11)	−0.05 (−0.12 to 0.02)
Oral medication	3.1	1.09 (0.80 to 1.48)	0.77 (0.54 to 1.08)	0.07 (−0.16 to 0.30)	0.03 (−0.02 to 0.08)
No reported treatment	1.8	1.31 (0.90 to 1.90)	1.62 (1.13 to 2.30)	−0.23 (−0.53 to 0.06)	−0.02 (−0.08 to 0.05)

TICS = telephone interview of cognitive status.

*Global score combines TICS, test of verbal fluency, delayed recall of TICS 10 word list, digit backwards test, immediate and delayed recalls of East Boston memory test.

†Adjusted for age at interview (years), highest attained education (registered nurse diploma, Bachelor's degree, Master's or Doctoral degree), history of high cholesterol (yes, no), history of high blood pressure (yes, no), use of vitamin E supplement (currently yes, no), age at menopause (<50, 50–52, ≥53 years), body mass index (<22, 22–24.9, 25–29.9, ≥30 kg/m²), cigarette smoking (current, past, never), antidepressant use (yes, no), alcohol intake (0, 1–4, 5–14, ≥15 g/day), use of aspirin (current use 1–5 times/week, use ≥6 times/week, no), use of other NSAID (current use, no), postmenopausal hormone use (currently yes, no), mental health index (0–52, 52–100), and energy-fatigue index (0–54, 55–100) from SF-36.

‡Data on medication use from questionnaire immediately before baseline cognitive assessment. Percentages do not total 100% as 0.8% who did not respond to medication question are not presented.

diet. Diabetes that can be controlled through diet may not be associated with poor cognition.[14] Thus, we have probably underestimated the effect of untreated diabetes. However, the increased odds of poor cognition associated with no treatment was similar across those with shorter and longer duration of diabetes (and duration is probably a good indicator of prevalence of dietary control), suggesting that our underestimate may be minimal.

What is already known on this topic

Many epidemiological studies have shown that type 2 diabetes increases the risk of cognitive decline, though most studies have been in men

Type 2 diabetes is associated with greater risk of cardiovascular disease in women than in men, and cardiovascular disease may increase the risk of cognitive decline

What this study adds

Women with type 2 diabetes have about 30% greater odds of poor cognitive function than those without diabetes, with a 50% increase after 15 years' of diabetes

Women with diabetes who did not report medical treatment had the highest risk of poor cognitive function and substantial cognitive decline

Women with diabetes who reported taking oral medication had a similar risk of cognitive decline as women without diabetes

Though our finding that insulin treatment was associated with poor cognitive performance is consistent with results of other studies of cognition,[8,14] it is difficult to draw conclusions; people with diabetes who use insulin all have longer

Originally published in *BMJ* 2004; **328**. Reproduced with permission.

duration of diabetes, worse control, and higher prevalence of hypoglycaemic attacks, rendering it hard to adjust appropriately for confounding. None the less, there is growing evidence directly linking insulin to cognitive impairment: chronic hyperinsulinaemia[10] and incremental increases in serum insulin concentration after a glucose load[13] predict diminished cognition in the absence of diabetes or glucose intolerance. Moreover, insulin degrading enzyme regulates concentrations of both insulin and amyloid β in the brain[27] and infusion of insulin into healthy humans increases amyloid β concentrations in the cerebrospinal fluid,[28] further supporting a direct association between insulin and cognition.

Finally, consistent with our findings of similar cognitive performance among women taking oral medication and those without diabetes, in a controlled trial of participants with type 2 diabetes, Testa and Simonson noted that improved glucose control with oral medications resulted in better cognitive acuity, memory, and orientation.[29] In addition, an observational study of Mexican-Americans with diabetes reported significantly less cognitive decline in those with medical treatment than without.[30] Thus, although physicians may avoid prescribing oral therapy for diabetes in older people, it may be important to their cognitive health.

Conclusions

In conclusion, we found worse cognitive function and accelerated cognitive decline among women with type 2 diabetes, which seemed to be ameliorated with oral hypoglycaemic treatment. Studies have established that, in apparently healthy people, even modest differences in cognition result in substantially increased risks of dementia over several years.[6] Prevention and control of type 2 diabetes in women could have critically important public health consequences.

Contributors: GL and FG led the study design; GL, JHK, and FG contributed to the interpretation and the analysis of the data; JHK conducted the analysis of the data. FG was responsible for obtaining funding for the study. All authors contributed to writing the manuscript and are joint guarantors.

Funding: Grants AG15424 and CA87969 from the National Institutes of Health. FG is partially supported by a New Scholars in Aging award from the Ellison Medical Foundation.

Competing interests: During the last five years GL has received honorariums for lectures from Pfeizer and Lilly Pharmaceutical. During the past five years FG has received honorariums or temporary consulting fees from Novo Nordisk, Schering-Plough, Novartis, Orion Pharma, and Wyeth Ayerst.

Ethical approval: This study was approved by the Institutional Review Board of Brigham and Women's Hospital, Boston, MA.

References

1 Ott A, Stolk RP, Van Harskamp F, Pols HA, Hofman A, Breteler MM. Diabetes mellitus and the risk of dementia: the Rotterdam study. *Neurology* 1999;53:1937–42.

2 Leibson CL, Rocca, WA, Hanson VA, Cha R, Kokmen E, O'Brien PC, et al. Risk of dementia among persons with diabetes mellitus: a population-based cohort study. *Am J Epidemiol* 1997;145:301–8.

3 Curb JD, Rodriguez BL, Abbott RD, Petrovitch H, Ross GW, Masaki KH, et al. Longitudinal association of vascular and Alzheimer's dementias, diabetes, and glucose tolerance. *Neurology* 1999;52:971–5.

4 Luchsinger JA, Tang MX, Stern Y, Shea S, Mayeaux R. Diabetes mellitus and risk of Alzheimer's disease and dementia with stroke in a multiethnic cohort. *Am J Epidemiol* 2001;154:635–41.

5 MacKnight C, Rockwood K, Awalt E, McDowell I. Diabetes mellitus and the risk of dementia, Alzheimer's disease and vascular cognitive impairment in the Canadian study of health and aging. *Dement Geriatr Cogn Disord* 2002;14:77–83.

6 Bozoki A, Giordani B, Heidebrink JL, Berent S, Foster NL. Mild cognitive impairments predict dementia in nondemented elderly patients with memory loss. *Arch Neurol* 2001;58:411–6.

7 Brookmeyer R, Gray S, Kawas C. Projections of Alzheimer's disease in the United States and the public health impact of delaying disease onset. *Am J Pub Health* 1998;88:1337–42.

8 Gregg EW, Yaffe K, Cauley JA, Rolka DB, Blackwell TL, Narayan KM, et al. Is diabetes associated with cognitive impairment and cognitive decline among older women? Study of Osteoporotic Fractures Research Group. *Arch Intern Med* 2000;160:174–80.

9 Knopman D, Boland LL, Mosley T, Howard G, Liao D, Szklo M, et al. Cardiovascular risk factors and cognitive decline in middle-aged adults. *Neurology* 2001;56:42–8.

10 Kalmijn S, Feskens EJ, Launer LJ, Stijnen T, Kromhout D. Glucose intolerance, hyperinsulinaemia and cognitive function in a general population of elderly men. *Diabetologia* 1995;38:1096–102.

11 Scott RD, Kritz-Silverstein D, Barrett-Connor E, Wiederholt WC. The association of non-insulin-dependent diabetes mellitus and cognitive function in an older cohort. *J Am Geriatr Soc* 1998;46:1217–22.

12 Fontbonne A, Berr C, Ducimetiere P, Alperovitch A. Changes in cognitive abilities over a 4-year period are unfavorably affected in elderly diabetic subjects: results of the epidemiology of vascular aging study. *Diabetes Care* 2001;24:366–70.

13 Stolk RP, Breteler MM, Ott A, Pols HA, Lamberts, SW, Grobbee DE, et al. Insulin and cognitive function in an elderly population. The Rotterdam study. *Diabetes Care* 1997;20:792–5.

14 Elias PK, Elias MF, D'Agostino RB, Cupples LA, Wilson PW, Silbershatz H, et al. NIDDM and blood pressure as risk factors for poor cognitive performance. The Framingham study. *Diabetes Care* 1997;20:1388–95.

15 Rodriguez-Saldana J, Morley JE, Reynoso MT, Medina CA, Salazar P, Cruz E, et al. Diabetes mellitus in a subgroup of older Mexicans: prevalence, association with cardiovascular risk factors, functional and cognitive impairment, and mortality. *J Am Geriatr Soc* 2002;50:111–6.

16 Nguyen HT, Black SA, Ray LA, Espino DV, Markides KS. Predictors of decline in MMSE scores among older Mexican Americans. *J Gerontol A Biol Sci Med Sci* 2002;57:M181–5.

17 Wu JH, Haan MN, Liang J, Ghosh D, Gonzalez HM, Herman WH. Impact of diabetes on cognitive function among older Latinos: a population-based cohort study. *J Clin Epidemiol* 2003;56:686–93.

18 Vanhanen M, Kuusisto J, Koivisto K, Mykkanen L, Helkala EL, Hanninen T, et al. Type-2 diabetes and cognitive function in a nondemented population. *Acta Neurol Scand* 1999;100:97–101.

19 Lindeman RD, Romero LJ, LaRue A, Yau CL, Schade DS, Koehler KM, et al. A biethnic community survey of cognition in

participants with type 2 diabetes, impaired glucose tolerance, and normal glucose tolerance: the New Mexico elder health survey. *Diabetes Care* 2001;24:1567–72.

20 Coker LH, Shumaker SA. Type 2 diabetes mellitus and cognition: an understudied issue in women's health. *J Psychosom Research* 2003;54:129–39.

21 Kang JH, Grodstein F. Regular use of nonsteroidal anti-inflammatory drugs and cognitive function in aging women. *Neurology* 2003;60:1591–7.

22 Brandt J, Spencer M, Folstein M. The telephone interview for cognitive status. *Neuropsychiatry Neuropsychol Behav Neurol* 1988;1:111–7.

23 National Diabetes Data Group. Classification and diagnosis of diabetes mellitus and other categories of glucose intolerance. *Diabetes* 1979;28:1039–57.

24 Expert Committee on the Diagnosis and Classification of Diabetes Mellitus. Report of the expert committee on the diagnosis and classification of diabetes mellitus. *Diabetes Care* 2000;suppl 1:S4–19.

25 Manson JE, Rimm EB, Stampfer MJ, Colditz GA, Willett WC, Krolewski AS, et al. Physical activity and incidence of non-insulin-dependent diabetes mellitus in women. *Lancet* 1991;338:774–8.

26 Vickers A, Altman D. Analysing controlled trials with baseline and follow-up measurements. *BMJ* 2001;323:1123–4.

27 Farris W, Mansourian S, Chang Y, Lindsley L, Eckman EA, Frosch MP, et al. Insulin-degrading enzyme regulates the levels of insulin, amyloid beta-protein, and the beta-amyloid precursor protein intracellular domain in vivo. *Proc Natl Acad Sci USA* 2003;100:4162–7.

28 Watson GS, Peskind ER, Asthana S, Purganan K, Wait C, Chapman D, et al. Insulin increases CSF Abeta42 levels in normal older adults. *Neurology* 2003;60:1899–903.

29 Testa MA, Simonson DC. Health economic benefits and quality of life during improved glycemic control in patients with type 2 diabetes mellitus: a randomized, controlled, double-blind trial. *JAMA* 1998;280:1490–6.

30 Wu JH, Haan MN, Liang J, Ghosh D, Gonzalez HM, Herman WH. Impact of antidiabetic medications on physical and cognitive functioning of older Mexican Americans with diabetes mellitus: a population-based cohort study. *Ann Epidemiol* 2003;13:369–76.

Originally published in *BMJ* 2004; **328**. Reproduced with permission.

UNIT 2

Incidence and prevalence rates

Aims

To understand the requirements for measuring incidence and prevalence accurately and how the sample size influences the precision in estimating these rates.

> **Learning objectives**
> On completion of this unit, participants will be able to:
> - distinguish between the terms incidence and prevalence and understand the situations in which each term can be used correctly;
> - calculate and interpret 95% confidence intervals around incidence and prevalence rates;
> - explain why estimates of incidence, remission and death are always lower than estimates of prevalence for a given population;
> - describe the types of bias that influence estimates of prevalence and incidence.

Background

In assessing the health status of a population, we are often interested in statistics such as how many people have a disease at a single point in time, the rate at which new cases occur or how many people die as the result of a certain illness. Calculating these statistics is vital for tracking whether disease rates are declining or increasing, and for assessing whether medical or population interventions are effective in promoting health and prolonging life. Tracking disease patterns can also lead to hypotheses about possible causal or preventive factors and knowledge of these factors can be vital for developing interventions that have the potential to lead to better health.

When estimating disease statistics, it is important that the population is carefully defined so that the statistics can be generalised to other populations with the same characteristics. A population is a section of society in which we may be interested, for example all children aged between 7 and 11 years in a defined rural region or all women aged over 60 years living in a local government area. When the population is too large to measure the characteristics of each person individually, a sample of the population is usually selected. If the sample is large enough and is selected randomly, then the characteristics of the sample are likely to be representative of the whole population and inferences to the 'true' rate of illness in the population can be made. The most reliable estimates of incidence and prevalence rates are obtained from large population samples in which a random, and therefore representative, sample is enrolled. Although there may be sampling error despite random sampling – that is, each sample may give a slightly different estimate or rate – sampling errors become smaller as the size of the sample increases. However, sometimes a study sample may be a convenience sample selected from a group of people who are readily available, for example people who attend a certain health care clinic or hospital. It is important to remember that a population who self-select themselves into a health care service may not be a representative sample of the population in which they live, that is, the population in a defined geographic region around the hospital.

The terms 'incidence' and 'prevalence' are used to describe the rate at which a condition occurs in a population sample. A common mistake in the reporting of frequency rates is to use these two terms interchangeably although they have entirely different meanings. For any given population, the term 'incidence' describes the number of new cases of the condition that occurred in a defined time period, whereas the term 'prevalence' describes the total number of cases with the condition at any point in time. The terms incidence and prevalence are usually applied to a specified time period, such as a 1-year or 5-year interval. Incidence rates are usually described directly in terms of the period in which they have been measured, for example as number of cases per year. However, when the total number of people who have a condition at one point in time, for example at birth, is measured, the term 'point prevalence' may be used. When the total number of people who have ever had the condition during a defined time is measured, the term 'cumulative prevalence' may be used.

Glossary

Term	Definition
Incidence	The number of new cases of a condition that develop in a population during a defined time period.
Prevalence	The total number of people in a population with a condition a given point in time.

To obtain reliable estimates of incidence or prevalence, a study must be carefully designed to minimise bias, especially selection, response and measurement bias. These types of bias lead to unreliable estimates of the 'true' rate of illness and they can occur regardless of the sample size. Selection bias occurs if the sample is not selected randomly or if the response rate is low and therefore the sample is unlikely to be representative of the population from which it was drawn. On the other hand, response bias occurs when participants self-select themselves into the study because of issues related to their health, for example the respondents may be healthier or they may have more interest in the illness being investigated than other members of the community who decline to participate. Response bias can have a significant influence on the frequency of responses to health care questions and the perceived associations between symptoms and exposures. Measurement bias, which includes reporting bias, ascertainment bias and poor recall of past illness events, can also influence estimates of incidence and prevalence because the outcome is not measured accurately. Bias is a major problem in research because it leads to incidence and prevalence rates being under-estimated or over-estimated, and therefore being inaccurate, and the magnitude or direction of the bias may not be known.

Measuring incidence and prevalence

To measure incidence, a cohort study is usually conducted in which a random sample of the population is enrolled and monitored over time. In such studies, new or incident cases are identified when they develop and, as such, they can be distinguished from previously existing, or prevalent, cases. On the other hand, to measure a prevalence rate, a cross-sectional study can be conducted in which a random sample of a population is enrolled from which all cases, whether incident or prevalent, are identified at a given point or period in time. As such, cross-sectional studies provide a useful 'snap-shot' of what is happening in a sample of the population at a single point in time, and are often used as a cheaper alternative to cohort studies for measuring trends in the health status of populations. However, to obtain precise estimates of prevalence rates, a high response rate of over 80% should be achieved in order to minimise the effects of selection bias.[1]

The prevalence of a condition in a given time period is the number of incident cases, plus the cases who were diagnosed (prevalent) prior to the time period, minus any deaths or remissions that have occurred. That is,

Prevalence = Incident cases + prior prevalent cases
　　　　　　　− (deaths + remissions)

Because the terms incidence and prevalence are used to describe rates of a condition in a population, it is essential that the study sample is sufficiently large to enable calculation of the rates with precision. When the condition is fairly common, incidence and prevalence rates are usually described as percentages, for example 10%. When the condition is rare, the rate is given as a number per unit of the population, for example 1 case per 10 000 or per 100 000 children. When a sample is not representative of the population, only the terms percentage, proportion or frequency should be used to describe disease rates.

Confidence intervals

Confidence intervals can be used to convey the precision with which an incidence or prevalence rate has been estimated. These intervals are calculated from a table, as shown in Table 2.1, in which number of participants with or without the condition of interest is shown as (a) disease present or (b) absent and in which 'N' is the total sample size. The incidence or prevalence rate is then calculated as a proportion of cases (p) in the sample, which is equal to a/N.

The 95% confidence intervals around an incidence or prevalence rate are an estimate of the range in which we are 95% certain that the true incidence or prevalence rate lies. If the incidence or prevalence rate (p) is between 5% and 95%, the standard error and the 95% confidence intervals can be calculated using the following formulae:

Incidence or prevalence (p) = a/N
Standard error (SE) = $\sqrt{(p\,(1-p)/N)}$
95% confidence interval = $p \pm (\text{SE} \times 1.96)$

The calculations are computed using proportions but both the incidence or prevalence rate (p) and the 95% confidence intervals can be converted into percentages simply by multiplying by 100. It can be seen from the formula that the standard error around an estimate will become smaller and therefore more precise as the sample size increases because the denominator is the square root of the sample

Table 2.1 Estimating incidence or prevalence

	Disease present	Disease absent	Total
Totals	a	b	N

size. Therefore, the 95% confidence intervals will become narrower to reflect this.

If the incidence or prevalence rate is very low, that is less than 5%, as in studies of rare diseases, the formula for calculating the confidence interval shown here does not approximate well and 'exact' confidence intervals based on a binomial distribution may be required. The importance of using exact confidence intervals is that they will not provide a negative rate, which would be an invalid value, for the lower interval. Exact confidence intervals are not symmetrical around estimates of incidence and prevalence as are the 95% confidence intervals calculated using the formulae above. Because the calculations of exact intervals are more complex, they are best computed using a dedicated statistical package such as the program EpiInfo (www.cdc.gov/EpiInfo).

Comparing groups

When comparing incidence or prevalence rates between two populations or groups, the degree of overlap between the 95% confidence intervals is a guide to whether the difference in rates is statistically significant. Thus, 95% confidence intervals are invaluable for making inferences about a P value when the P value is not reported.[2,3] Figure 2.1 shows three prevalence rates and their 95% confidence intervals. If the intervals do not overlap, as between population samples A and C, the rate of disease is significantly different between the two groups. When these two rates are compared using a chi-square test (as described in Unit 3), the P value is highly significant at <0.0001. If there is a large degree of overlap, as between population samples B and C where the top of the interval for group C is close to the summary statistic for group B, the two rates are not significantly different. The P value for this comparison is 0.4. If there is some overlap but the rate for one population sample is not within the

Table 2.2 Rules for reporting rates as percentages

Rule	Example
Report percentages to one decimal place if the sample size is larger than 100	In the sample of 320 children, 10.9% had asthma
Report percentages with no decimal places if the sample size is between 20 and 100	In the sample of 32 children, 9% had asthma
Do not use percentages if the sample size is less than 20	In the sample of 16 children, 2 had asthma

confidence interval of the other, as between groups A and B, the difference may be significant. When these two groups are compared, the P value is statistically significant at 0.048.

Reporting

When reporting incidence and prevalence rates, it is important that the correct number of decimal places is used so that only the precision that is provided by the sample size is implied. The rules for reporting rates as percentages are shown in Table 2.2. When rates are reported as proportions, only one decimal place is used if the sample is less than 100, otherwise two decimal places are used.[4] To avoid multiple decimal places for low rates, the denominator can be changed, for example a rate of 0.0062% can be reported as 6.2 cases per 100 000 children.

TAKE HOME LIST

- Estimates of incidence and prevalence rates can be influenced by selection, response or measurement bias.

- Confidence intervals can be used to indicate the precision with which an incidence or prevalence rate has been estimated.

- The degree of overlap of the 95% confidence intervals between two groups is a guide to whether the difference in rates is statistically significant.

Reading and questions
Reprint

Langemo D, *et al.* A quick overview on measuring pressure ulcer prevalence and incidence. Adv Skin Wound Care 2007; 20(12):642–644. (See p. 25.)

After reading Unit 2 and the reprint by Langemo *et al.* (2007), answer the following questions:

1 What is a cross-sectional study?
2 What is the difference between incidence and prevalence rates?

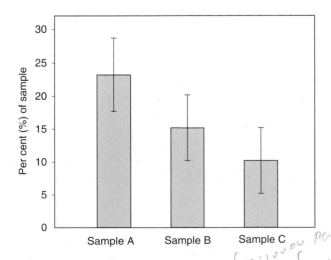

Figure 2.1 Bar chart showing estimates of prevalence with 95% confidence intervals.

Table 2.3 Prevalence of asthma in children aged 8–11 years living in Belmont, Australia

	1982		1992		2002	
	Prevalence	95% CI	Prevalence	95% CI	Prevalence	95% CI
Total number	*718*		*914*		*810*	
Asthma diagnosed	9.1%	7.0, 11.2	38.3%	35.1, 41.4	31.0%	27.8, 34.2
Wheeze in last 12 months	10.4%	8.2, 12.7	28.6%	25.6, 31.5	23.7%	20.8, 26.7
Recent use of asthma medication	9.6%	7.5, 11.0	28.1%	25.2, 31.1	23.2%	20.3, 26.1

3 What conditions need to be met for a prevalence rate to be generalised to the population?

4 Why do cohort studies provide an ideal study design for estimating incidence rates?

5 What types of bias can influence estimates of incidence and prevalence rates?

6 How can bias be minimised?

Worked example

Set article 1

Toelle BG, Ng K, Belousova E, Salome CM, Peat JK, Marks GB. Prevalence of asthma and allergy in schoolchildren in Belmont, Australia: three cross sectional surveys over 20 years. BMJ 2004;328:386–387. (See p. 27.)

It is sometimes important to know whether the prevalence of an illness has increased or decreased in recent years. This is often measured by conducting repeat cross-sectional studies over time as shown in the article by Toelle *et al.* (2004). To measure whether the prevalence of asthma had increased in a region of Australia, three cross-sectional studies were conducted in 1982, 1992 and 2002 in which all children aged between 8 and 11 years old in schools within a defined region were asked to participate. Table 2.3 shows the prevalence rates of three of the outcomes measured. Although the 95% confidence intervals were not included in the article, they can be easily calculated from the numerators and denominators reported using the formulae given in this Unit and are shown in Table 2.3.

The article does not report *P* values for between-year comparisons, but the significance of the differences between years can be inferred from the 95% confidence intervals shown in Table 2.3. The prevalence rates in 1992 are more than 10% higher than in 1982, with a wide gap between confidence intervals indicating that the increase between 1982 and 1992 would be highly significant, probably at *P* < 0.0001. In contrast, the prevalence rates for 2002 are lower than in 1992. The prevalence rates for 1992 are outside the 95% confidence intervals for 2002 indicating a marginally significant decrease in prevalence, probably with a *P* value of 0.05 or slightly lower, reflecting the smaller magnitude of the differences.

The authors conclude that the trajectory of an increasing prevalence of asthma between 1982 and 1992 has not continued. In the comment section of the article, it is reported that estimates of the rates were more reliable in 1982 when the response rate was 88% and in 1992 when the response rate was 86.9%, than in 2002 when the response rate was lower at 66.3%. In 2002, there is a greater possibility of selection bias as a result of the lower response rate, and therefore a definitive conclusion that the prevalence of asthma decreased significantly between 1992 and 2002 would not be warranted. However, the authors provide evidence that the prevalence rates in 2002 were likely to have been over-estimated rather than under-estimated and therefore that the prevalence of asthma had not continued to increase further. Providing evidence of the direction of selection bias helps to validate the conclusions. Nevertheless, the extent to which increased asthma awareness has influenced the results is not known and it is possible that some of the large increase in prevalence between 1982 and 1992 could be explained by ascertainment and reporting bias following wide scale asthma awareness campaigns during that period.

Quick quiz

After reading the set article by Toelle *et al.* (2004), tick the correct answer for each of the following questions.

1 What type of study is reported in this article:
  (a) a longitudinal follow-up study;
  (b) a series of cross-sectional surveys;
  (c) three different case-control studies;
  (d) an ongoing ecological study.

2 The differences in prevalence rates between 1982 and 1992 were:
  (a) large and significant;
  (b) large and non-significant;
  (c) small and significant;
  (d) small and non-significant.

3 The differences in prevalence rates between 1992 and 2002 were:

(a) large and significant;

(b) large and non-significant;

(c) small and significant;

(d) small and non-significant.

4 The prevalence rates in 2002 could have been influenced by:

(a) confounding, because the sample was selected randomly;

(b) asthma awareness programmes conducted since 1982;

(c) measurement error, because methods changed over the study period;

(d) selection bias, because the response rate was lower.

Critical appraisal

Work through the critical appraisal checklist below to review the article by Toelle *et al.* (2004) and decide whether the interpretations of their results are valid.

Exercise

Set article 2

Judd A, Hickman M, Jones S, McDonald T, Parry JV, Stimson GV, Hall AJ. Incidence of hepatitis C virus and HIV among new injecting drug users in London: prospective cohort study. BMJ 2005; 330:24–25. (See p. 29.)

Using the set article by Judd *et al.* (2005) complete Table 2.4 by calculating:

- the prevalence of antibodies to hepatitis C virus if the number of cases identified in the sample had been 90, 150 or 165 instead of 187;
- the 95% confidence intervals for each sample size.

Table 2.4 Prevalence rates and 95% CI

	Number positive	Total number	Prevalence (95% CI)
Prevalence rate 1	187	428	43.7 (38.9–48.5)
Prevalence rate 2	90	428	
Prevalence rate 3	150	428	
Prevalence rate 4	165	428	

Critical appraisal checklist for an article reporting incidence or prevalence

A. Study design	
1. What is the design of the study?	
2. Was the sample randomly selected?	
3. Was the response rate adequate?	
4. Which patient or population group do the results generalise to?	
B. Statistical methods	
5. Have the terms incidence and/or prevalence been used correctly?	
6. Was the denominator used appropriate?	
7. Are 95% confidence intervals reported?	
C. Results	
8. How precise were the measured rates as indicated by the confidence intervals?	
9. Are the between-group comparisons that are made valid?	
D. Interpretation	
10. Are the results interpreted correctly?	

Note that in the formula given earlier in this Unit, p is a proportion, e.g. 0.4. To convert the values into a prevalence rate expressed as a percentage, first calculate the prevalence and 95% confidence intervals using proportions and then multiply by 100.

- If the four prevalence rates had been collected at yearly intervals over a 4-year period, what inferences could be made about significant differences between them by comparing the confidence intervals?

References

1. Evans SJ. Good surveys guide. BMJ 1991;302:302–303.
2. Berry G. Statistical significance and confidence intervals. Med J Aust 1986;144:618–619.
3. Altman D. Confidence intervals in research evaluation. ACP J Club 1992;116:A28–A29.
4. Lang TA, Secic M. Rules for presenting numbers in text. In: How to report statistics in medicine. Philadelphia, Pennsylvania: American College of Physicians, 1997; pp 339–341.

RESEARCH FORUM

A quick overview on measuring pressure ulcer prevalence and incidence

Diane Langemo, PhD, RN, FAAN, Julie Anderson, PhD, RN, CCRC, Darlene Hanson, MS, RN, Susan Hunter, MSN, RN, Patricia Thompson, MS, RN

Pressure ulcers remain a significant concern in the acute care, long-term care, rehabilitation, and, to a somewhat lesser extent, home care and hospice settings. Determining how many individuals are admitted with a pressure ulcer and/or develop a pressure ulcer after admission can be motivating for an agency both internally and externally. Internally, this information provides each facility with a better perspective on the scope of the problem and allows wound care providers to compare these rates with those of similar facilities. The data also allow each facility to evaluate its individual pressure ulcer prevention and intervention efforts.[1]

Defining prevalence and incidence

Prevalence is a measure of the proportion of a group that has a pressure ulcer at any given time. The time frame may be a given day (point prevalence) or during a specific time period of a week, month, quarter, or year (period prevalence). Prevalence can be viewed as a snapshot of a situation. The current trend is measuring agency-acquired prevalence, or the number of individuals who developed a pressure ulcer post-admission and who are present at the time of the prevalence audit.

Incidence is a measure of the proportion of a group who is pressure ulcer–free at the outset, but who develops a pressure ulcer over a given time frame. Incidence reflects the nosocomial problem of pressure ulcer development and, in essence, is a more accurate and sensitive indicator of quality.

Both prevalence and incidence are calculated as a proportion or fraction, with both a numerator and denominator. The numerator represents a pressure ulcer case or patient with an ulcer, rather than an individual ulcer. Each individual, whether he or she has 1 or 3 pressure ulcers, is only counted 1 time. The denominator of the fraction represents the number of individuals who are at risk for pressure ulcer development in a given population. An individual is at risk if he or she has a likelihood of developing a pressure ulcer if exposed to pressure ulcer risk factors. Thus, anyone admitted with a pressure ulcer is eliminated from the incidence study.

University of North Dakota College of Nursing, Grand Forks, ND

Diane Langemo *Chester Fritz Distinguished Professor Emeritus*
Julie Anderson *Associate Professor*
Darlene Hanson *Clinical Associate Professor*
Susan Hunter *Associate Professor*
Patricia Thompson *Clinical Assistant Professor*

The equations for prevalence and incidence follow along with an example calculation:

Prevalence rate

Number of patients with a pressure ulcer on the day of data collection
Number of patients in the facility who are included in data collection × 100
   Example: 10
   $\frac{10}{120} \times 100 = 12\%$

Incidence rate

Number of at-risk patients who developed pressure ulcers in the time period
Number of at-risk patients admitted during time period × 100
   Example: 05
   $\frac{05}{100} \times 100 = 5\%$

Issues in measuring pressure ulcer prevalence and incidence

When measuring pressure ulcer prevalence and incidence, it does not matter how many ulcers a patient has, the individual is measured/counted only once. The patient is only counted 1 time to represent the pressure ulcer problem accurately. The numerator represents the total number of patients with a pressure ulcer. Second, patients who are included in the denominator are those at risk for developing the disease (pressure ulcer). Consequently, outpatient surgery patients, routine obstetric care patients, and ambulatory psychiatric patients are not generally included in the prevalence or incidence audit. Some facilities choose to include all pressure ulcers in a study, whereas others elect to include only stages II through IV pressure ulcers. Including Stage I pressure ulcers presents the most accurate picture. The specific criteria used must be included in the reporting.

Prevalence rates may be influenced by admission policies and vice versa. For example, prevalence includes pressure ulcers that developed before admission to the facility; thus, a high rate may be reflective of admission policies. Conversely, a facility willing to admit a patient with a pressure ulcer may be penalized. For example, the admission could reflect a higher pressure ulcer prevalence rate when the facility is actually opening its doors to all patients.

To measure incidence, the clinician follows up patients over a given period that is long enough to accurately represent the

---

Originally published in *Advances in Skin and Wound Care* 2007; **20**(12): 642–644. Reproduced with permission.

problem. If a short time is used, the incidence rate may be artificially low. Conversely, if the time frame is unduly long, the rate may be uncharacteristically high. Generally, 1 month or 1 quarter is recommended. Incidence rates are generally lower than prevalence rates; thus, comparing the 2 presents difficulties. Clinicians should not attempt to compare incidence rates measured by different methods.

Conclusions

In summary, although both prevalence and incidence are measures of the frequency of a problem, each provides a different perspective on the scope of the problem. As clinical practice moves from a clinically based to a scientifically based model, providers are meeting the challenge of scientifically documenting the extent of the pressure ulcer problem through prevalence and incidence studies.[2]

References

1 Gallagher SM. Outcomes in clinical practice: pressure ulcer prevalence and incidence studies. Ostomy Wound Manage 1997; 43:28–35.
2 Frantz RA. Measuring prevalence and incidence of pressure ulcers. Adv Wound Care 1997;10(1):21–4.

Originally published in *Advances in Skin and Wound Care* 2007; **20**(12): 642–644. Reproduced with permission.

Prevalence of asthma and allergy in schoolchildren in Belmont, Australia: three cross sectional surveys over 20 years

Brett G Toelle, Kitty Ng, Elena Belousova, Cheryl M Salome, Jennifer K Peat, Guy B Marks

We have previously shown that the prevalence of asthma in Australian primary schoolchildren increased substantially between 1982 and 1992.[1] Similar increases have been reported in studies of children of different ages and from various geographical regions, spanning periods up to the mid-1990s.[2] It is not known whether this trend has continued during the late 1990s and early 2000s. We therefore conducted a third cross sectional study in the same population that was surveyed previously.[1] We report here on prevalence trends over the latter 10 year period.

Participants, methods, and results

We conducted all studies during June and July in primary schools in and around Belmont, a coastal suburb some 150 km north of Sydney, Australia. We invited all children in years 3, 4, and 5 (ages 8–11 years) at selected schools to participate and studied only children who had parental consent. Parents completed a questionnaire about symptoms, diagnosis, and treatment of asthma and other allergic illnesses. We used a histamine challenge test to measure airway hyperresponsiveness and assessed atopy by skin prick tests to house dust, *Dermatophagoides farinae, D pterronyssinus,* ryegrass, cockroach, cat, *Alternaria tenuis* (Hollistier-Stier, Spokane, WA, USA). Questionnaires and tests were the same as in 1992.[1] The data collected in 1982 are not directly comparable because only 8–10 year old children were included and some equipment was different[1]. Owing to a low initial response rate in 2002 a single page anonymous questionnaire was issued to parents who had not consented to their child's participation in the clinical tests. The limited data from this questionnaire have been included.

In 2002 we initially enrolled 627 children (292 (46.6%) boys), representing 51.3% of the eligible sample of 1222. A further 183 participants subsequently provided a questionnaire, yielding an overall sample of 810 children (399 (49.3%) boys), represent 66% of the eligible sample. The response rate in 2002 was lower than in previous surveys (table). Between 1992 and 2002 the prevalence of diagnosed asthma, recent wheeze, and use of asthma medication decreased significantly (table). However, the prevalence of hay fever, eczema, atopy, airway hyperresponsiveness, or current asthma (defined as recent wheeze plus airway hyperresponsiveness) did not change significantly. These trends contrast with the substantial rise in the prevalence of most of these indicators during the period 1982 to 1992.[1]

Comment

These results provide evidence that the trajectory of increasing prevalence of asthma has not continued. A potential limitation is the possibility of selection bias arising from a lower response rate in 2002 compared with 1992. In the 2002 survey the prevalence of asthma symptoms was higher in the initial responders than in the responders in the second phase (data not shown). It seems reasonable to assume that non-responders were more similar to the responders in the second phase than the initial responders,[4] and some empirical evidence supports this.[5] If this is the case then the prevalence estimates for 2002 are likely to be overestimates for the population. This direction of potential bias tends to strengthen our conclusion that the prevalence of asthma has not increased further during the period 1992 to 2002.

Although it is good news that the trajectory of increasing asthma prevalence has halted in the locality we studied, it remains to be seen how generalisable and sustained this new trend is. Uncertainty remains about the extent to which fluctuations in asthma prevalence over the past two decades can be attributed to changes in awareness of asthma. The explanation for the reduction in prevalence remains as elusive as the explanation for the initial increase.

University of Sydney, Woolcock Institute of Medical Research, Box M77 Missenden Road Post Office, Camperdown, NSW 2050, Australia

Brett G Toelle *senior research officer,*
Kitty Ng *research scientist*
Elena Belousova *research scientist*
Cheryl M Salome *research fellow*
Guy B Marks *honorary associate professor*

Department of Paediatrics and Child Health, University of Sydney

Jennifer K Peat *associate professor*

Address for correspondence: B G Toelle (email: bgt@woolcock.org.au)

(*Accepted 16 October 2003*)

Contributors: BGT collected data, conducted data analysis, and wrote the manuscript. KN coordinated the study, collected data and reviewed the manuscript. EB collected data, designed the database, checked accuracy of the data, and reviewed the manuscript. CMS participated in all three surveys, collected data, and reviewed the manuscript. GBM collected data, interpreted the data, and co-wrote the manuscript. JKP assisted with interpretation of the data and reviewed the manuscript.

Changes in prevalence of atopy and asthma in primary school children, Belmont, New South Wales, Australia, 1982 to 2002. Values are numbers (percentages) unless otherwise indicated

	1982* (n = 816)	1992† (n = 1052)	2002† (n = 1222)	1992 to 2002 Absolute % increase (95% CI‡)
Participants (response rate)	718 (88.0)	914 (86.9)	810 (66.3)	
Asthma diagnosed	65/718 (9.1)	348/909 (38.3)	249/804 (31.0)	−7.3% (−11.8% to −2.8%)
Recent use of asthma medicine	69/718 (9.6)	256/910 (28.1)	185/798 (23.2)	−4.9% (−9.0% to −0.8%)
Recent use of inhaled steroids	NA	112/910 (12.3)	59/591 (10.0)	−2.3% (−5.5% to 0.9%)
Wheeze in the past 12 months§	75/718 (10.4)	259/907 (28.6)	189/795 (23.7)	−4.9% (−9.1% to −0.7%)
No. of attacks of wheeze in the past 12 months:				
<4	57/718 (7.9)	106/905 (11.7)	80/783 (10.2)	−1.5% (−4.5% to 1.5%)
≥4	18/718 (2.5)	144/905 (15.9)	92/783 (11.8)	−4.1% (−7.4% to −0.8%)
Hay fever	147/718 (20.5)	310/908 (34.1)	309/804 (38.4)	4.3% (−0.3% to 8.9%)
Eczema	146/718 (20.3)	222/908 (24.4)	198/800 (24.8)	0.4% (−3.7% to 4.5%)
Parental asthma ever	129/718 (18.0)	248/891 (27.8)	218/571 (38.2)	10.4% (5.5% to 15.4%)
Skin prick test positive¶		356/906 (39.3)	216/597 (36.2)	−3.1% (−8.1% to 1.9%)
Airway hyperresponsiveness**				
All participants	65/718 (9.1)	180/891 (20.2)	108/550 (19.6)	−0.6% (−4.8% to 3.6%)
In non-atopic participants		40/540 (7.4)	35/353 (9.9)	2.5% (−1.3% to 6.3%)
In atopic participants		139/347 (40.1)	71/192 (37.0)	−3.1% (−11.7% to 5.7%)
Current asthma††	32/718 (4.5)	110/889 (12.4)	62/549 (11.3)	−1.1% (−4.5% to 2.3%)

NA = Not available.

*Data from[3] and relating to children aged 8–10 years only.

†Data for children aged 8–11 years in the 1992 and the current (2002) study.

‡Ranges that exclude zero are significant at the 5% level.

§Includes a positive response to either wheeze or exercise wheeze in the past 12 months.

¶ Any allergen skin prick test mean wheal diameter ≥3 mm. 1982 data not presented because of methodological differences with 1992 and 2002 data.

**Provoking dose of histamine to cause a 20% fall in forced expiratory volume at 1 second <3.91 µmol.

†† Recent wheeze and airway hyperresponsiveness.

Funding: Australia Health Management Group.

Competing interests: None declared.

Ethical approval: Human Ethics Committee of the University of Sydney.

References

1 Peat JK, van den Berg RH, Green WF, Mellis CM, Leeder SR, Woolcock AJ. Changing prevalence of asthma in Australian children. BMJ 1994;308:1591–6.

2 Peat JK, Li J. Reversing the trend: Reducing the prevalence of asthma. J Allergy Clin Immunol 1999;103:1–10.

3 Britton WJ, Woolcock AJ, Peat JK, Sedgwick CJ, Lloyd DM, Leeder SR. Prevalence of bronchial hyperresponsiveness in children: the relationship between asthma: the relationship between asthma and skin reactivity to allergens in two communities. Int J Epidemiol 1986;15:202–9.

4 Drane JW Imputing nonresponses to mail-back questionnaires. Am J Epidemiol 1991;134:908–12.

5 de Marco R, Verlato G, Zanolin E, Bugiani M, Drane JW. Nonresponse bias in EC respiratory health survey in Italy. Eur Respir J 1994;7:2139–45.

Incidence of hepatitis C virus and HIV among new injecting drug users in London: prospective cohort study

Ali Judd, Matthew Hickman, Steve Jones, Tamara McDonald, John V Parry, Gerry V Stimson, Andrew J Hall

In England, the low prevalence of HIV among injecting drug users during the 1990s was attributed in part to the introduction of harm reduction interventions in the late 1980s. Also, the prevalence of hepatitis C virus in the late 1990s was thought to be relatively low compared with other countries, at around 40% overall and 15% among those who had been injecting drugs for less than six years.[1] We carried out a prospective cohort study of new injecting drug users in London to estimate the incidence of hepatitis C virus and HIV.

Participants, methods, and results

In 2001, we recruited from community settings mainly in London, but also in Brighton, 428 injecting drug users who were aged below 30 years or had been injecting for six years or fewer. All had injected in the previous four weeks and could provide addresses for follow up. They completed interviewer administered questionnaires and provided oral fluid specimens and optionally dried capillary blood spots for testing for antibodies to hepatitis C virus and HIV using published methods.[2,3] They were followed up 12 months later. We calculated incidence using standard person time methods.

Most of the participants (91%) were recruited in London. The mean (SD) age was 27.4 (5.3) years, and 29% of the participants were women. Three fifths (61%) of the sample

Centre for Research on Drugs and Health Behaviour, Department of Primary Care and Social Medicine, Imperial College London, London W6 8RP

Ali Judd *research associate*
Matthew Hickman *senior lecturer*
Steve Jones *researcher*

Gerry V Stimson *emeritus professor*

Sexually Transmitted and Blood Borne Virus Laboratory, Health Protection Agency London

Tamara McDonald *research scientist*
John V Parry *deputy director*

Infectious Disease Epidemiology Unit, London School of Hygiene and Tropical Medicine, London

Andrew J Hall *professor*

Correspondence to: A Judd
(email: a.judd@imperial.ac.uk)

(Accepted 7 September 2004)

at baseline had been injecting for less than four years, and the median frequency of injecting was 2.5 times a day. Most (71%) mainly injected opiates, although just over half (53%) had injected cocaine or crack in the previous year. Participants reported high levels of injecting risk behaviour, with 24% at baseline reporting injecting in the previous four weeks with needles and syringes used by someone else, and 53% sharing injecting paraphernalia. The baseline prevalence of antibody to hepatitis C virus was 44% and of antibody to HIV was 4% (table).

The overall follow up rate was 70%, and we found no difference between those followed up and those lost to follow up for sociodemographic characteristics or injecting risk behaviour. The incidence of antibody to hepatitis C virus was 41.8 cases per 100 person years and of antibody to HIV was 3.4 cases per 100 person years (see table).

Comment

The incidence of hepatitis C virus in England is high and of HIV higher than expected. These findings are corroborated by ongoing surveillance data, and suggest that transmission may have recently increased.[1] Injecting drug users in London have a higher incidence of hepatitis C virus than those in many cities worldwide, and an incidence of HIV comparable to that among men who have sex with men attending clinics for sexually transmitted infection in London.[4]

Possible explanations for the rising incidence include changes in patterns of injecting drug use, with greater injection of crack and injecting risk behaviour in newer injecting drug users than in those injecting in the early to mid-1990s. In addition there may have been increases in the size of the population of injecting drug users over and above any increase in protective interventions. Recent estimates suggest that current syringe distribution in London provides one new needle per injecting drug user every two days and that fewer than one in four are in drug treatment at any one time.[5] Specific targets to prevent bloodborne viruses among injecting drug users have been absent from the UK government's drug strategy in the past five years, and there has been little targeted health education or prevention campaigns. Increasing the coverage of syringe exchange and provision of drug treatment is only part of the solution. Innovative strategies are required, specific to hepatitis C virus and to HIV, to change behaviour and to deliver health education messages and harm reduction strategies early enough to make a difference.

Originally published in *BMJ* 2005; **330**: 24–5. Reproduced with permission.

Prevalence and incidence of hepatitis C virus and HIV antibody among new injecting drug users in London, 2001–3

Viral antibodies	Baseline		Follow up	
	No positive/total	Prevalence (95% CI)	No. of seroconversions/total (mean follow up time)	Incidence rate per 100 person years
Hepatitis C virus	187/428	43.7 (38.9 to 48.5)	53/151 (372 days)	41.8 (31.9 to 54.7)
HIV	18/428	4.2 (2.5 to 6.6)	9/273 (360 days)	3.4 (1.8 to 6.6)

What is already known on this topic

Injecting drug users are at high risk of acquiring HIV, hepatitis C virus, and other bloodborne infections

What this study adds

The incidences of hepatitis C virus and HIV among new injecting drug users in London are 41.8 and 3.4 cases per 100 person years, respectively

Current drug policy is failing to maintain historical levels of protection from bloodborne viruses among this high risk group

We thank the interviewers and participants; Greg Holloway for his significant contribution to the fieldwork; Sheila Bird, David Goldberg, Adrian Renton, Tim Rhodes, Avril Taylor, and advisory group members for their ongoing advice. Matthew Hickman is funded through a Department of Health Public Health Career Scientist award. The Centre for Research on Drugs and Health Behaviour is core funded by the Department of Health.

Contributors: AJ, MH, SJ, JP, GVS, and AJH designed and conducted the cohort study. TMcD conducted the laboratory testing, overseen by JVP. AJ undertook the statistical analysis; she is guarantor for the paper. All authors contributed to the writing of the paper.

Funding: Policy research programme of the Department of Health. The views expressed are those of the authors and not necessarily those of the Department of Health. The funding source had minor involvement in the study design, through attendance at steering group meetings.

Competing interests: None declared.

Ethical approval: This study received ethical approval from Hammersmith, Queen Charlotte's and Chelsea and Acton Hospitals research ethics committee.

References

1 Health Protection Agency, Scottish Centre for Infection and Environmental Health, National Public Health Service for Wales, Communicable Disease Surveillance Centre Northern Ireland, Centre for Research on Drugs and Health Behaviour, Unlinked Anonymous Surveys Steering Group. *Shooting up: infections among injecting drug users in the United Kingdom 2002.* London: HPA, 2003.

2 Judd A, Parry J, Hickman M, McDonald T, Jordan I, Lewis K, et al. Evaluation of a modified commercial assay in detecting antibody to hepatitis C virus in oral fluids and dried blood spots. *J Med Virol* 2003;71:49–55.

3 Connell JA, Parry JV, Mortimer PP, Duncan J. Novel assay for the detection of immunoglobulin G antihuman immunodeficiency virus in untreated saliva and urine. *J Med Virol* 1993;41:159–64.

4 Murphy G, Charlett A, Jordan LF, Osner N, Gill ON, Parry JV. HIV incidence appears constant in men who have sex with men despite widespread use of effective antiretroviral therapy. *AIDS* 2004;18:265–72.

5 Hickman M, Higgins V, Hope VD, Bellis MA, Tilling K, Walker A, et al. Injecting drug use in Brighton, Liverpool, and London: best estimates of prevalence and coverage of public health indicators. *J Epidemiol Community Health* 2004;58:766–71.

Originally published in *BMJ* 2005; **330**: 24–5. Reproduced with permission.

UNIT 3

Comparing proportions

Aims

To understand how to determine whether the frequency of an outcome is significantly different between treatments or exposure groups, and how to estimate whether there has been a significant increase or decrease in the frequency of a condition over time or over incremental exposure groups.

Learning objectives

On completion of this unit, participants will be able to:
- decide whether appropriate percentages and chi-square statistics have been used to describe the results;
- choose the correct chi-square value to describe the relationship between categorical outcome and explanatory variables;
- distinguish between clinically important and statistically significant effects;
- interpret tests for measuring trends in an outcome over time or over incremental exposures.

Background

We often want to test whether the frequency of a condition is significantly different between two or more groups, such as groups who receive different treatments or who have been exposed to different environmental factors. For example, we may want to test whether symptoms are less frequent in a group that has received a new treatment compared to a group that has received standard treatment. Alternatively, we may want to test whether children who are breast-fed have fewer respiratory infections than children who are formula-fed. For these types of research questions, in which both the outcome and exposure variables can be classified into categories such as the presence or absence of symptoms, a chi-square statistic is used to test whether there is good evidence that the exposure and outcome variables are related. The *P* value obtained from a chi-square test indicates the probability that a difference in the outcome rate between exposure groups has occurred by chance.

Table 3.1 Contingency table for estimating chi-square values

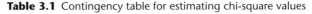

	Disease present	Disease absent	Total
Exposure present	a	b	a + b
Exposure absent	c	d	c + d
Total	a + c	b + d	Total

Cross-tabulations

In Unit 2, we discussed the methods that can be used to describe the rate of an illness in a population sample as either an incidence or prevalence rate. In this Unit, we use the term 'frequency' to describe the number of cases with the outcome of interest that occur in a given exposure category. When exploring a relationship between two categorical variables, the data should first be summarised using a contingency table or cross-tabulation as shown in Table 3.1. The contingency table shown is called a 2×2 table because there are two categories for each of the disease (column) and exposure (row) variables. However, contingency tables can be larger when either the outcome or the exposure has more than two categories, for example, a 2×3 or a 3×3 table.

In clinical and epidemiological research, the exposure is conventionally displayed as the rows and the outcome as the columns. For example, in Table 3.1, the exposure, for example the receipt of a new treatment (present, absent) forms the rows and the outcome, that is the disease or symptoms (present, absent) forms the columns. In this way, the people with the outcome of interest are displayed in the left-hand column and the people in whom the outcome is absent are in the right-hand column. Similarly, people who are exposed to the factor of interest are displayed in the first row of the table and people who are not exposed in the second row.

Presenting the exposure and outcome variables as shown in Table 3.1 is the conventional format used in most clinical epidemiology text books, and is standard for tables from which other statistics, such as measures of agreement or diagnostic statistics, are computed. However, the rows and columns in the table will be reversed on computer output when a statistics program is used if the outcome and

31

exposure variables are conventionally coded by assigning 'no' a number that is numerically lower than 'yes', for example no = 0 and yes = 1, or no = 1 and yes = 2. Obviously, the order of coding has no effect on the association between the variables, the percentages in the table or on the chi-square test. However, coding in this way does ensure that the direction of other measures of association, such as odds ratios or relative risks as described in Unit 4, are correctly calculated so that their interpretation is intuitive.

The data from a study to examine the effect of exposure to environmental tobacco smoke on the prevalence of respiratory infection in early life in 1200 children are shown in Table 3.2. Exposure was defined as having a parent who smoked and the disease was defined as having been treated for bronchitis by a doctor or at a hospital during the first two years of life. Table 3.2 shows that 300/1200 or 25.0% of children were exposed to parental smoking and 135/1200 or 11.3% had been treated for bronchitis. In tables such as this, the percentages across the rows help to interpret the association between the two variables because they provide an estimate of effect. The row percentages show that 15.0% of children who were exposed to parental smoking had treatment for bronchitis compared to 10.0% of children who were not exposed. A chi-square test is used to assess whether this 5% difference in the rate of bronchitis between the two groups is statistically significant or has arisen by chance. The *P* value indicates the strength of association between the exposure variable (parental smoking) and the outcome variable (treatment for bronchitis).

Table 3.2 Association between exposure to tobacco smoke and bronchitis in early life

	Bronchitis	No bronchitis	Total
Parental smoker	45 (15.0%)	255 (85.0%)	300 (100.0%)
Parental non-smoker	90 (10.0%)	810 (90.0%)	900 (100.0%)
Total	135 (11.3%)	1065 (88.8%)	1200 (100.0%)

For the data presented in Table 3.2, the Pearson's chi-square value is 5.63 and *P* = 0.018, indicating that children who have a parent who smokes have a significantly higher rate of being treated for bronchitis than children who are not exposed to parental smoking.

Chi-square tests

The internal cells of a contingency table show the number of people in each of the disease/exposure groups. When using a chi-square test, each person must be included in the table once only. Sometimes a person may be represented in a data set more than once, for example if they have been studied on two or more occasions for a reason such as being re-admitted to hospital or having measurements taken from both legs. If a person has two or more records in the data file, then only one record can be used in a chi-square analysis and a decision needs to be made about which record to use, for example data collected on either the first or the second occasion. Inclusion of a person more than once in a chi-square analysis would violate one of the assumptions of the test, which is that all observations are independent.

Chi-square tests are easily calculated using a statistics package or a program available on the Internet, for example Simple Interactive Statistical Analysis (SISA) at http://home.clara.net/sisa. Most statistical packages print out a range of different chi-square values for 2 × 2 tables. As shown in Table 3.3, the correct statistic to use depends on both the sample size and the expected count in each cell of the contingency table. The expected counts are the numbers that would be expected in each cell if the null hypothesis of no association between the two variables was true.[1]

Although a chi-square value is easily obtained by using a statistics package, an understanding of how the statistic is computed helps in its interpretation. The calculation of Pearson's chi-square value is relatively simple. Firstly, the 'expected' count for each cell in the contingency table is calculated by multiplying the row total by the column total for the cell and dividing this number by the sample size. For Table 3.1, the expected count in cell '*a*' would be $(a + b) \times (a + c)/$Total. Each cell count is simply the number predicted

Table 3.3 When to use each chi-square value

Statistic	Description	Application
Pearson's chi-square	Approximation for large sample sizes	Used when the sample size is very large, say over 1000. At least 80% of the cells should have an expected count greater than 5.
Continuity correction	Adjusted for small sample sizes	Used when the sample size is smaller, say less than 1000. This statistic is only available for 2 × 2 tables.
Fisher's exact test	Used when the count in one or more cells is low	Used when one or more cells in a 2 × 2 table have a small expected count that is less than 5.
Chi-square trend (also called Linear-by-linear)	Trend test	Used to test for a trend in the frequency of the outcome across an ordered exposure variable.

by the probability of exposure and the probability of disease in the sample.

The Pearson's chi-square value is calculated by summing the deviations between the observed and expected counts in each cell as follows:

Pearson chi-square = Sum (Observed count
$$- \text{Expected count})^2/\text{Expected count}$$

Expected count

As for many statistics, the deviations between the observed and expected values are squared to remove the influence of negative values that would balance out the positive values if the deviations were summed without being squared. Obviously, if the expected counts are close to the observed counts, the chi-square will be close to zero and will be non-significant. The larger the difference between the observed and expected counts, the more likely the chi-square value will become statistically significant, indicating a very low probability that the association has occurred by chance and that there is good evidence that the exposure and the disease are related.

Pearson's chi-square is an approximate statistic based on the assumption of a very large sample size. However, other chi-square values that are adjusted for smaller sample sizes are available. If the expected number in any cell of the contingency table is less than 5, a Fisher's exact test should be used rather than a Pearson's chi-square test.

Glossary	
Term	**Definition**
Chi-square test	A statistic used to test whether the rate of an outcome is significantly different between two or more exposure groups. The test provides a probability that the outcome and the exposure are independent.
Chi-square test for trend	A statistic used to test whether there is a linear trend for an outcome to increase or decrease over the range of an ordered categorical exposure variable.

Chi-square trend tests

To decide whether an outcome and an exposure are significantly related in a dose–response manner, a chi-square trend test can be used to measure whether the rate of the outcome increases or decreases significantly over time, or as the exposure increases or decreases. A chi-square trend test is used in a situation in which the outcome is binary and the exposure is an ordered categorical variable.

A chi-square trend test differs from other chi-square tests in the calculation of 'degrees of freedom'. The degrees of freedom for any test is the effective sample size used to determine

the *P* value, and is calculated as the sample size minus the number of parameters used in calculating the statistic. For chi-square, the degrees of freedom are the number of rows minus 1, multiplied by the number of columns minus 1. The smaller the number of degrees of freedom, the more significant the *P* value will be for the same chi-square value. A chi-square trend test is a more powerful statistic than Pearson's chi-square statistic for a table that is 3 × 2 or larger because it is based on only one degree of freedom, rather than the number of exposure categories minus 1. Also, if most of the variation between groups is due to the trend, then the trend test will give a much smaller and therefore more significant *P* value than Pearson's chi-square.[2]

When using a chi-square trend test, the exposure needs to be presented in at least three ordered categories. For example, the exposure could be time (say years presented as 1974, 1984 and 1994) or a dietary factor such as vitamin C intake (coded as low, medium or high). The chi-square trend test then indicates whether the slope of the line through the frequency estimate in each exposure category is significantly different from zero, that is, whether it is significantly different from a horizontal line, which would indicate no trend. Figure 3.1 shows four frequencies of a theoretical outcome estimated over time with the trend line displayed. The trend appears important because the line shows that the estimated frequency has risen from approximately 9% in 1975 to approximately 18% in 2005, that is, by approximately 3% every 10 years. A chi-square trend test will indicate whether the slope of this line is significantly different from zero or has arisen by chance. For Figure 3.1, if the group studied in each year had a sample size of 500, the chi-square value for the trend would be 14.47 which, with 1 degree of freedom, would give a *P* value of <0.01 indicating a significant trend for the outcome to linearly increase over time.

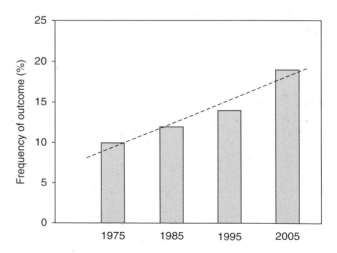

Figure 3.1 Frequency of an illness (or outcome) across ordered exposure categories.

TAKE HOME LIST

- For Pearson's and a continuity corrected chi-square, at least 80% of the cells in the contingency table must have an expected count greater than 5.

- The *P* value from a chi-square test is influenced by the sample size. The smaller the sample size, the less significant the *P* value will be for the same chi-square value.

- A chi-square test for trend can be used when the exposure has three or more ordered categories.

- For the same chi-square value, a chi-square test for trend is more powerful than a Pearson's chi-square test because it has fewer degrees of freedom, and therefore will have a lower *P* value.

Reading and questions
Set article

Miranda-Filho DB, Ximenes RAA, Barone AA, Vaz VL, Vieira AG, Albuquerque VMG. Randomised controlled trial of tetanus treatment with antitetanus immunoglobulin by the intrathecal or intramuscular route. BMJ 2004;328:615–618. (See p. 37.)

In the article by Miranda-Filho *et al.* (2004) the clinical progression of tetanus is measured in a randomised controlled trial. Patients in an intensive care unit were randomised to one of two treatment groups and received anti-tetanus immunoglobulin by either the intrathecal and intramuscular route (new treatment group) or the intramuscular route (control group). There were 58 patients in the treatment group and 62 in the control group and therefore the sample size is moderately large for a single centre study.

In the results section of the article, the first statistical result that the authors report is that the patients in the treatment group showed better clinical progression as measured by grade of tetanus than patients in the control group with a chi-square trend *P* value of 0.0052.

After reading the article, answer the following questions.

1 Using the values presented in Table 3 in the article, roughly sketch the percentage of patients in the study and control group with grade III or IV tetanus over the 10-day period to create a figure similar to Figure 3.1. Has the chi-square trend value been used in a classical way?

2 The most important clinical outcomes, that is, complications and mortality, are reported in Table 5 in the article. What is the difference in per cent with complications, respiratory infection, respiratory failure and death between the new treatment (study) group and the control treatment group? How would you interpret the *P* values?

3 In Table 5 in the article, it can be seen that there is more than a 50% reduction in mortality between the new treatment (study) group (mortality 7%) and the control group (mortality 16%) but the *P* value is 0.197. Why do you think the *P* value is so large?

4 Would you reach the same conclusions that the authors have reached about the effectiveness of the treatment in reducing complications?

Worked example

In the article by Miranda-Filho *et al.* (2004) the authors refer to Table 3 and state that up to 10 days after admission most patients in the treatment group had grade I or II disease and most patients in the control group had grade III or IV disease. However, no statistics are presented to indicate whether these rates of outcome in the two groups are significantly different.

To calculate the *P* value for the difference in outcomes between treatment groups so that we can be certain of the statistical significance, a 2 × 2 contingency table can be created from Table 3 in the article using grade of tetanus at day 2 and extrapolating the numbers as shown in Table 3.4. In this article, treatment group is the exposure and grade of tetanus is the outcome. For this exercise, we will calculate Pearson's chi-square, although if using a statistics package a continuity chi-square would be the most appropriate statistic because the sample size is less than 1000.

In tables such as this, to estimate the effect size and aid in the interpretation of the *P* value, it is useful to compare the percentage of participants with the outcome of interest in each of the groups. In Table 3.4, it can be seen that 25% of the participants in the treatment (study) group have grade III–IV tetanus on day 2 compared to 49% of the control group – a 24% difference in severe disease. The Pearson's chi-square value for the table can be calculated from the formula shown in this Unit either using a calculator or an Excel spreadsheet, as shown in Table 3.5.

Note that the observed minus the expected counts (*O − E*) for each cell are of the same magnitude with equal signs for opposite quarters of Table 3.4. When calculating the chi-square value, this is a good cross-check that the calculations are correct. If any of the cells have an expected count

Table 3.4 Grade of tetanus on day 2 by treatment group

	Grade III or IV tetanus	Grade I or II tetanus	Total
Treatment (study) group	14 (25%)	42 (75%)	56
Control group	27 (49%)	28 (51%)	55
Total	41	70	111

Table 3.5 Calculation of Pearson's chi-square using Excel

Observed (O)	Row total	Column total	Total sample size	Expected (E)	$O - E$	$(O - E)^2/E$
14	56	41	111	20.7	−6.7	2.16
42	56	70	111	35.3	6.7	1.27
27	55	41	111	20.3	6.7	2.20
28	55	70	111	34.7	−6.7	1.29
					Sum	6.91

Table 3.6 Calculation of Pearson's chi-square when sample size is theoretically reduced to 25 per group

Observed (O)	Row total	Column total	Total sample size	Expected (E)	$O - E$	$(O - E)^2/E$
6	25	18	50	9.0	−3.0	1.00
19	25	32	50	16.0	3.0	0.56
12	25	18	50	9.0	3.0	1.00
13	25	32	50	16.0	−3.0	0.56
					Sum	3.13

of less than 5, then a Fisher's exact test would be more appropriate than a chi-square test.

The chi-square value, which is the sum of the $(O - E)^2/E$ terms, is 6.91. For a 2 × 2 table with 1 degree of freedom, consulting a chi-square table in a statistics book shows that a chi-square value of 3.84 indicates $P = 0.05$, a value of 6.63 indicates $P = 0.01$ and a value of 10.83 indicates $P < 0.001$. Thus, the chi-square value of 6.91 indicates that the difference of 49%−25% (or 24%) in frequency of grade III or IV tetanus between treatment groups is significant with a P value of less than 0.01. Thus, we can conclude that there is a very small probability that the difference between groups has arisen by chance and reject the null hypothesis that there is no difference between the groups. That is, there is good evidence of a relationship between treatment and severity of tetanus.

The chi-square value is, however, heavily dependent on the sample size. If the sample size had been only 25 patients in each group, but with the same percentages in categories and difference in rates between the groups, the numbers shown in Table 3.6 would be obtained. The chi-square value would equal 3.13 and the P value would be greater than 0.05 and therefore not significant. As discussed in Unit 1, clinically important differences between groups may not be statistically significant when the sample size is small, and clinically unimportant differences between groups are likely to be statistically significant when the sample size is large. Thus, it is essential that P values are interpreted in the context of both the sample size and the clinical importance of the difference in frequencies of outcomes between the groups.

Exercise

Using the article by Miranda-Filho *et al.*(2004) construct a 2 × 2 contingency table for the comparison of tetanus grade I–II vs tetanus grade III–IV at 6 days after onset of treatment and calculate the Pearson chi-square value.
- Is the Pearson's chi-square value statistically significant and value consistent with the difference in severity rates between treatment groups?
- If the number of patients enrolled was 25 in each group with approximately the same percentages and rates as day 6, would the difference in severity rates between groups on day 6 still be statistically significant? Would this result lead you to change the conclusion drawn by the authors?

Quick quiz

Tick the correct answer for each of the following questions.

1 When the total sample size is 78 patients and all cells of the contingency table have an expected count greater than 5, which statistical test should be used to examine the association between two categorical variables?
 (a) Pearson's chi-square;
 (b) Continuity corrected chi-square;
 (c) Fisher's exact chi-square;
 (d) Linear-by-linear chi-square.

Critical appraisal checklist for an article that compares prevalence rates between groups	
A. Study design	
1. What is the design of the study?	
2. Were the sampling/recruitment techniques appropriate?	
3. What are the strengths of this study?	
4. Can we be confident that each patient is included only once in each comparison?	
B. Statistical methods	
5. Are the correct terms used to describe frequencies?	
6. Are the correct statistics reported?	
C. Results	
7. Are the outcomes clinically important?	
8. How large was the effect of the treatment/exposure?	
9. Are 95% confidence intervals used to make the size of the differences between exposure groups clear?	
D. Interpretation	
10. Which patient or population group do the results generalise to?	
11. How are the results relevant to clinical practice?	
12. Have the effects been interpreted correctly?	

2 The expected counts indicate the number that would be expected in each cell if:
(a) the data had come from a random population sample;
(b) the sample characteristics were similar to the general population;
(c) the rate of exposure and illness in the population was the same as in the sample;
(d) the exposure has a clinically important effect on the outcome.

3 It is appropriate to use a Pearson's chi-square test when:
(a) the number of observed counts in each cell is larger than 5;
(b) the data have been randomly selected from the population;
(c) the outcome variable has a continuous distribution;
(d) both variables are categorical and each person appears in the data set once only.

4 A chi-square test for trend indicates that:
(a) the exposure rate increases with increasing outcome rates;

(b) a regression line can be drawn through the estimates;
(c) the prevalence of an illness increases over time;
(d) an outcome rate changes significantly with increasing exposure.

Critical appraisal

Work through the critical appraisal checklist to review the article by Miranda-Filho et al. (2004) and decide whether the results warrant a change in clinical practice.

References

1. Bland JM. The chi-square test for association. In: An introduction to medical statistics. Oxford: Oxford University Press, 1996; pp 225–235.
2. Altman DG. Ordered categories. In: Practical statistics for medical research. London: Chapman & Hall, 1996; pp 261–265.

Randomised controlled trial of tetanus treatment with antitetanus immunoglobulin by the intrathecal or intramuscular route

Demócrito de Barros Miranda-Filho, Ricardo Arraes de Alencar Ximenes, Antônio Alci Barone, Vicente Luiz Vaz, Aderbal Gomes Vieira, Valéria Maria Gonçalves Albuquerque

Abstract

Objective To evaluate the effect of intrathecal therapy with human antitetanus immunoglobulin on clinical progression of and mortality from tetanus.

Design Randomised controlled trial.

Setting Intensive care unit of a university hospital, Pernambuco, Brazil.

Participants 120 patients with tetanus allocated to antitetanus immunoglobulin by either the intrathecal and intramuscular route (n = 58) or the intramuscular route (n = 62; control group).

Main outcome measures Clinical progression of disease, duration of hospital stay, duration of occurrence of spasms, complications, respiratory infection, respiratory failure or mechanical ventilation, duration of respiratory assistance, and mortality.

Results Patients in the treatment group showed a better clinical progression than those in the control group (x^2 for trend 7.752, P = 0.005; difference in proportion of patients with improvement 20%, 95% confidence interval 4% to 35%). The duration of occurrence of spasms, hospital stay, and respiratory assistance were all shorter in patients the treatment group: respectively, 14.96, 0.0001 (difference in proportion of patients with spasms lasting ≤10 days 36%, 18% to 55%); 4.56, 0.03; and 6.56, 0.01 (proportion of patients who needed assistance for ≤10 days 69.2% in the treatment group and 30.8% in the control group (difference 38%, 12% to 65%)).

Conclusion Patients treated with antitetanus immunoglobulin by the intrathecal route show better clinical progression than those treated by the intramuscular route.

Introduction

Tetanus is a universal public health problem, with around one million cases a year and a mortality between 6% and 60%.[1] Over the past 30 years only nine randomised controlled trials have studied the prevention and treatment of tetanus.[2] Recent advances in treating tetanus are ascribed to the more frequent and effective use of aggressive treatments that utilise tracheotomy, artificial paralysis, and artificial respiration.[2–4]

Treating tetanus by neutralising the toxin is still controversial, especially dosage and route of administration.[5–15]

A meta-analysis of intrathecal therapy was inconclusive in adults.[16] We evaluated the effect of such therapy on clinical progression of and mortality from tetanus.

Methods

Our study sample was patients with tetanus admitted to the intensive care unit of the Oswaldo Cruz University Hospital, Recife, Brazil. Potential participants were aged 12 or more and had secondary sex characteristics. They were randomised to receive antitetanus immunoglobulin by either

doi 10.1136/bmj.38027.560347.7C

Department of Clinical Medicine, Faculty of Medical Sciences, University of Pernambuco, Santo Amaro, 50100.130, Recife, Pernambuco, Brazil

Demócrito de Barros Miranda-Filho *reader in infectious diseases*
Ricardo Arraes de Alencar Ximenes *reader in infectious diseases*
Vicente Luiz Vaz *lecturer in infectious diseases*
Valéria Maria Gonçalves Albuquerque *senior lecturer in infectious diseases*

Institute of Tropical Medicine Faculty of Medicine, University of São Paulo, 05.403-000, São Paulo, SP, Brazil

Antônio Alci Barone *reader in infectious diseases*

Oswaldo Cruz University Hospital, University of Pernambuco

Aderbal Gomes Vieira *consultant in infectious diseases*

Correspondence to: D B Miranda-Filho, Rua Cosme Bezerra, 85/107, Iputinga 50.670.310, Recife, Pernambuco, Brazil (email: demofilho@uol.com.br)

(Accepted 22 December 2003)

Originally published in *BMJ* 2004; **328**: 615. Reproduced with permission.

the intrathecal and intramuscular routes (treatment group) or the intramuscular route (control group).

Sample size calculations

Our sample size was based on two outcomes: disease progression and mortality.[17] Clinical progression was based on the study by Gupta and coworkers, where 6% of patients worsened after treatment compared with 21% in the control group.[7] Assuming an α of 5% and a β of 20% (80% power), we needed 112 patients, 56 in each group.

In the past 15 years, mortality from tetanus at our hospital has been up to 35%.[18] Taking previous studies as reference, we estimated a reduction in mortality to 18%.[5,7,8] Assuming an α of 5% and a β of 40% (60% power), we needed 132 patients, 66 in each group.

Data collection

After obtaining written informed consent, we randomised participants to either the treatment group or the control group. Randomisation was based on blocks of 20, and treatment allocation was concealed in sealed envelopes. We classified tetanus as grade 1, trismus, dysphagia, and generalised rigidity with no spasms; grade 2, mild and occasional spasms; grade 3, severe and recurrent spasms—usually triggered by minor or imperceptible stimuli; and grade 4, features of grade 3 and overactivity of the sympathetic nervous system.[19] Meetings were held weekly to discuss and verify these criteria. The grade was recorded on admission.[20,21] Using a standardised form we collected data on clinical progression and outcome of each case, as well as re-evaluations as outpatients. The occurrence of spasms was recorded daily on another form.

Although blinding effectively minimises bias, placebo would be unethical in our study. We therefore used several approaches to minimise observation bias: the doctors who classified the disease were rotated on alternate days for 10 days after patients were admitted; the clinical stage was recorded on a form devoid of information on treatment or previous classifications; treatment allocation was known only by certain members of the research team; and regular meetings were held to discuss problems.

For intrathecal therapy, we used 1000 IU of a lyophilised human immunoglobulin, free of preservatives to avoid irritating the meninges and the need for corticosteroids. The immunoglobulin was diluted in distilled water to a volume of 4 ml, injected by lumbar, or preferably suboccipital, puncture after removal of the corresponding volume of cerebrospinal fluid. Both groups received 3000 IU of immunoglobulin with preservative by the intramuscular route. All patients were treated according to the standardised protocol.

Data processing and analysis

We used EPI INFO 6.0 for analyses and we made double entries. The frequency of each outcome was compared by χ^2 test or relative risks with 95% confidence intervals. For ordered categories we used the χ^2 test for linear trend. The t test was used for mean comparisons. Participants who failed to undergo the therapeutic procedure were analysed according to the group to which they were allocated.

Results

From July 1997 to July 2001 we recruited 120 patients; 58 were allocated to the treatment group and 62 to the control group (figure). Potential confounders were similarly distributed between the groups (table 1).

Three patients refused to participate. They were treated in accordance with normal routine and were eventually discharged from hospital. In two patients it proved technically difficult to achieve suboccipital or lumbar puncture; they received treatment by the intramuscular route only, but for analyses they were considered in the intrathecal group. We excluded one patient randomised to each group owing to misclassification of diagnosis: one had herpes virus meningitis and the other muscular rigidity due to metoclopramide.

The treatment group showed better clinical progression than the control group (χ^2 for trend 7.82, P = 0.0052; table 2). Most of the participants were classified with either grade I or II disease. Up to 10 days after admission most patients in the treatment group had grade I or II disease and most patients in the control group had grade III or IV disease (table 3).

We excluded 23 patients on the basis of spasms: 17 had none during hospital stay, five died during the period that spasms occurred, and in one the record of daily spasms was mislaid. The study group had shorter duration of occurrence of spasms (χ^2 for trend 14.96, P = 0.0001; table 4). Among the 106 patients who survived, duration of hospital stay varied from 2 to 80 days. The treatment group had a shorter duration of hospital stay (4.56, 0.03; table 4); a smaller proportion had complications during this time, although the difference was not significant (P = 0.071; table 5).

Respiratory infection was the most common complication. It occurred less frequently in the treatment group, although the difference was not significant (P = 0.073; table 5). The relative risk of patients developing respiratory failure that

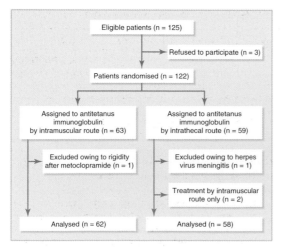

Trial profile

Originally published in *BMJ* 2004; **328**: 615. Reproduced with permission.

Table 1 Baseline characteristics of patients treated for tetanus by the intramuscular route (control group) or intrathecal route

Characteristic	No. (%) in control group (n = 62)	No. (%) in study group (n = 58)
Male	52 (84)	53 (91)
Age (years):		
12–30	21 (34)	14 (24)
31–50	18 (29)	24 (41)
51–70	18 (29)	13 (22)
>70	5 (8)	7 (12)
Incubation period (days)*:		
≤10	32 (52)	38 (66)
>10	21 (34)	18 (31)
Unknown	9 (15)	2 (3)
Period of onset (hours)*:		
≤48	30 (48)	30 (52)
>48	24 (39)	18 (31)
Unknown	1 (2)	2 (3)
With no progression to spasms	7 (11)	8 (14)
Time between start of symptoms and admission (hours)*:		
≤36	15 (24)	18 (32)
>36	47 (76)	39 (68)
Prognostic classification†:		
1A	7 (11)	9 (12)
2A	23 (37)	20 (35)
3A	32 (52)	29 (50)
Clinical grade on admission:		
I	24 (39)	21 (36)
II	23 (37)	23 (40)
III	15 (24)	13 (22)
IV	—	1 (2)

*Cut-off points based on Miranda-Filho et al.[21]

†According to Armitage and Clifford.[20] Prognostic classification based on time elapsed between beginning of symptoms and admission and spasms at admission; improved prognostic from 1A to 3A.

Table 2 Clinical progression of patients treated for tetanus by the intramuscular route (control group) or intrathecal route

Clinical progression	No. (%) in control group (n = 60)	No. (%) in study (n = 58)	P value*
Improvement	10 (17)	21 (36)	χ^2 = 7.752; 0.005
Stabilisation and improvement	13 (22)	15 (26)	
Deterioration†	37 (62)	22 (38)	

*χ^2 for linear trend.

†Smaller risk of deterioration or death within first 10 days in study group (relative risk 0.6, 95% confidence interval 0.4 to 0.9).

required artificial respiration was smaller in the treatment group than in the control group, but the difference was not significant (P = 0.094; table 5). However, the difference in the duration of respiratory assistance among 50 patients in both groups (six died during respiratory assistance) was significant (χ^2 for trend 6.56, P = 0.01; see table 4).

The relative risk of death was smaller among patients in the treatment group, although the difference was not significant (P = 0.2). The wide confidence interval (0.78 to 7.05) suggests that the sample size was too small to detect a difference of this magnitude (table 5).

In general, all results showed improvement among patients in the treatment group. Differences were not significant for mortality and complications only.

Five patients had mild headache during the intrathecal procedure. In only one did this continue after the flow rate of the

Originally published in *BMJ* 2004; **328**: 615. Reproduced with permission.

drug was reduced and the procedure finished; the headache stopped after 500 mg dipirona was given intravenously. We observed no meningeal irritation or meningitis among patients given intrathecal therapy. Among the 106 patients

who were discharged, 64 returned to the outpatient clinic for a check up, in accordance with the study protocol. Of these, 37 belonged to the treatment group; they had no side effects.

Fourteen patients died during the study. The cause of death was not determined in seven, four died from septicaemia or septic shock, one died in an anoxic coma after prolonged cardiorespiratory arrest, one died from respiratory infection, and one died from acute respiratory failure. Half of these patients died within 10 days of admission. The others died between days 16 and 89. No particular pattern was observed for deaths.

Discussion

Patients treated for tetanus with human antitetanus immunoglobulin by the intrathecal route show better clinical progression than patients treated by the intramuscular route. They also showed fewer complications, particularly respiratory ones, and needed less intervention if they did and had a shorter duration of occurrence of spasms.

The use of mortality as an indicator of treatment response is common in evaluating therapeutic measures in tetanus. Indicators of morbidity and disease progression have been used in several studies.[5–8,11,12,14,22] We monitored disease progression by grade of tetanus.[19] Grade I and II predominated in the treatment group and grade III and IV predominated in the control group. Such differences were perceptible in the early stages of hospital stay and may be attributed to intrathecal therapy.

To our knowledge no studies have compared the duration of occurrence of spasms.[5–8,11–15,22] Spasm is easily identified and a relatively reliable indicator. The duration of occurrence of spasms was shorter among patients in the treatment group.

Table 3 Severity of tetanus within 10 days of admission. Values are numbers (percentages) of patients

Days after admission	Grade of tetanus			
	I	II	III	IV
Day 2:				
Control	15 (27)	13 (24)	19 (35)	8 (15)
Study	20 (36)	22 (39)	13 (23)	1 (2)
Day 4:				
Control	10 (19)	13 (25)	20 (38)	10 (19)
Study	19 (36)	23 (43)	9 (17)	2 (4)
Day 6:				
Control	11 (21)	12 (23)	17 (33)	12 (23)
Study	18 (39)	21 (46)	7 (15)	—
Day 8:				
Control	9 (18)	16 (31)	17 (33)	9 (18)
Study	23 (52)	16 (36)	05 (11)	—
Day 10:				
Control	9 (21)	11 (26)	17 (40)	6 (14)
Study	22 (56)	10 (26)	5 (13)	2 (5)

82 patients were evaluated on day 10, 20 had been discharged, seven had died, and 11 missed appointments.

Table 4 Duration of occurrence of spasms and hospital stay and need for respiratory assistance in patients treated for tetanus by the intramuscular route (control group) or intrathecal route

Duration (days) of outcome	Control group	Study group	P value*
Permanence of spasms:	n = 51	n = 46	
≤10	14 (32)	30 (68)	14.96; 0.0001†
11–20	18 (62)	11 (38)	
>20	19 (80)	5 (21)	
Hospital stay:	n = 52	n = 54	
≤15	14 (27)	23 (43)	4.56; 0.03‡
16–30	17 (33)	19 (35)	
>30	21 (40)	12 (22)	
Respiratory assistance:	n = 30	n = 20	
≤10	4 (31)	9 (70)	6.56; 0.01§
11–20	12 (63)	7 (37)	
>20	14 (78)	4 (22)	

*χ^2 for linear trend.
†P = 0.001 (t test).
‡P = 0.13 (t test).
§P = 0.01 (t test).

Originally published in *BMJ* 2004; **328**: 615. Reproduced with permission.

Table 5 Complications and mortality in patients treated for tetanus by the intramuscular route (control group) or intrathecal route

Outcome	Control group (n = 62)	Study group (n = 58)	Relative risk (95% CI)	P value
Complications	46 (74)	33 (57)	1.30 (1.00 to 1.70)	0.071
No complications	16 (26)	25 (43)		
Respiratory infection	42 (68)	29 (50)	1.35 (0.99 to 1.85)	0.073
No respiratory infection	20 (32)	29 (50)		
Respiratory failure or mechanical ventilation	34 (55)	22 (38)	1.45 (0.97 to 2.16)	0.094
No respiratory failure or mechanical ventilation	28 (45)	36 (62)		
Died	10 (16)	4 (7)	2.34 (0.78 to 7.05)	0.197
Did not die	52 (84)	54 (93)		

Duration of hospital stay was also shorter in the treatment group, which agrees with previous studies.[8,12,22]

What is already known on this topic

Neutralisation of tetanus toxin as part of tetanus therapy is still controversial, especially the dosage and route of administration

A meta-analysis of intrathecal therapy with antitetanus immunoglobulin was inconclusive in adults

What this study adds

Giving antitetanus immunoglobulin by the intrathecal route shows several clinical benefits

Patients treated by the intrathecal route had a better disease progression than those treated by the intramuscular route

Complications from tetanus, especially respiratory ones, are often followed by death.[21,23] Studies have shown benefits on respiratory complications from intrathecal therapy. In one study, treated patients needed artificial respiration less and for shorter duration than controls.[14] In another, tracheotomy and mechanical ventilation were less likely to be needed by patients with mild tetanus.

Over half of the patients in our study had some type of complication, such as respiratory infection or respiratory failure, most often in the control group. Although the differences were not statistically significant, in both cases the probability was close to the cut-off point. Patients in the treatment group who did require artificial respiration needed less assistance than those in the control group. The difference was statistically significant.

Fourteen of our 120 patients died; 10 had undergone conventional treatment and four intrathecal therapy. Although the difference was not statistically significant, the result is in the same direction as those for all other outcomes compared. It is possible that the sample was too small to study mortality, as suggested by the large confidence interval.

To calculate our sample size we chose the outcome of reduction in mortality. During the early stage of data collection the intensive care unit was created and mortality from tetanus decreased from 35% to almost 12%. This may have had made it more difficult to show a statistically significant difference between the groups.

An analysis of the causes of death, the circumstances in which it occurred, and the time from admission to death did not provide any important information with which to compare the two groups. Seven of the 14 deaths occurred suddenly and the cause was not determined; similar proportions have been reported elsewhere.[1,23,24]

Contributors: DBMF, RAAX, and AAB conceived and designed the study, analysed and interpreted the data, and drafted the article. VLV, AGV, and VMGA helped conceive the study and collect and interpret the data. DBMF will act as guarantor for the paper. The guarantor accepts full responsibility for the conduct of the study, had access to the data, and controlled the decision to publish.

Funding: This study was funded by the Foundation of Support to Science and Technology of the State of Pernambuco, Health Foundation Amaury de Medeiros and Health Secretariat of the State of Pernambuco-Northeast Project; National Center of Epidemiology and National Health Foundation and Health Ministry of Brazil.

Ethical approval: This study was approved by the national ethics committee.

References

1 Bleck TP. Clostridium tetani (tetanus). In: Mandell GL, Bennett JE, Dolin R, eds. *Mandell, Douglas, and Bennett's principles and practice of infectious diseases.* Philadelphia: Churchill Livingstone, 2000;2537–43.

2 Thwaites CL, Farrar JJ. Preventing and treating tetanus. The challenge continues in the face of neglect and lack of research. *BMJ* 2003;326:117–8.

3 Edmondson RS, Flowers MW. Intensive care in tetanus: management, complications and mortality in 100 cases. *BMJ* 1979; 1:1401–4.

4 Harding-Goldson HE, Hanna WJ. Tetanus: a recurring intensive care problem. *J Trop Med Hyg* 1995;98:179–84.

5 Sanders RKM, Martyn B, Joseph R, Peacock ML. Intrathecal antitetanus serum (horse) in the treatment of tetanus. *Lancet* 1977;1:974–7.

6 Vakil BJ, Armitage P, Clifford RE, Laurence DR. Therapeutic trial of intracisternal human tetanus immunoglobulin in clinical tetanus. *Trans R Soc Trop Med Hyg* 1979;73:579–83.

Originally published in *BMJ* 2004; **328**: 615. Reproduced with permission.

7 Gupta PS, Goyal S, Kapoor R, Batra VK, Jain BK. Intrathecal human tetanus immunoglobulin in early tetanus. *Lancet* 1980;2:439–40.

8 Keswani NK, Singh AK, Upadhyana KD. Intrathecal tetanus anti-toxin in moderate and severe tetanus. *J Indian Med Assoc* 1980;75:67–9.

9 Rossano C, Giugliano F. Prime esperienze e risultati terapeutici con immunoglobuline umane antitetaniche per via subaracnoidea. *Minerva Anestesiol* 1970;36:725–7.

10 Ildirim I. Intrathecal treatment of tetanus with antitetanus serum and prednisolone mixture. In: International Conference on Tetanus, São Paulo. Pan American Health Organisation - Scient public 1972;253:119–26.

11 Veronesi R, Bizzini B, Hutzler RU, Focaccia R, Mazza CC, Feldman C, et al. Eficácia do tratamiento do tétano com antitoxina tetânica por via raquideana e/ou venosa. Estudo de 101 casos, com pesquisa sobre a permanência da gamaglobulina humana - F(ab)^2 -no líqüor e no sangue. *Revista brasileira Clínica e Terapêutica* 1980;9:301–19.

12 Sun KO, Chan YW Cheung RTF, So PC, Yu YL, Li PCK Management of tetanus: a review of 18 cases. *J R Soc Med* 1994;87:135–7.

13 Gallais, H. Intérêt de l'administration intrathécale de sérum antitétanique et de corticoïdes pour le treatment du tétanos déclaré. *La Nouvelle Presse médicale* 1977;6:571.

14 List WF. The immediate treatment of tetanus with high doses of human tetanus antitoxin. *Nofallmedizin* 1981;7:731 –3.

15 Thomas PP, Crowell EB, Mathew M. Intrathecal anti-tetanus serum (ATS) and parenteral betamethasone in treatment of tetanus. *Trans R Soc Trop Med Hyg* 1982;76:620–3.

16 Abrutyn E, Berlin JA. Intrathecal therapy in tetanus, a meta-analysis. *JAMA* 1991;266:2262–7.

17 Friedman LM, Furberg CD, Demets DL. *Fundamentals of clinical trials,* 3rd ed. St Louis, MI: Mosby, 1996.

18 Miranda Filho DB, Ximenes RAA, Bernardino SN, Escarião AG. Caracterização epidemiológica do tétano no estado de Pernambuco no período de 1981 a 1995. Resumos do IX Congresso Brasileiro de Infectologia; 1996; Aug 25–9; Recife. Sociedade Brasileira de Infectologia.

19 Miranda Filho D, Ximenes R, Barone A, Vaz V, Vieira. Classificação clínica de pacientes com tétano para monitoramento da resposta a medidas terapêuticas. *Braz J Infect Dis* 2003;7(suppl 1):S18.

20 Armitage P, Clifford R. Prognosis in tetanus: use of data from therapeutic trial. *J Infect Dis* 1978;138:1–8.

21 Miranda Filho DB, Ximenes RAA, Bernardino SN, Escarião AG. Identification of risk factors for death from tetanus in Pernambuco, Brazil. A case control study. *Rev Inst Med Trop Sao Paulo* 2000;42:333–9.

22 Agarwal M, Thomas K, Peter JV, Jeyaseelan L, Cherian AM. A randomised double-blind sham controlled study of intrathecal human anti-tetanus immunoglobulin in the management of tetanus. *Natl Med J India* 1998;11:209–12.

23 Barone AA, Raineri HC, Ferreira JM. Tétano: aspectos epidemiológicos, clínicos e ter-apêuticos. Análise de 461 casos. *Rev Hosp Clin Fac Med Sao Paulo* 1976;31:215–25.

24 Udwadia FE, Lall A, Udwadia ZF, Sekhar M, Vora A. Tetanus and its complications: intensive care and management experience in 150 Indian patients. *Epidemiol Infect* 1987;99:675–84.

Originally published in *BMJ* 2004; **328**: 615. Reproduced with permission.

UNIT 4
Relative risk and odds ratio

Aims

To understand the statistical methods used to estimate the magnitude of an association between two binary variables, and to calculate the likelihood that a person will have an outcome if exposed to a risk factor of interest, such as a new treatment or an environmental exposure.

Learning objectives

On completion of this unit, participants will be able to:
- define the terms relative risk and odds ratio;
- identify when a relative risk or odds ratio should be used;
- calculate a relative risk and an odds ratio from a 2 × 2 table;
- explain why an odds ratio is often called a 'poor man's relative risk';
- convert estimates of risk into estimates of protection, and vice versa;
- understand how to interpret confidence intervals around a relative risk or odds ratio.

Background

In health research and in clinical practice, we are often interested in identifying whether a health outcome, such as the presence of a disease, is related to exposure to a potential risk factor. The statistics of relative risk and odds ratio are valuable methods for estimating the strength of such a relationship when the two variables are binary, such as disease (present/absent) and potential risk factor (present/absent). These statistics describe the probability or odds that people who are exposed to a factor will have the outcome of interest compared to people who are not exposed. The exposure could be any factor, such as an environmental agent or a newly developed treatment. Whereas chi-square tests measure the probability that the outcome and exposure are related (see Unit 3), relative risk and odds ratios describe the risk or likelihood that the outcome is

Table 4.1 Contingency table to measure the relationship between an outcome and an exposure to a risk factor

	Outcome present (cases)	Outcome absent (controls)	Total
Exposure present	a	b	a + b
Exposure absent	c	d	c + d
Total	a + c	b + d	N

different between the exposed and non-exposed groups. The difference between relative risk and odds ratios lies in the ways in which they are calculated and can therefore be interpreted. Although an odds ratio is frequently interpreted as have the same meaning as that of relative risk,[1] this is often not the case.

How to calculate relative risk and an odds ratio

To calculate whether an outcome and an exposure are related, the counts for each category are summarised in a 2 × 2 contingency table as shown in Table 4.1. This table is the same as the contingency table shown in Unit 3 for calculating chi-square values.

Risk refers to the probability of an event or outcome occurring, such as the risk of infection, death or cure. For example, vaccination of newborn babies has reduced the risk of infections such as hepatitis B. Risk is calculated as the number of people with the outcome divided by the total number of people. Relative risk is calculated as the ratio of the prevalence (probability) of the outcome in the exposed group compared to the prevalence (probability) of the outcome in the non-exposed group as follows:

$$\text{Relative risk (RR)} = \frac{a/(a+b)}{c/(c+d)}$$

The advantage of relative risk is that it has an intuitive interpretation. A relative risk of 2 indicates that the prevalence of the outcome (present) in the exposed group

43

is twice as high as the prevalence of the outcome (present) in the unexposed group. That is, people in the exposed group are two times more likely than people in the non-exposed group to have the disease, indicating that the exposure confers a risk for disease. A relative risk of 0.5 would indicate that the prevalence of the outcome (present) in the exposed group is half that of the prevalence of the outcome (present) in the unexposed group, that is, the exposure confers protection against disease. Obviously, a relative risk of 1 indicates equal risk in the two exposure groups and that the outcome is not related to the exposure.

The 'odds' are the probability of an event occurring divided by the probability of that event not occurring. The probability of the event not occurring is 1 minus the probability of the event occurring. An odds ratio is then the odds of an event occurring in one group divided by the odds of an event occurring in another group. An odds ratio can be calculated from Table 4.1 as follows:

$$\text{Odds ratio (OR)} = \frac{(a/b)}{(c/d)}$$

The odds ratio is a way of representing probability that is especially familiar to betting, but perhaps not to most people in health care research.[2] An odds ratio is not only less intuitive to interpret than relative risk, but the interpretation is dictated by the study design. In most studies, the odds ratio describes the odds of the outcome occurring in the exposed group compared to the odds of the outcome occurring in the non-exposed group. For example, an odds ratio of 2 indicates that the odds of the disease occurring in the exposed group are twice that of the odds of the disease occurring in the non-exposed group. An odds ratio equal to 1 indicates that the odds of the outcome are equally likely in both the exposed and non-exposed groups. That is, there is no relationship between the exposure and the outcome.

The interpretation of odds ratios from case-control studies is slightly different. In case-control studies, the odds ratio describes the odds that the cases have been exposed compared to the odds that the controls have received the same exposure. Thus, an odds ratio of 2 would indicate that the odds of exposure in the cases was twice as high as the odds of exposure in the controls. Case-control studies are often conducted because the outcome of interest is rare. For rare outcomes, a cross-sectional or cohort study would have to be very large to enrol sufficient cases to measure risk accurately. The probability needed to compute relative risk can only be estimated accurately from a representative population sample, and thus the odds ratio offers a method of estimating an approximate relative risk in case-control studies in which a convenience method of selecting the sample is used.[3]

Glossary

Term	Definition
Risk	The probability of an event or outcome occurring, such as the risk of infection, death or cure.
Relative risk	Ratio of the probability of the outcome occurring in the exposed group, divided by the probability of the outcome occurring in the non-exposed group.
Odds	The probability of an event (p) occurring, divided by the probability of that event not occurring ($1 - p$).
Odds ratio	Ratio of the odds of the outcome occurring in one group, divided by the odds of the outcome occurring in another group.

When to use a relative risk or odds ratio

Clearly, the advantage of using relative risk is that it has a more direct and intuitive interpretation than an odds ratio. In practice, the decision of which statistic is most appropriate to use largely depends on the study design and whether an adjustment for the effects of other risk factors needs to be made.

Relative risk indicates the increased risk of a person having a disease if they are exposed to a factor of interest. Because this statistic relies on the probability of the outcome in the sample being the same as the probability of the outcome in the population, relative risk can only be used when the sample has been selected randomly or when a representative sample has been enrolled. Random samples are often enrolled in cross-sectional studies and in some cohort studies and clinical trials. In non-random samples, such as in case-control studies in which the proportion of people with disease depends on the sampling process, the probability of disease will be altered by the selection criteria and therefore the relative risk will not represent the population risk. Thus, relative risk should only be calculated from a sample that has the same characteristics as the population from which it is drawn, and in which the proportion of people with the outcome represents the population prevalence rate of the disease.

The odds ratio indicates the odds of a person having a disease if they are exposed to a factor of interest compared to the odds if not exposed. This statistic has the advantage that it can be calculated regardless of the sampling method or whether the rate of disease in the sample is similar to the rate in the population. Thus, odds ratios can be calculated from data collected in case-control studies in which the proportion of people with the disease is usually very different from the prevalence of the disease in the population.

For this reason, odds ratios allow direct comparisons of effect between different study designs, and odds ratios from studies such as cohort and case-control studies can be compared and combined. This can be important, for example, when comparing results from different clinical trials or when meta-analysis is used to summarise the results from several studies. Although relative risks can be compared and combined in the same way, they must always be generated from studies in which a random population sample is enrolled, so that the frequency of the outcome in the sample is approximately the same as the prevalence in the population.

When an odds ratio is calculated directly from a 2 × 2 table, it is called an 'unadjusted' odds ratio. However, odds ratios can be adjusted for the effects of other related exposures by using logistic regression, in which case the summary estimates are called 'adjusted' odds ratios. This is important because exposures are often related. For example, exposures that are associated with personal choice, such as smoking and exercise, are often related in that the prevalence of smoking in people who exercise infrequently is often higher than in people who exercise regularly.[4] Exposures that are related to one another and that are also related to the outcome are called confounders. Confounding often occurs because people self-select themselves into related exposure groups. Logistic regression is a multivariate modelling technique that is used to separate out the independent effects of related exposures.

In general, odds ratios should not be used to estimate the relative risk. When the relative risk is more than 1, indicating a risk from exposure, an odds ratio will overestimate the relative risk.[5] Conversely, when the relative risk is less than 1, indicating benefit or protection from exposure, the odds ratio will overestimate the protective value of the exposure when compared to a relative risk calculated from the same sample.[5] The difference between the odds ratio and the relative risk value becomes larger when either the exposure or the disease is relatively common in the sample. Only when the outcome of interest in the study population is infrequent, that is less than 10%, does the odds ratio approximate to the relative risk.[5] Because the odds ratio does not always approximate to the relative risk, it can be a misleading statistic if generalised to a population setting.[6] However, a counter view is that odds ratios are only misleading when they are applied as though they were a relative risk.[7]

Confidence intervals

The calculations of confidence intervals for both relative risk and odds ratios are more complicated than for percentages and mean values in that they are based on logarithms[2] and are therefore best obtained using a dedicated statistics program. But, as for other summary statistics, the confidence intervals show the range in which we are 95% certain that the true relative risk or odds ratio in the population lies. The confidence intervals around estimates of relative risk

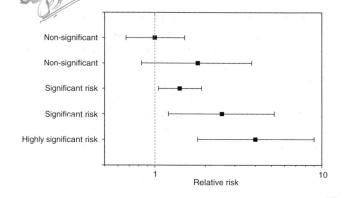

Figure 4.1 Relative risk and interpretation of 95% confidence intervals.

and odds ratios are only symmetrical around the summary statistic when the results are expressed in logarithmic units, and they are asymmetrical when the results are converted back into linear units.

Confidence intervals are an important aid in interpreting the clinical importance and statistical significance of relative risks and odds ratios. For both statistics, a value of 1 indicates no risk or no association. Therefore, a relative risk that is greater than 1 with a 95% confidence interval that does not cross the line of unity indicates a significant positive association between exposure and outcome of interest, with the outcome more likely in the exposed group. Conversely, if the relative risk is less than 1 and the 95% confidence interval does not cross the line of unity, this indicates a significant negative association between exposure and outcome of interest, with the outcome more likely in the non-exposed group.

Figure 4.1 shows five relative risks with their 95% confidence intervals. If the confidence interval crosses the line of no risk (unity), we can be fairly certain that the estimate is not significant at the $P < 0.05$ level no matter how large the relative risk. On the other hand, a relative risk with a 95% confidence interval that does not cross the line of unity will be statistically significant at the $P < 0.05$ level even though the relative risk may be small. Although relative risks are shown in Figure 4.1, the same principles apply to interpreting odds ratios and their 95% confidence intervals.

Clearly, relative risks and odds ratios need to be interpreted in terms of the size of the estimate, the clinical importance of the effect size, and the precision indicated by the width of the confidence intervals. When estimating the clinical importance, the severity of the outcome and the rate of exposure in the community must also be considered. If an exposure is rare, then a small relative risk or odds ratio will only be clinically important if the outcome has severe health consequences because few people will be affected. However, a small relative risk or odds ratio will be clinically important if the outcome is not severe but if many people are exposed. For example, the odds ratio for Australasian children to have symptoms of asthma (wheeze) if exposed to a mother who smokes is very small at 1.3.[8] However, approximately 25% of mothers smoke so that, across the population, many thousands of children will have symptoms of asthma as a result of exposure. Although symptoms of wheeze rarely require tertiary treatment, the burden on children and on the primary health care system as a result of exposure will be clinically important.

TAKE HOME LIST

- Both relative risks and odds ratios should be interpreted in terms of both their magnitude and their 95% confidence intervals.

- A relative risk larger than 1 with a 95% confidence interval that does not cross the line of unity indicates that the prevalence of the outcome is significantly higher in the exposed group.

- A relative risk or odds ratio with a 95% confidence interval that crosses the line of unity indicates that there is no association between the outcome and exposure.

- In a case-control study, an odds ratio larger than 1 with a 95% confidence interval that does not cross the line of unity indicates that the odds of the exposure is significantly greater in the cases than in the controls.

- In general, odds ratios should not be used to estimate relative risk. When the frequency of the outcome of interest is less than 10%, the odds ratio will be close to the relative risk.

Further reading and questions
Reprints

Altman DG, Deeks JJ, Sackett DL. Odds ratios should be avoided when events are common. BMJ 1998; 317:1318. (See p. 49.)
Davies HTO, Crombie IK, Tavakoli M. When can odds ratios mislead? BMJ 1998; 316:989–991. (See p. 50.)

After reading the reprints, answer the following questions.
1 Why have odds ratios become popular statistics to describe the strength of a relationship?
2 What is the difference between an odds ratio and a relative risk?
3 What is the interpretation of a relative risk that is less than 1?
4 Why is the relative risk not in the centre of its confidence interval on a linear scale?
5 In what situation is the odds ratio a poor estimate of the relative risk?

Set article

Diggle L, Deeks J. Effect of needle length on incidence of local reactions to routine immunisation in infants age 4 months: randomised controlled trial. BMJ 2000; 321:931–933. (See p. 53.)

Table 4.2 Association between redness and needle size in infants

	Redness present	Redness absent	Total
Long, thin (23 G, 25 mm) needle	21	32	53
Short, wide (25 G, 16 mm) needle	34	23	57
Total	55	55	110

Worked example

Reducing local reactions for infants who undergo routine vaccinations is important for both medical practitioners and parents. The set article by Diggle and Deeks (2000) compares rates of reactions in infants immunised with two different sizes of needles. The 2 × 2 table for redness at 6 hours can be reconstructed from the article as shown in Table 4.2 with redness as the outcome of interest and exposure present being the long, thin needle.

The relative risk and odds ratio can then be calculated as follows:

$$\text{Relative risk (RR)} = \frac{(21/53)}{(34/57)} = \frac{0.40}{0.60} = 0.66$$

$$\text{Odds ratio (OR)} = \frac{(21/32)}{(34/23)} = \frac{0.66}{1.48} = 0.44$$

The probability of having redness is 21/53, or approximately 40%, in the children with whom a long, thin needle is used and is 34/57, or approximately 60%, in children with whom a short, wide needle is used. Both the relative risk and the odds ratio are less than 1 indicating a protective effect, that is, indicating that long, thin needles are associated with less redness at 6 hours than short, wide needles. The results published in the article show that at 6 hours the relative risk of 0.66 has a 95% confidence interval of 0.45–0.99. This confidence interval does not cross the line of unity (no effect) and is therefore consistent with a significant P value of 0.007.

Obviously if exposure to a factor is protective then absence of exposure to the factor confers a risk, and therefore the calculations above also indicate that short, wide needles increase the risk of redness occurring. Estimates of protection can be converted into risk simply by reciprocating them. Figure 4.2 shows an estimate of risk plotted on a logarithmic scale, and the same estimate when converted into a protective factor by reciprocation. The two estimates

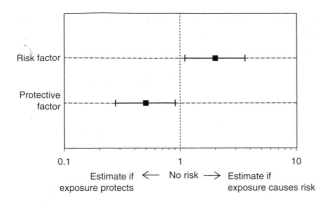

Figure 4.2 Converting estimates of risk and their 95% confidence intervals from risk to protection, or vice versa.

are symmetrical around the line of no risk (unity) because one is simply the inverse of the other.

By reciprocating the relative risk, we can calculate that the risk of redness at 6 hours conferred by a short, wide needle is 1/0.66 or 1.51 indicating that an extra 51% of infants will have redness when this type of needle is used. This estimate is a direct comparison of the approximate probability of redness of 60% in the group in which short, wide needles were used compared to the probability of 40% in the group in which long, thin needles were used. Similarly, the reciprocated odds ratio is 1/0.44 or 2.27. The difference between the relative risk and odds ratio shows how the odds ratio over-estimates the relative risk, in this case showing greater odds of an adverse reaction to short, wide needles than relative risk, because approximately half of the infants are exposed and the rate of redness is fairly common in each group.

Exercise

Using the paper by Diggle and Deeks (2000), reconstruct the 2 × 2 tables for redness at 1, 2 and 3 days and calculate the relative risks and odds ratios as both protection and risk to complete Table 4.3.

After completing Table 4.3, answer the following questions.
1 For risk, what can you infer from the estimates of relative risk and odds ratio over time?
2 Does the difference between the estimates of relative risk and odds ratio vary with the frequency of the outcome?
3 Why do you think this happens?

Critical appraisal

Work through the critical appraisal checklist to review the set article by Diggle and Deeks (2000) and decide whether

Table 4.3 Relative risk and odds ratios for redness over 3 days

Redness	Protection		Risk	
	Relative risk	Odds ratio	Relative risk	Odds ratio
6 hours	0.66	0.44	1.51	2.27
1 day				
2 days				
3 days				

the results warrant a change in the immunisation guidelines used by doctors and nurses.

Quick quiz

Tick the correct answer for each of the following questions.

1 An odds ratio that indicates risk and an odds ratio of the same magnitude that indicates protection:
(a) need to be calculated from different samples;
(b) can be converted by changing the plus or minus sign, or vice versa;
(c) would have confidence intervals that do not cross the line of unity;
(d) are the inverse of one another.

2 An odds ratio over-estimates the relative risk if:
(a) the relative risk is large;
(b) the sample is not randomly selected;
(c) the outcome of interest is common;
(d) the disease is rare.

3 A relative risk can be used when:
(a) the frequency of illness is the same as the population prevalence;
(b) a large sample of consecutive hospital patients is enrolled;
(c) the study has been designed with cases and matched controls;
(d) people who are exposed to the factor of interest are unlikely to have the illness.

4 In case-control studies, an odds ratio is used because:
(a) it is a close approximation of the relative risk;
(b) it will have smaller 95% confidence intervals than the relative risk;
(c) the sample size is usually smaller than in population studies;
(d) the rate of illness does not approximate to the population prevalence.

Critical appraisal checklist for an article reporting estimates of risk

A. Study design	
1. What is the design of the study? *RC*	
2. Was the sample randomly selected? *Yes lond*	
3. Who do the results generalise to? *Local Commn*	
B. Statistical methods	
4. Are the proportions of patients with the outcome in the exposed and non-exposed groups reported? *No*	
5. Has a relative risk or odds ratio been used correctly? *Yes*	
6. Are the explanatory factors presented consistently as risk factors or protective factors?	
7. Are confidence intervals included and do they help in interpreting the P values?	✓
8. Is more than one exposure presented and, if so, are all of the exposures independent exposure factors?	✓
C. Results	
9. Are the outcomes clinically relevant?	✓
10. How large was the effect of the exposures?	
11. How precise were the measures of effect as indicated by the confidence intervals?	
D. Interpretation	
12. How relevant are the results to clinical practice?	
13. Have the effects been interpreted correctly?	

References

1. Katz KA. The (relative) risks of using odds ratio. Arch Dermatol 2006;142:761–764.
2. Bland JM, Altman DG. The odds ratio. BMJ 2000;320:1468.
3. Altman DG. The odds ratio. In: Practical statistics for medical research. London: Chapman & Hall, 1996; pp 268–271.
4. Peat JK, Mellis CM, Williams K, Xuan W. Confounders. In: Health science research. A handbook of quantitative methods. Sydney: Allen and Unwin, 2001; pp 92–97.
5. Zhang J, Yu KF. What's the relative risk? A method of correcting the odds ratio in cohort studies of common outcomes. JAMA 1998;280:1690–1691.
6. Sackett D, Deeks J, Altman DG. Down with odds ratios! Evidence-Based Med 1996;1:164–166.
7. Cook TD. Up with odds ratios! A case for odds ratios when outcomes are common. Acad Emerg Med 2002;9:1430–1434.
8. Peat JK. Can asthma be prevented? Evidence from epidemiological studies of children in Australia and New Zealand in the last decade. Clin Exp Allergy 1998;28:261–265.

LETTERS

Odds ratios should be avoided when events are common

Douglas G Altman, Jonathon J Deeks, David L Sackett

EDITOR—A news item stated that "a review article written by authors with affiliations to the tobacco industry is 88 times more likely to conclude that passive smoking is not harmful than if the review was written by authors with no connection to the tobacco industry."[1] We are concerned that readers may have interpreted this huge effect at face value. The proportions being compared (which were not given in the news item) were 29/31 (94%) and 10/75 (13%). The relative risk here is 7, which indicates a strong association but is an order of magnitude lower than the reported odds ratio of 88.[2] This value is correct but is seriously misleading if presented or interpreted as meaning that the relative risk that affiliated authors would draw favourable conclusions was 88, as it was in this news item.

The odds ratio is valuable in case-control studies where events are usually rare and the relative risk cannot validly be estimated directly. In prospective studies interpretation of the odds ratio as an approximation to the relative risk becomes unreliable when events are common, and thus its use for prospective studies, especially randomised trials and systematic reviews, has been criticised.[3,4] The distortion is especially large when the event rate is high in only one group, as in this example. The odds ratio should not be interpreted as an approximate relative risk unless the events are rare in both groups (say, less than 20–30%).

The odds ratio remains especially useful when researchers need to adjust for other variables, for which logistic regression is the usual approach. While such analyses are valid, when the objective is to communicate study results to an audience unfamiliar with the relation between odds ratios and relative risks, surely it makes no sense also to report the relative risk when this differs markedly from the odds ratio.

References

1 Wise J. Links to tobacco industry influences review conclusions. *BMJ* 1998; 316: 1554. (23 May.)
2 Barnes DE, Dero LA. Why review articles on the health effects of passive smoking reach different conclusions. *JAMA* 1998; 279: 1566–1570. [Abstract/Free Full Text.]
3 Sackett DL, Deeks JJ, Altman DG. Down with odds ratios! *Evidence-Based Med* 1996; 1: 164–166.
4 Deeks JJ. When can odds ratios mislead? *BMJ* 1998; 317: 1155–1156. [Free Full Text]. (25 October.)

ICRF/NHS Centre for Statistics in Medicine, Institute of Health Sciences, Oxford OX3 7LF

Douglas G Altman, *Director*
Jonathon J Deeks, *Statistician*

NHS R&D Centre for Evidence-Based Medicine, John Radcliffe Hospital, Oxford OX3 9DU

David L Sackett, *Professor*

(*Accepted 7 November 1998*)

Originally published in *BMJ* 1998; **317**: 1318. Reproduced with permission.

When can odds ratios mislead?

Huw Talfryn Oakley Davies, Iain Kinloch Crombie, Manouche Tavakoli

Odds ratios are a common measure of the size of an effect and may be reported in case-control studies, cohort studies, or clinical trials. Increasingly, they are also used to report the findings from systematic reviews and meta-analyses. Odds ratios are hard to comprehend directly and are usually interpreted as being equivalent to the relative risk. Unfortunately, there is a recognised problem that odds ratios do not approximate well to the relative risk when the initial risk (that is, the prevalence of the outcome of interest) is high.[1,2] Thus there is a danger that if odds ratios are interpreted as though they were relative risks then they may mislead.

The advice given in many texts is unusually coy on the matter. For example: "The odds ratio is approximately the same as the relative risk if the outcome of interest is rare. For common events, however, they can be quite different."[3] How close is "approximately the same," how uncommon does an event have to be to qualify as "rare," and how different is "quite different"?

This short note quantifies the discrepancy between odds ratios and relative risks in different circumstances, and assesses whether such a discrepancy may seriously mislead if an odds ratio is used as an estimate of the relative risk.

Odds and risk

There is a problem with odds: unlike risks, they are difficult to understand. The risk of an event happening is simply the number of those who experience the event divided by the total number of people at risk of having that event. It is usually expressed as a proportion or as a percentage. In either case the meaning is usually clear.

In contrast, the odds of an event is the number of those who experience the event divided by the number of those who do not. It is expressed as a number from zero (event will never happen) to infinity (event is certain to happen). Odds are fairly easy to visualise when they are greater than one, but are less easily grasped when the value is less than one. Thus

Department of Management, University of St Andrews, St Andrews KY16 9AL

Huw Talfryn Oakley Davies, *lecturer in health care management*
Manouche Tavakoli, *lecturer in health and industrial economics*

Department of Epidemiology and Public Health, University of Dundee, Ninewells Hospital and Medical School, Dundee DD1 9SY

Iain Kinloch Crombie, *reader in epidemiology*

Correspondence to: Dr Davies
(email: hd@st-and.ac.uk)

(Accepted 24 February 1998)

Summary points

If the odds ratio is interpreted as a relative risk it will always overstate any effect size: the odds ratio is smaller than the relative risk for odds ratios of less than one, and bigger than the relative risk for odds ratios of greater than one

The extent of overstatement increases as both the initial risk increases and the odds ratio departs from unity

However, serious divergence between the odds ratio and the relative risk occurs only with large effects on groups at high initial risk. Therefore qualitative judgments based on interpreting odds ratios as though they were relative risks are unlikely to be seriously in error

In studies which show reductions in risk (odds ratios of less than one), the odds ratio will never underestimate the relative risk by a greater percentage than the level of initial risk

In studies which show increases in risk (odds ratios of greater than one), the odds ratio will be no more than twice the relative risk so long as the odds ratio times the initial risk is less than 100%

odds of six (that is, six to one) mean that six people will experience the event for every one that does not (a risk of six out of seven or 86%). An odds of 0.2 however seems less intuitive: 0.2 people will experience the event for every one that does not. This translates to one event for every five non-events (a risk of one in six or 17%).

A second problem with odds is that, although they are related to risk, the relation is not straightforward. The table shows the odds for various risks. For risks of less than about 20% the odds are not greatly dissimilar to the risk, but as the risk climbs above 50% the odds start to look very different.

Relative risks and odds ratios

The relative risk of one group compared with another is simply the ratio of the risks in the two groups. Thus the relative risk tells us how much risk is increased or decreased from an initial level. Again it is readily understood: a relative risk of 0.5 shows that the initial risk has been halved; a relative risk of 3 shows that the initial risk has been increased threefold.

The odds ratio is calculated in a similar way: it is simply the ratio of the odds in the two groups of interest. We know that if the odds ratio is less than one then the odds (and therefore

Originally published in *BMJ* 1998; **316**: 989–91. Reproduced with permission.

Table 1 Comparing risks and odds

Risk	Odds
0.05 or 5%	0.053
0.1 or 10%	0.11
0.2 or 20%	0.25
0.3 or 30%	0.43
0.4 or 40%	0.67
0.5 or 50%	1
0.6 or 60%	1.5
0.7 or 70%	2.3
0.8 or 80%	4
0.9 or 90%	9
0.95 or 95%	19

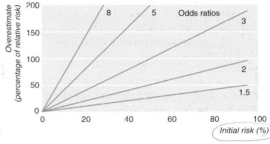

Figure 1 Amount by which odds ratios of <1 underestimate relative risk, for different odds ratios and different levels of initial risk.

Figure 2 Amount by which odds ratios of >1 overestimate relative risk, for different odds ratios and different levels of initial risk.

the risk too) has decreased, and if the odds ratio is greater than one then they have increased. But by how much? How do we interpret an odds ratio of, say, 0.5 or an odds ratio of 3? A lack of familiarity with odds means that many people have no intuitive feel for the size of the difference when expressed in this way.

When the risks (or odds) in the two groups being compared are both small (say less than 20%) then the odds will approximate to the risks and the odds ratio will approximate to the relative risk. Then interpretation is easy. But as the risk in either group rises above 20% the gap between the odds ratio and the relative risk will widen. A recent article in *Bandolier* concluded that "as both the prevalence [initial risk] and the odds ratio increase, the error in the approximation quickly becomes unacceptable."[2] But is this the case? In what circumstances will interpreting an odds ratio as though it were a relative risk lead to serious errors in interpretation?

Odds ratio as an approximation of relative risk

When faced with an odds ratio, we want to know the discrepancy between that odds ratio and the relative risk. Figures 1 and 2 show the extent to which the reported odds ratio underestimates or overestimates the relative risk for different odds ratios and a given level of initial risk (see appendix for calculations).

Figure 1 shows the underestimation of the relative risk by the odds ratio in studies that report odds ratios of less than one (typically studies of benefit from treatment or exposure). Even with initial risks as high as 50% and very large reductions in this risk (odds ratios of about 0.1), the odds ratio is only 50% smaller than the relative risk (0.1 for the odds ratio compared with a true value for the relative risk of 0.2). In fact, the discrepancy between the odds ratio and the true relative risk will never be greater than the initial risk (see appendix for proof).

Figure 2 shows the discrepancy between the odds ratio and the relative risk for studies which report odds ratios of greater

than one (typically studies showing harm). Although large discrepancies between the odds ratio and the relative risk are possible, the odds ratio overstates the relative risk by less than 50% for a wide range of both initial risks and effect sizes. For initial risks of 10% or less, even odds ratios of up to eight can reasonably be interpreted as relative risks; for initial risks up to 30% the approximation breaks down when the effect size gives odds ratios of more than about three. As a conservative rule of thumb, if the initial risk multiplied by the odds ratio is less than 100% then the odds ratio will overestimate the relative risk by less than twofold.

Does the discrepancy influence our interpretation?

The figures show that the odds ratio will always exaggerate the size of the effect compared with a relative risk. That is, if the odds ratio is less than one then it is always smaller than the relative risk. Conversely, if the odds ratio is greater than one then it is always bigger than the relative risk. Thus interpreting an odds ratio as though it were a relative risk could mislead us into believing that an effect size is bigger than is actually the case.

Crucially, however, large discrepancies are seen for only large effect sizes. Suppose an odds ratio of, say, 0.2 reflects a true relative risk of 0.4. Such a discrepancy is unlikely to alter your view: this is a large reduction in risk whichever way

Originally published in *BMJ* 1998; **316**: 989–91. Reproduced with permission.

Example of use of odds ratios

The fortnightly review by Dennis and Langhorne, "So stroke units save lives: where do we go from here?" (*BMJ* 1994;309:1273–7) reported outcomes after stroke (death or living in an institution) for patients managed in specialist stroke units compared with patients managed on general medical wards. Specialist stroke units had the better outcomes, with a reported odds ratio of 0.66. The authors advised that an "odds ratio of < 1.0 indicates that outcome of care in a stroke unit is better," and concluded that "patients with stroke treated in specialist units were less likely to die than those treated in general medical wards." No further guidance was given on interpreting the quoted odds ratio.

Because the frequency of a poor outcome was very high (about 55%) there might be concern that the odds ratio is a poor estimate of the relative risk. In fact, the odds ratio of 0.66 corresponds to a relative risk of 0.81—that is, the odds ratio underestimates the relative risk by just 19%. In other words, interpreting the odds ratio as a relative risk suggests a reduction in deleterious outcomes after stroke (death or living in an institution) of about a third compared with a more likely true reduction of about a fifth. Clearly, in either case this represents a substantial reduction in poor outcomes for a patient group with a large initial risk.

you look at it. This is particularly so as large discrepancies occur only when the initial risk is high and thus even modest changes in the relative risk will mean substantial gains. So, for studies which show reductions in risk, the odds ratio is unlikely to mislead: either it will be close in value to the relative risk or it represents a substantial effect for groups at high initial risk. Thus any qualitative judgment is unaltered by the discrepancy between the odds ratio and the relative risk (see box).

The same logic holds for studies which show increases in risk. The discrepancy between the odds ratio and the relative risk becomes large only when there are large effects (a twofold or threefold increase in risk) for groups already at a large initial risk. Although the odds ratio may diverge quite sharply from the relative risk, by the time it does so the message conveyed by the different measures is the same: these are large effects.

Of course, although qualitative judgments may be unaltered by the odds ratio deviating from the relative risk, quantitatively we can still be led astray. Thus if we are interested in assessing the impact of interventions quantitatively (for example, for a cost effectiveness analysis) then, for larger initial risks and substantial odds ratios, the actual relative risk should still be calculated.

Conclusion

The difference between the odds ratio and the relative risk depends on the risks (or odds) in both groups. So for

any reported odds ratio, the discrepancy between that odds ratio and the relative risk depends on both the initial risk and the odds ratio itself. This is possibly why textbooks are coy about giving a single figure for risk beneath which it is acceptable to interpret odds ratios as though they were relative risks.

Odds ratios may be non-intuitive in interpretation, but in almost all realistic cases interpreting them as though they were relative risks is unlikely to change any qualitative assessment of the study findings. The odds ratio will always overstate the case when interpreted as a relative risk, and the degree of overstatement will increase as both the initial risk increases and the size of any treatment effect increases. However, there is no point at which the degree of overstatement is likely to lead to qualitatively different judgments about the study. Substantial discrepancies between the odds ratio and the relative risk are seen only when the effect sizes are large and the initial risk is high. Whether a large increase or a large decrease in risk is indicated, our judgments are likely to be the same—they are important effects.

Appendix: Calculation of discrepancy between odds ratios and relative risks

If the proportions of subjects experiencing an event in two groups are P_1 (initial risk) and P_2 (post-intervention risk) then the relative risk is P_2/P_1 and the odds ratio is $(1 - P_1)/(1 - P_2) \times$ relative risk. Simple algebra leads this multiplier to be recast as $1 - P_1 + (P_1 \times$ odds ratio$)$. However, it is convenient to express the discrepancy between the odds ratio and the relative risk as a proportion of the relative risk. Therefore, for studies in which the odds ratio is < 1, 1 minus this multiplier is the discrepancy $(P_1 - (P_1 \times$ odds ratio$))$. For studies in which the odds ratio is > 1, the multiplier minus 1 gives the discrepancy $((P_1 \times$ odds ratio$) - P_1)$. Figures 1 and 2 plot these discrepancy values (as percentages) for various initial risks and odds ratios.

Contributors: The ideas contained in this paper arose from discussions between HTOD and IKC and were clarified in debate with MT. HTOD wrote the first draft of the manuscript, which was edited by IKC and MT. HTOD is guarantor for the article.

Conflict of interest: None.

References

1 Sinclair JC, Bracken MB. Clinically useful measures of effect in binary analyses of randomized trials. *J Clin Epidemiol* 1994; 47:881–9.
2 Deeks J. Swots corner: what is an odds ratio? *Bandolier* 1996;3(3):6–7.
3 Altman DG. *Practical statistics for medical research*. London: Chapman and Hall, 1991.

Originally published in *BMJ* 1998; **316**: 989–91. Reproduced with permission.

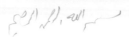

Effect of needle length on incidence of local reactions to routine immunisation in infants aged 4 months: randomised controlled trial

Linda Diggle, Jonathan Deeks

Abstract

Objective   To compare rates of local reactions associated with two needle sizes used to administer routine immunisations to infants.

Design   Randomised controlled trial.

Setting   Routine immunisation clinics in eight general practices in Buckinghamshire.

Participants   Healthy infants attending for third primary immunisation due at 16 weeks of age: 119 infants were recruited, and 110 diary cards were analysed.

Interventions   Immunisation with 25 gauge, 16 mm, orange hub needle or 23 gauge, 25 mm, blue hub needle.

Main outcome measures   Parental recordings of redness, swelling, and tenderness for three days after immunisation.

Results   Rate of redness with the longer needle was initially two thirds the rate with the smaller needle (relative risk 0.66 (95% confidence interval 0.45 to 0.99), P = 0.04), and by the third day this had decreased to a seventh (relative risk 0.13 (0.03 to 0.56), P = 0.0006). Rate of swelling with the longer needle was initially about a third that with the smaller needle (relative risk 0.39 (0.23 to 0.67), P = 0.0002), and this difference remained for all three days. Rates of tenderness were also lower with the longer needle throughout follow up, but not significantly (relative risk 0.60 (0.29 to 1.25), P = 0.17).

Conclusions   Use of 25 mm needles significantly reduced rates of local reaction to routine infant immunisation. On average, for every five infants vaccinated, use of the longer needle instead of the shorter needle would prevent one infant from experiencing any local reaction. Vaccine manufacturers should review their policy of supplying the shorter needle in vaccine packs.

Introduction

As part of the UK childhood immunisation schedule, infants routinely receive diphtheria, pertussis, and tetanus (DPT) vaccine and *Haemophilus influenzae* type b (Hib) vaccine at 2, 3, and 4 months.[1] Nationally available guidelines advise practitioners to administer primary vaccines to infants by deep subcutaneous or intramuscular injection using either a 25 or 23 gauge needle but give no recommendation regarding needle length.[1] The question of optimum needle length for infant immunisation has not previously been addressed in

Britain, despite calls from nurses for evidence on which to base immunisation practice. We conducted a randomised controlled trial of the two needle sizes currently used by UK practitioners to determine whether needle size affects the incidence of redness, swelling, and tenderness.

Participants and methods

Participants

Eight of 11 general practices approached in Buckinghamshire agreed to participate in the study. Practice nurses recruited healthy infants attending routine immunisation clinics. Parents received written information about the study when attending for the second primary vaccination and were asked if they wished to participate when they returned for the third vaccination. The only exclusion criteria were those normally applicable to a child receiving primary immunisations.[1] We obtained ethical approval from the local ethics committee.

Interventions

Infants were allocated to receive their third primary immunisation with either the 25 gauge, 16 mm needle or the 23 gauge,

Oxford Vaccine Group, University Department of Paediatrics, John Radcliffe Hospital, Oxford OX3 9DU

Linda Diggle *senior research nurse*

ICRF/NHS Centre for Statistics in Medicine, Institute of Health Sciences, University of Oxford, Oxford OX3 7LF

Jonathan Deeks *senior medical statistician*

Correspondence to: L Diggle
(email: linda.diggle@paediatrics.oxford.ac.uk)

(*Accepted 22 September 2000*)

Originally published in *BMJ* 2000; **321**: 931–33. Reproduced with permission.

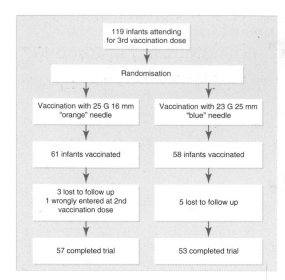

Flow chart describing randomisation sequence

25 mm needle according to a computer generated blocked randomisation scheme stratified by practice. Allocations were concealed in sequentially numbered opaque envelopes opened once written parental consent was obtained. Practice nurses were instructed verbally, by demonstration and in writing, to use the technique of injecting into the anterolateral thigh, stretching the skin taut and inserting the needle at a 90° angle to the skin.[2] The right thigh was used, with the needle inserted into the skin up to the hub.

Outcomes

Parents recorded redness, swelling, and tenderness in a diary for three days after immunisation. The size of swelling and redness were measured with a plastic ruler, while the child's reaction to movement of the limb or to touch of the site was graded with a standard scale. We supplied parents with a prepaid envelope to return the diary, and we contacted parents by telephone if return was delayed.

At the start of the trial all practices were using the 0.5 ml mix of Pasteur-Merieux DPT/Hib vaccine. However, a change in national vaccine supply necessitated a switch to the 1.0 ml mix of Evans DPT and Wyeth Lederle Hib-Titer. Blocked randomisation ensured that the numbers receiving each vaccine were evenly distributed between the groups.

Statistical analysis

In order to detect clinically important relative differences of 25% in tenderness and 30% in redness and swelling, we estimated that 250 infants should be recruited for the study to have 80% power of detecting differences at the 5% significance level. In January 2000, problems with vaccine supply necessitated the temporary nationwide replacement of the whole cell component of the combined DPT/Hib vaccine with acellular pertussis vaccine.[3] As this vaccine has a different local reactogenicity profile, we decided to stop the trial early.

We used χ^2 tests to compare the proportions of children with each local reaction at 6 hours and 1, 2, and 3 days after immunisation. We compared differences in the size of reaction using a χ^2 test for trend.

Results

Of the 119 children recruited to the study, 61 were randomised to the 16 mm needle group and 58 to the 25 mm needle group (see figure). Nine were not included in the analysis (four in the 16 mm needle group and five in the 25 mm group): diaries were not returned for eight, while the ninth was mistakenly included in the study at the second vaccination. Inclusion of this child did not materially affect the results. The two groups had similar baseline characteristics (see table).

Over half of the infants vaccinated with the 16 mm needle subsequently experienced redness and swelling (table). The rate of redness with the 25 mm needle was initially two thirds the rate with the 16 mm needle (relative risk 0.66 (95% confidence interval 0.45 to 0.99)), and, by the third day, this had decreased further to a seventh (relative risk 0.13 (0.03 to 0.56)). Similarly, rates of swelling after injection with the longer needle were initially around a third of those after use of the smaller needle (relative risk 0.39 (0.23 to 0.67)), and this difference was maintained for all three days. These differences were statistically significant. Tenderness was less frequent and, although the rates of tenderness were also lower with the longer needle throughout follow up, the differences were not significant (table).

Discussion

This study showed that both redness and swelling were significantly reduced when the 23 gauge, 25 mm, blue hub needle was used instead of the 25 gauge, 16 mm, orange hub needle to administer the third dose of diphtheria, pertussis, and tetanus and *Haemophilus influenzae* type b vaccines to infants. The differences suggest that, for every three to five infants vaccinated with the longer rather than the shorter needle, one case of redness and one of swelling would be prevented.

The needles compared in this study are those most commonly used in general practice.[4] As they differed in both length (16 v 25 mm) and bore (25 v 23 gauge), we cannot know which of these factors determined the observed differences in the rates of redness and swelling. However, previous studies comparing injections given at different depths (subcutaneous versus intramuscular) with the same gauge needle have shown similar differences in local reactions.[5, 6] We suggest that the length of the longer needle used in our study ensured that the vaccine reached the thigh muscle in 4 month old infants.

Originally published in *BMJ* 2000; **321**: 931–33. Reproduced with permission.

Baseline characteristics of 4 month old infants and rate of local reactions to immunisation over three days by needle used for vaccination. Values are numbers (percentages) of infants unless stated otherwise

Local reaction	Size of needle		Difference between longer and shorter needle	
	23 G, 25 mm (n = 53)	25 G, 16 mm (n = 57)	Relative risk (95% CI); P value	Test for trend
Baseline characteristics				
Mean (SD) weight (kg)*	6.7 (0.9)	6.8 (0.9)		
Age at vaccination (weeks):				
16–17	37 (70)	36 (63)		
18–19	11 (21)	16 (28)		
≥20	5 (9)	5 (9)		
Sex				
Male	34 (64)	30 (53)		
Female	19 (36)	27 (47)		
Site of injection:				
Left leg	13 (25)	12 (21)		
Right leg	40 (75)	45 (79)		
Vaccine type†:				
0.5 ml	8 (15)	8 (14)		
1.0 ml	45 (85)	49 (86)		
Local reactions				
Redness:				
At 6 hours	21 (40)	34 (60)	0.66 (0.45 to 0.99); P = 0.04	P = 0.007
At 1 day	15 (28)	36 (63)	0.45 (0.28 to 0.72); P = 0.0002	P < 0.0001
At 2 days	5 (9)	22 (39)	0.24 (0.10 to 0.60); P = 0.0004	P = 0.0004
At 3 days	2 (4)	16 (28)	0.13 (0.03 to 0.56); P = 0.0006	P = 0.001
Swelling:				
At 6 hours	12 (23)	33 (58)	0.39 (0.23 to 0.67); P = 0.0002	P = 0.0009
At 1 day	15 (28)	36 (63)	0.45 (0.28 to 0.72); P = 0.0002	P = 0.0001
At 2 days	10 (19)	29 (51)	0.37 (0.20 to 0.69); P = 0.0005	P = 0.0007
At 3 days	7 (13)	23 (40)	0.33 (0.15 to 0.70); P = 0.001	P = 0.002
Tenderness:				
At 6 hours	9 (17)	16 (28)	0.60 (0.29 to 1.25); P = 0.17	P = 0.4
At 1 day	4 (8)	8 (14)	0.54 (0.17 to 1.68); P = 0.3	P = 0.4
At 2 days	0	3 (5)	0 (not estimable); P = 0.09	P = 0.4
At 3 days	0	1 (2)	0 (not estimable); P = 0.3	P = 0.2
Any local reaction	33 (62)	48 (84)	0.74 (0.58 to 0.94); P = 0.009	

*Weight missing for three infants.
†0.5 ml vaccine = Pasteur Merieux DPT/Hib. 1 ml vaccine = Evans DPT reconstituting Wyeth Lederle HibTiter.

What is already known on this topic

Most infants experience local reactions to routine vaccinations

Previous local reactions have been cited by parents as a disincentive to further vaccinations

National guidelines on immunisation do not specify a preferred needle length

What this study adds

Local reactions are significantly reduced by use of the 23 gauge, 25 mm, blue hub needle rather than the 25 gauge, 16 mm, orange hub needle supplied by vaccine manufacturers

Although our study was not blinded, parents were not told which needle was used to vaccinate their child. We believe that if knowledge of needle allocation introduced bias into the results, it would be less likely that such bias would be in the direction of the longer needle.

These findings are of clinical importance for those involved in administering infant immunisations. In the United Kingdom, where routine vaccines are currently supplied with the shorter needle, a change in the manufacturing process is now required. Any factor that can reduce the rates of adverse reactions in childhood vaccinations has the potential to improve parental acceptance of vaccines[7] and would be welcomed by practitioners.

Originally published in *BMJ* 2000; **321**: 931–33. Reproduced with permission.

We thank the parents and babies involved in the study, and the following practice nurses at Buckinghamshire surgeries for recruiting infants and administering immunisations: Lyn Hurry, Waddesdon; Lyn Murphy, Whitehill; Carol Gill, Aston Clinton; Judith Brown, Meadowcroft; Cesca Carter, Wendover; Nicky Oliver, Oakfield; Chris Mildred, Wing; Clare Stroud, Tring Road. We also thank Professor Richard Moxon and Drs Paul Heath, Jim Buttery, Jodie McVernon, Jenny MacLennan, and Karen Sleeman from the Oxford Vaccine Group for helpful advice and support and Dr Ann Mulhall for research supervision.

Contributors: LD conceived and planned the study, recruited and trained practice nurses, managed data collection, wrote the first draft of the paper, and is guarantor for the study. JD advised on design, produced the randomisation scheme, and undertook all analyses. Both authors had input into the final manuscript.

Funding: This study was funded by the Smith and Nephew Foundation through the award of a nursing research scholarship.

Competing interests: None declared.

References

1 Department of Health. *Immunisation against infectious diseases.* London: HMSO, 1996.

2 World Health Organisation. *Immunisation in practice. Module 8. During a session: giving immunisations.* Geneva: WHO, 1998. (www.who.int/vaccines-documents/DoxTrng/H4IIP.htm (accessed 3 October 2000).)

3 Department of Health. *Current vaccine issues: action update.* London: DoH, 1999. (Professional letter PL/CMO/99/5.)

4 Diggle L. A randomised controlled trial of different needle lengths on the incidence of local reactions when administering the combined injection of diphtheria/pertussis/tetanus (DPT) and Haemophilus influenzae type b (Hib) to infants at 4-months of age [dissertation]. London: Royal College of Nursing Institute, 1999.

5 Mark A, Carlsson R, Granstrom M. Subcutaneous versus intramuscular injection for booster DT vaccination of adolescents. *Vaccine* 1999;17:2067–72.

6 Scheifele DW, Bjornson G, Boraston S. Local adverse effects of meningo-coccal vaccine. *Can Med Assoc J* 1994;150:14–5.

7 Lieu T, Black S, Ray G, Martin K, Shinefield H, Weniger B. The hidden costs of infant vaccination. *Vaccine* 2000;19:33–41.

Originally published in *BMJ* 2000; **321**: 931–33. Reproduced with permission.

UNIT 5
Clinical trials

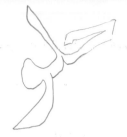

Aims

To understand the different types of clinical trials, the different ways in which the data from clinical trials can be analysed, and the role of a data and safety monitoring committee in conducting a clinical trial.

> ### Learning objectives
> On completion of this unit, participants will be able to:
> - understand and identify different types of clinical trials;
> - judge the value of intention-to-treat, treatment received and interim analyses;
> - describe the role of data and safety monitoring committees;
> - calculate event rates in treatment and control groups;
> - understand the meaning of number-needed-to-treat.

, Time for Event

Background
Clinical trials

A clinical trial is a prospective study that is designed to measure whether a new treatment has benefits over and above either a sham/control treatment or an existing treatment that is considered standard best care. In clinical trials, volunteer participants are enrolled to assess whether the new treatment is safe and efficacious, that is, confers benefit under ideal conditions, or effective, that is, confers benefit under routine clinical practice or community health care conditions. A clinical trial can be used to ascertain whether a new treatment is better than existing treatment, or whether an existing treatment can be used effectively in a different way or in a different group of patients. Most clinical trials are used to evaluate drug therapies, but clinical trial designs are also appropriate for evaluating other forms of health care such as allied health practices or different methods of patient management. The new 'treatment' may be an environmental intervention, such as a new dietary guideline, a change in exercise habits or avoidance of an environmental exposure rather than a drug therapy.

Table 5.1 Classification of clinical trials

Term	Definition
Phase I trial	Initial trial of a new treatment to assess safety and feasibility in a small group of volunteers who do not have the disease or patients with symptoms.
Phase II trial	A clinical trial to measure efficacy, that is, the effect of a treatment under ideal conditions, in patients with the disease.
Phase III trial	Large randomised controlled trial or multi-centre study to measure effectiveness in the community, that is, the effect of a treatment in general clinical practice.
Phase IV surveillance	Post-marketing survey to measure rare adverse events.

The different phases of clinical trials are usually classified according to their purpose as shown in Table 5.1. Initially, the safety and effects of using a new treatment are usually established by animal studies. Following the results of these studies, a Phase I trial may be conducted to establish the safety of using a new treatment in a small group of say 20–30 volunteers who may not necessarily have the symptoms that the new therapy is intended to treat. This type of study is used to evaluate side effects and pharmacological properties of drugs, such as safe dosage levels. After volunteer studies are completed, Phase I trials involving a small group of participants who have the disease may also be conducted. These types of trials in selected groups of participants help to ensure that a new treatment or intervention is safe and feasible for testing in the general community.

Following the success of a Phase I trial, a Phase II clinical trial may be conducted in a larger group of say 30–100 participants who have the disease. Phase II trials are conducted to establish the efficacy of the new treatment under controlled conditions. In Phase II trials, toxicity is often evaluated and the benefits and harms of a new treatment under ideal clinical management are assessed. When the main aim is to investigate the efficacy of newly developed treatment, Phase II trials may include a control group of participants who receive an inactive placebo or sham treatment and who therefore do not receive current standard care.

Phase II trials are often conducted in participants who are carefully diagnosed and who are selected as being likely to adhere to the new treatment regimen. Participants are usually required to follow a precise protocol and they are often closely monitored and receive more regular and personalised attention than can usually be provided in medical settings in the community. New treatments are initially tested in this way because if they do not confer a benefit under ideal treatment conditions then it is unlikely that they will have efficacy in less controlled settings such as general practice.

Once safety and efficacy are established, a more rigorous Phase III evaluation can be undertaken in a much larger number of participants to measure the effectiveness of the new treatment or intervention in the general community or in routine clinical practice. Phase III trials are used to measure whether a treatment does more good than harm under usual health care conditions in which factors such as misdiagnosis or poor participant compliance may occur. Phase III trials are always comparative, that is, participants receiving the new treatment are compared to a control group of participants who receive 'current best practice' treatment or a placebo treatment. However, it is unethical for an inactive placebo treatment to be used in the community when there is evidence that 'current best practice' confers a benefit. An important research concept is that practitioners must be in a position of equipoise, that is, they have no clear evidence that the current best practice treatment confers benefit, before a placebo can be used as the control group treatment in a Phase III evaluation.[1]

In Phase II and III studies, participants are randomly allocated to study groups to minimise the effects of confounders on the study results.[2] Thus, the trial is called a randomised controlled trial, where 'randomised' describes the random allocation of participants to a group so that each participant has an equal chance of receiving either treatment. The term 'controlled' describes the inclusion of a comparison or control group who receive standard best care treatment or a placebo. The process of randomisation balances the effects of both known and unknown confounders between the groups and, because of this, randomised controlled trials provide the most reliable and rigorous study design for collecting a high level of evidence of the efficacy or effectiveness of an intervention. Experimental randomised controlled trials are superior to observational study designs because the effects of both bias and confounding on the study results can be minimised.

In clinical trials, bias can occur if participants suspect which treatment they will be allocated to receive or are aware of the treatment they are receiving. Researchers who are responsible for recruitment and who are aware of upcoming treatment allocations could route participants to a certain treatment. Thus, adequate allocation concealment, that is, participants and study personnel being unaware of upcoming treatment allocations, will prevent selection and confounding bias before randomisation occurs and until allocation. In addition, participants may decline to enrol or may withdraw if they believe they will be in a specific group such as the control group. Participants who are aware of the treatment they are receiving often assume that the new treatment will be better than standard best treatment[3] and this may influence reporting of their symptoms or perception of the effect of their illness on their quality of life. In addition, awareness by study personnel of the group to which participants have been allocated may influence data recording practices simply because of the expectation that the new treatment will confer benefits. To avoid reporting and observer bias, both participants and researchers should be blinded (sometimes called 'masked') to treatment status, that is, have no knowledge of the assigned treatment following randomisation.

If both researchers and participants are aware of treatment status, the trial is called an 'open label' trial. If one party is aware of treatment status, the trial is called 'single blinded'. Trials in which both participants and researchers are unaware of treatment status are generally called 'double-blind' trials. It has been suggested that the term 'double-blind' is ambiguous because the definition of this term varies. In some clinical trials reported as double blind, participants or researchers may not be blinded and more than two parties may be blinded. Other parties involved in the study, such as the pharmacist and statistician, should be blinded to treatment status in addition to the participants and the researchers to avoid bias.

Although a blinded design is preferred because it minimises observer and reporting bias, blinding is not always possible. In most surgical trials it would be both unethical and impractical for control group participants to undergo surgery and have an incision to mimic the treatment delivered in the active group.[4] When it is not possible to blind the observers to group status, objective outcome measurements, such as lung function or biochemical tests, that are unlikely to be influenced by observer bias are preferred. In evaluating the results from a randomised controlled trial, details of who was blinded and how blinding was achieved should be appraised.

Following Phase III studies, Phase IV studies that involve post-marketing surveillance are often conducted to monitor any adverse rare or long-term effects of the treatment in the population over a longer time period than previously established in Phase III studies. Phase IV surveillance is used after a treatment has shown to be effective and marketing approval has been obtained from regulatory authorities, such as the Therapeutic Goods Administration (TGA) or the Food and Drug Administration (FDA). However, post-marketing surveillance can be inefficient and there have been cases in which long periods have elapsed and many adverse events have occurred before drugs have been withdrawn from use.[5]

Power and sample size

The sample size for a clinical trial needs to be large enough so that the smallest clinically valuable difference between groups reaches statistical significance.[6] Prior to conducting a trial, the treatment effect between groups that would be required for the experimental treatment to be regarded as more beneficial than the control or existing 'best practice' treatment should be specified. It is critical that the sample size is large enough to ensure that estimates of benefit have not arisen by chance and to provide precision, that is, 95% confidence intervals around outcome measures that are acceptably small in each group. In estimating sample size, it is important to consider the power of a study, that is, the probability of detecting a meaningful difference if one exists. The power of a study will increase as the sample size increases. However, an under-powered study in which a clinically important difference between groups will fail to reach statistical significance (a type II error) needs to be balanced against an over-powered study in which a small clinically unimportant difference between groups will become statistically significant (a type I error) as discussed in Unit 1.

Clinical trials with a small sample size may be unethical because their hypothesis cannot be properly tested. However, many small trials are conducted as preliminary studies to provide essential evidence that a larger trial is warranted. On the other hand, clinical trials with an overly large sample size may also be unethical because they require many more participants to be enrolled than are needed to test the study hypothesis. Limiting the sample size can be of prime importance if adverse outcomes are expected. In a review of mortality rates in two clinical trials, it was thought that hundreds of patients who were not needed to test the study hypotheses had been enrolled, and that over 50 deaths could have been prevented if the studies had been limited to smaller but adequate sample sizes.[7]

Intention-to-treat and as-treated analyses

The primary analyses from randomised controlled trials should be conducted using 'intention-to-treat' analyses. Intention-to-treat analyses are designed to maintain the balance of both known and unknown confounders between groups that the randomisation process was intended to ensure. Thus, an intention-to-treat analysis requires that all participants be maintained in the group to which they were initially allocated regardless of any subsequent events, such as withdrawal from the study, not using the treatment, departing from the study protocol or choosing other treatments. In addition, participants should be included in intention-to-treat analyses even if their final outcome value was not collected, for example if they were lost to follow-up or chose to withdraw. In this way, an intention-to-treat analysis provides an unbiased estimate of the effectiveness of a new treatment under the normal conditions of medical practice.

When critically appraising the results from a clinical trial, it is important to ascertain whether an intention-to-treat analysis was appropriately and adequately applied, because some studies fail to do this.[8] When applying the intention-to-treat principle, participants should be analysed in the study groups they were randomised to regardless of compliance, withdrawal or protocol deviations. An intention-to-treat analysis can only be conducted when complete outcome data for all randomised participants are available. One way to assess whether the term 'intention-to-treat' has been used appropriately is by ascertaining how many participants had missing outcome data and how these missing outcomes were dealt with. Imputation is often used to replace missing values, for example by replacing the missing value by carrying the last value forward or by replacing with a mean value. These methods are not ideal but do maintain the benefits conferred by randomisation. In using these methods, an intention-to-treat analysis provides a conservative estimate of the treatment effect.[9]

Analyses that are considered secondary to intention-to-treat analyses include an 'available-case analysis', in which data are analysed for only the participants in whom the final study outcomes were collected. In addition, 'treatment-received' (also called 'as-treated') analyses are commonly conducted in which participants are regrouped according to the treatment they actually received irrespective of the group to which they were allocated. Available-case and treatment-received analyses provide estimates of the treatment effect under more optimal conditions of compliance, but the results are likely to be influenced by the effects of confounders and will often provide a more optimistic treatment effect than intention-to-treat analyses.

Interim analyses

The term 'interim analysis' is used to describe any data analysis that is conducted before all of the participants have completed the study. Even though interim analyses can be conducted without breaking the randomisation code, they should be planned before the study begins and should be undertaken as rarely as possible. An important purpose of an interim analysis is to decide whether a trial should be stopped early to protect the safety of the participants. If a treatment has a high rate of adverse outcomes, an interim analysis can help to ensure that current participants will not continue in a trial any longer than is needed to test the study hypothesis, and that future participants will not receive an inferior treatment.

Another common use for an interim analysis is to make an internal validation of the adequacy of the planned final sample size, and to recalculate the sample size required if the treatment difference is smaller than expected. If the treatment effect is smaller than expected, then larger numbers of participants will be required to show a statistically significant difference between groups. However, if the treatment difference is larger than expected, it is usual to maintain the initial sample size calculation rather than stopping the trial early to ensure precision

Glossary

Term	Definition
Intention-to-treat analysis	All participants are analysed in the group to which they were allocated, regardless of subsequent events such as non-compliance or withdrawal from the study. This provides a conservative estimate of treatment effect that is not influenced by confounders.
Available-case analysis	Only participants with final study outcomes are included in the data analysis, but participants are maintained in the group to which they were allocated. The results may be influenced by bias and confounders.
Treatment-received-analysis	Participants are re-grouped according to the treatment they actually received, irrespective of the treatment to which they were allocated. Using this method, there is no control of confounders.

around the estimates, and because a large effect that occurs when the sample size is small may be an early random event.

Interim analyses can play an important part in managing a clinical trial, but undertaking this type of analysis too early when the sample size is small, or too frequently, increases the chance of finding a false-positive interim result.[10] More importantly, if the people in the research team are not blinded to the results of the interim analyses, there is a potential for observer bias to be introduced into future data collection as a result of expectation of effect, especially if they are not blinded to the treatment status of participants. Thus, interim analyses should be planned carefully and only performed under controlled conditions in which everyone in the research team is blinded to the results. This process helps to maintain the scientific integrity of the study and helps to ensure the validity of the study results.

Data and safety monitoring committees

The primary objective of a data and safety monitoring committee (DSMC) is to ensure the safety of trial participants by providing a process for the ongoing review of study events and study outcomes that is independent of the research team, steering committee and trial sponsors.[11,12] A DSMC can play an important part in managing a randomised controlled trial. The committee is usually comprised of three to five members – often including a clinician, a statistician, a pharmacologist and/or an ethicist. The people on the DSMC should be the only people who can be unblinded to the otherwise blinded aspects of the study.

The DSMC members should meet at scheduled intervals, but the study team may call a meeting of the DSMC if any concerns about safety arise during the trial. In monitoring safety and efficacy indicators, a DSMC can recommend either stopping, continuing or modifying the trial at any point.[13] Ideally, a DSMC should be appointed in Phase III studies, but not all trials require a DSMC and considerations such as the duration of study, type of treatment and potential adverse events influence decisions about whether a DSMC needs to be appointed.

If a DSMC is appointed, the committee must have access to original data including the treatment the participants were assigned to receive. These data provide more immediate information than can be provided by aggregated data that can mask a high adverse event rate in one group if the adverse event rate in the other group is low.[7] In addition to reviewing adverse and unexpected events, the DSMC should also have the responsibility of planning, conducting and acting on any interim analyses. The advantages of appointing an independent DSMC is that the ethical conduct of the trial can be ensured without any compromise to scientific integrity.

Number-needed-to-treat

When deciding how to apply the results of a randomised controlled trial to decision making in a clinical setting, it is often important to have treatment objectives. For this, the number of people who need to receive a new treatment to prevent one adverse event occurring can be a useful statistic. This statistic, which is called number-needed-to-treat (NNT), provides an absolute measure of treatment effect. As such, NNT may have a more practical value in a clinical setting than statistics such as a chi-square, *P* value or a relative risk, which only indicate the extent to which the new treatment and the outcome are related to one another. In clinical practice, NNT also provides a more practical estimate of effect than an odds ratio, which only shows the odds of an outcome if a patient receives the new treatment compared to the odds if the control treatment is received (see Unit 4).

Glossary

Term	Definition
Number-needed-to-treat (NNT)	The number of people who need to receive a new treatment to prevent one adverse event occurring.
Control event rate (CER)	The frequency of the outcome in the control (current best practice treatment or placebo) group.
Experimental event rate (EER)	The frequency of the outcome in the experimental (new treatment) group.
Absolute risk reduction (ARR)	The reduction in risk (probability of the outcome) that is conferred by the new treatment.

Table 5.2 Contingency table of data from a randomised controlled trial

	Adverse event present	Adverse event absent	Total
New treatment group	a	b	$a + b$
Control treatment group	c	d	$c + d$
Total	$a + c$	$b + d$	Total

To calculate NNT, the two binary variables that represent the outcome groups and the treatment groups are displayed in a 2×2 contingency table similar to Table 3.1 shown in Unit 3. In Table 5.2, a 2×2 contingency table is used, except the outcome (adverse event present or absent) and exposure (new treatment group vs control treatment group) are re-labelled to be consistent with the terms used in a clinical trial.

The frequency of the outcome in the new treatment group is the row proportion $a/(a + b)$ and is called the experimental event rate (EER). Similarly, the frequency of the outcome in the control group is the corresponding row proportion $c/(c + d)$ and is called the control event rate (CER). If the EER is less than the CER this suggests a potential benefit from the new treatment. For calculating NNT, both the EER and the CER are calculated as proportions rather than percentages. From these proportions, the absolute risk reduction (ARR), that is, the reduction in risk that is conferred by the new treatment, can be calculated. The ARR is simply the absolute difference in frequency rates between the two study groups as follows:

Experimental event rate (EER) $= a/(a+b)$
Control event rate (CER) $= c/(c+d)$
Absolute risk reduction (ARR) $=$ CER−EER

and the NNT is the reciprocal of the ARR and can be calculated as:

Number needed to treat (NNT) $= 1/$ARR

Thus if the ARR is low, say 0.1, indicating that is there is little difference in the frequency of the outcome between the control and new treatment groups, then the NNT will be large at 1/0.1, or 10, indicating that 10 people will need to receive the new treatment to prevent one adverse event occurring. Conversely, if the ARR is higher, say 0.3, indicating a larger difference in the frequency of the outcome between the control and new treatment groups, the NNT will be smaller at 1/0.3, or approximately 3, indicating that only 3 people need to receive the new treatment to prevent one adverse event occurring. Obviously, for translating this statistic into use in clinical practice, NNT is rounded to a whole number. The size of the NNT that is clinically important, such as the number of children who need to undergo surgery to prevent one adverse outcome or the number of people who need to receive a new drug to prevent one coronary event, depends on the nature of the treatment and the severity of the outcome and can only be judged by experts in the field.

TAKE HOME LIST

- Randomising participants to study groups balances both known and unknown confounders between the study groups.

- In randomised controlled trials, blinding the participants, observers, pharmacists and statisticians to treatment status helps to minimise both observer and reporting bias.

- Randomised controlled trials provide the most rigorous study design for collecting a high level of evidence of the efficacy or effectiveness of a new treatment.

- The roles of a data and safety monitoring committee are to ensure the safety of participants and to plan, conduct and act on any interim analyses.

Reading and questions
Reprints
Altman DG. Randomisation: essential for reducing bias. BMJ 1991; 302:1481–1482. (See p. 64.)
Heritier SR, Gebski VJ, Keech AC. Inclusion of patients in clinical trial analysis: the intention to treat principle. Med J Aust 2003; 179:438–440. (See p. 66.)

After reading the reprints, answer the following questions.
1 What methods are best used to randomly allocate participants to study groups and why?
2 What methods are used to reduce bias in clinical trials?
3 How can allocation concealment be achieved?
4 What are the advantages and disadvantages of using intention-to-treat analyses?
5 Why are treatment-received analyses often reported and what are their limitations?

Worked example
Set article
Miranda-Filho DB, Ximenes RA, Barone AA, Vaz VL, Vieira AG, Albuquerque VMG. Randomised controlled trial of tetanus treatment with antitetanus immunoglobulin by the intrathecal or intramuscular route. BMJ 2004; 328:615–618. (See p. 37.)

The paper by Miranda-Filho *et al.* (2004), which was included as the set article in Unit 3, reports on the clinical progression of tetanus as measured in a randomised controlled trial. Participants in an intensive care unit were randomised to receive one of two treatment groups, that is, anti-tetanus immunoglobulin by either the intrathecal and intramuscular route (new treatment or study group) or the intramuscular route (control group). At day 4, there were 53 participants remaining in both the treatment study group and the control group. This sample size is moderately large for a single centre study.

Using the data shown in Table 3 of the article at day 4, the ARR for reduction of tetanus from grade III–IV to grade I–II is the event rate in control group (30/53) subtracted from the event in the study group (11/53), which is 0.57 − 0.21, or 0.36. The NNT is therefore 1/0.36 or 2.78 which can be rounded to 3. This indicates that three people need to receive anti-tetanus immunoglobulin by the intrathecal and intramuscular route to prevent one person remaining in grade III–IV tetanus on day 4.

In the article, Table 3 also shows that at day 10, there were 43 participants remaining in the control group and 39 in the new treatment group. At this time point, the ARR for reduction of tetanus from grade III–IV to grade I–II at day 10 is 23/43 − 7/39 which is 0.53 − 0.18, or 0.35. The NNT is therefore 1/0.35 which can be rounded to 3. The NNT at day 10 is the same as day 4. Although NNT can be influenced by the time at which the outcome is measured, the NNT in this study has remained stable from 4 to 10 days after admission.

Exercise

In the set article by Miranda-Filho *et al.* (2004) (see p. 37), use Table 5.2 and the formulas presented in this unit to calculate NNT for complications, respiratory infection, respiratory failure or mechanical ventilation and death, presented in Table 5 of the article, and complete Table 5.3.

After completing Table 5.3, answer the following questions.
- How do the NNT values compare and which NNT value would be the most important for deciding which treatment to use?
- In the study, there were 10 deaths in the control group and 4 deaths in the new treatment group. If the reverse had happened, that is, there were 10 deaths in the new treatment group compared to 4 in the control group, what would the NNT be?

Table 5.3 ARR and NNT for complications and mortality for tetanus by intrathecal and intramuscular route or the intramuscular route

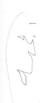

Outcome	CER	EER	ARR	NNT
Complications	0.74	0.57	0.17	6
Respiratory infection	0.68	0.50	0.18	6
Respiratory failure or mechanical ventilation	0.55	0.38	0.17	6
Death	0.16	0.07	0.09	11

- What type of analyses does the paper report (intention-to-treat, available-case analysis or treatment-received)? How does this influence how you would interpret the results?

Quick quiz

Tick the correct answer for each of the following questions:

1 What type of trial is reported in the Miranda-Filho *et al.* (2004) article?
 (a) Phase I
 (b) Phase II
 (c) Phase III
 (d) Phase IV ✓

2 When the CER and EER are equal, indicating no treatment effect, what value will the NNT take?
 (a) Negative
 (b) Zero
 (c) Positive
 (d) Infinity ✓

3 What does a data and safety monitoring committee (DSMC) do?
 (a) Monitor the ways in which the outcome and safety data are collected.
 (b) Report adverse events to the ethics committee.
 (c) Advise on procedure if an adverse event occurs.
 (d) Provide statistical assistance with analyses.

4 Why is sample size important in clinical trials?
 (a) With a large sample size, the effects of confounding are minimised.
 (b) An adequate number is needed to show a clinically important treatment effect.
 (c) Large clinical trials reduce bias and therefore provide more reliable results.
 (d) Results from trials with a large sample size are more ethical.
 (e) Larger numbers of participants tend to increase treatment differences between groups.

Critical appraisal

It is essential to critically appraise results reported from trials to decide whether they are valid before applying the information in clinical practice.[14] Work through the critical appraisal checklist to review the set paper by Miranda-Filho *et al.* (2004) and decide whether the results warrant a change in clinical practice and, if so, in which group of patients.

Critical appraisal checklist for an article that reports the results of a randomised clinical trial

A. Study design	
1. What phase is the study design (I, II, III or IV)?	
2. Was the trial properly randomised?	
3. Was the treatment compared to standard best treatment or to a placebo treatment?	
4. Have precise details of the new treatment intervention been given?	
5. Is the sample size adequate?	
6. Do the results reported constitute an interim analysis and how might this affect the ongoing trial?	
7. Was a data and safety monitoring committee appointed?	
B. Statistical methods	
8. Is NNT reported?	
9. Was the statistician blinded to group status?	
10. Was an intention-to-treat analysis conducted?	
C. Results	
11. Are the baseline characteristics of the groups comparable?	
12. Are compliance rates in each group reported?	
13. Are the primary outcomes clinically important?	
14. Are important adverse events reported?	
D. Interpretation	
15. Which patient or population group do the results generalise to?	
16. Have the results been interpreted appropriately?	

References

1. Freedman B. Equipoise and the ethics of clinical research. N Engl J Med 1987;317:141–145.
2. Altman DG. Randomisation: essential for reducing bias. BMJ 1991;302:1481–1482.
3. Forder PM, Gebski VJ, Keech AC. Allocation concealment and blinding: when ignorance is bliss. Med J Aust 2005;182:87–89.
4. Solomon MJ, McLeod RS. Surgery and the randomised controlled trial: past, present and future. Med J Aust 1998;169:380–383.
5. Fontanarosa PB, Rennie D, DeAngelis CD. Postmarketing surveillance – lack of vigilance, lack of trust. JAMA 2004;292:2647–2650.
6. Moher D, Dulberg CS, Wells GA. Statistical power, sample size, and their reporting in randomised controlled trials. JAMA 1994;272:122–124.
7. Freeman BD, Danner RL, Banks SM, Natanson C. Safeguarding patients in clinical trials with high mortality rates. Am J Respir Crit Care Med 2001;164:190–192.
8. Hollis S, Campbell F. What is meant by intention to treat analyses? Survey of published randomised controlled trials. BMJ 1999;319:670–674.
9. Heritier SR, Gebski VJ, Keech AC. Inclusion of patients in clinical trial analysis: the intention-to-treat principle. Med J Aust 2003;179:438–440.
10. Pocock S, White I. Trials stopped early: too good to be true? Lancet 1999;353:943–944.
11. Wilhelmsen L. Role of the data and safety monitoring committee (DSMC). Stat Med 2002;21:2823–2829.
12. Meinert CL. Clinical trials and treatment effects monitoring. Control Clin Trials 1998;19:515–522.
13. Pocock SJ. When to stop a clinical trial. BMJ 1992;305:235–240.
14. Greenhalgh T. How to read a paper: Papers that report drug trials. BMJ 1997;315:480–483.

RANDOMISATION

Essential for reducing bias

Douglas G Altman

In the past year the *BMJ* has rejected several otherwise satisfactory studies for publication because of faulty randomisation. How can researchers avoid this fate for their papers?

Randomisation is one of many statistical ideas that have permeated medical research but are imperfectly understood. Its use is most familiar in controlled trials, where patients are given one of two or more treatments chosen at random. The purpose is to eliminate possible biases that may lead to systematic differences between the treatment groups — in particular to eliminate any influence on the allocation of treatment by the investigator (either subconscious or deliberate).

Random does not mean the same as haphazard: random allocation in a clinical trial means that all patients have the same chance of receiving any particular treatment (and in most cases each treatment is equally likely). Patients should be entered into a trial before their allocation to a particular treatment is known. A common misconception exists that allocation based on, for example, odd or even dates of birth or hospital numbers is random. These systematic allocation methods, however, clearly violate the requirement that all patients have the same chance of receiving each treatment. Alternate allocation does not in principle suffer from such problems, but there is a risk of abuse because the investigator's knowledge of the next treatment may lead to some patients being excluded from the trial[1] — making this method inadvisable. Trials using these inferior methods of allocation are not aceptable to the *BMJ*.

Even with proper randomisation a risk of bias exists when the investigators are aware of the treatment awaiting the next patient to be entered into the trial. Better to use a method of allocation that aims to remove the problems of bias — such as by telephone to a randomisation centre, by the pharmacy, or by a secure system of sequentially numbered opaque sealed envelopes. These are the considerations that underlie the requirement to provide information about the method of randomisation in the statistical checklist used by the *BMJ's* statistical referees.[2]

Exclusion of some of the randomised patients from the analysis of a controlled trial, for whatever reason, will destroy the unbiased comparison of treatments. This is the reason for the recommendation to analyse all randomised patients in the groups they were allocated to, even if some did not receive the intended treatment (an "intention to treat" analysis). For controlled trials, it is desirable for the groups receiving each treatment to be as similar as possible. Simple randomisation does not guarantee this for any particular trial, especially if the sample is small.[3] Imbalance may be greatly reduced by using stratified randomisation.[1]

In some circumstances randomisation is not possible, either for ethical reasons or because few patients are willing to be randomised. An unrandomised study of concurrent groups treated differently on the basis of clinical judgment or patient preference, or both, will need careful analysis to take account of differing characteristics of the patients and may still be of doubtful value. Failure to use randomisation when it could be used may fatally compromise the credibility of research, as happened in a study of periconceptional vitamin supplementation.[4]

Randomisation is also valuable in other types of research. In surveys it may not be practicable to contact the whole target population. A representative subset can be chosen by random sampling, whereby each person is equally likely to be selected. A low response rate will negate the advantage of random selection because of the strong possibility that those who respond are a biased subset. Thus it is more sensible to put resources into trying to get complete information from a random sample than to get poor data from the whole population of interest.[5] Random sampling is feasible only when there is a list of all members of the relevant population. A sample survey can be made more representative of the population by stratified sampling — for example, to preserve the age-sex distribution.

Likewise, in case-control and cohort studies it may not be feasible to investigate all of the people of interest — again, random samples should be taken. Randomisation also has a place in laboratory experiments — for example, when locating samples on a 6×6 plate in an automatic analyser. Comparative experiments on animals should also use random selection of animals rather than using those most easily caught.[6]

In all types of study the use of randomisation means that no systematic bias is introduced and the samples selected should be representative of the populations of interest. Once the principles are understood, random selection or allocation is straightforward, using tables of random numbers or a random number generator on a computer.[1] The use of randomisation does not obviate the need for care in other aspects

Head, Medical Statistical Laboratory,
Imperial Cancer Research Fund,
London WC2A 3PX

Originally published in *BMJ* 1991; **302**: 1481–82. Reproduced with permission.

of the design and analysis of research. For example, though randomised controlled trials are widely agreed to yield the most reliable scientific information, careless or inappropriate analysis may lead to misleading conclusions. The standard of statistics in published reports of clinical trials can be greatly improved.[7,8]

References

1 Pocock SJ. *Clinical trials: a practical approach.* Chichester: John Wiley, 1983.

2 Anonymous. *Guidelines for writing papers. BMJ* 1991;302:40–2.

3 Altman DG. A fair trial? *BMJ* 1984;289:336–7.

4 Smithells RW, Sheppard S, Schorah CJ, *et al.* Possible prevention of neural-tube defects by periconceptional vitamin supplementation. *Lancet* 1980;i:339–40.

5 Evans SJW. Good surveys guide. *BMJ* 1991;302:302–3.

6 Anonymous. *Guidelines on the care of laboratory animals and their use for scientific purposes. IV. Planning and design of experiments.* London: Laboratory Animals Science Association and Universities Federation for Animal Welfare, 1990.

7 Altman DG, Doré CJ. Randomisation and baseline comparisons in clinical trials. *Lancet* 1990;335:149–53.

8 Gotzsche PC. Methodology and overt and hidden bias in reports of 196 double-blind trials of non-steroidal antiinflammatory drugs in rheumatoid arthritis. *Controlled Clin Trials* 1989;**10**:31–56.

Originally published in *BMJ* 1991; **302**: 1481–82. Reproduced with permission.

Inclusion of patients in clinical trial analysis: the intention-to-treat principle

Stephane R Heritier, Val J Gebski and Anthony C Keech

1: CONSORT checklist of items to include when reporting a trial

Selection and topic	Item no.	Descriptor
Numbers analysed	16	Number of participants (denominator) in each group included in each analysis, and whether the analysis was by "intention to treat". State results in absolute numbers (eg, 10/20, not 50%).

2: Advantages and limitations of an intention-to-treat (ITT) analysis

Advantages
- Retains balance in prognostic factors arising from the original random treatment allocation
- Gives an unbiased estimate of treatment effect
- Admits non-compliance and protocol deviations, thus reflecting a real clinical situation

Limitations
- Estimate of treatment effect is generally conservative because of dilution due to non-compliance
- In equivalence trials (attempting to prove that two treatments do not differ by more than a certain amount), this analysis will favour equality of treatments
- Interpretation becomes difficult if a large proportion of participants cross over to opposite treatment arms

Requirements for an ideal ITT analysis
- Full compliance with randomised treatment
- No missing responses
- Follow-up on all participants

ITT analysis is highly desirable unless:
- There is overwhelming justification for a different analysis policy (eg, an unacceptably high proportion of ineligible participants — those without the disease under study, for whom there is no potential benefit from the intervention. In these circumstances a "quasi" ITT approach (in which ineligible patients are excluded) is more appropriate.

Determining the sample of participants to be analysed is a crucial step in reporting clinical trials. For such analyses, the gold standard is the "intention-to-treat" principle. The question of which participants are included in the analysis appears as Item 16 of the CONSORT statement (Box 1)[1]

Intention-to-treat (ITT)

Analysis by ITT is a strategy that compares the study groups in terms of the treatment to which they were randomly allocated, irrespective of the treatment they actually received or other trial outcomes. Regardless of protocol deviations and participant compliance or withdrawal, analysis is performed according to the assigned treatment group.[2,3]

Random allocation aims to ensure that trial participants' risk factors that may affect the outcome under investigation are balanced between the allocated treatments. This is to ensure that any differences in outcomes observed between groups are actually a result of the trial interventions. Importantly, there can be no guarantee that participants from each group who do not comply with the allocated treatment have the same risk-factor profile. Any analysis other than an ITT analysis (eg, one that excludes non-compliant participants) will potentially compromise the balance of these factors and introduce bias into the treatment comparisons.

Thus, the ITT strategy generally gives a conservative estimate of the treatment effect compared with what would be expected if there was full compliance. By accepting that non-compliance and protocol deviations are likely to occur in actual clinical practice,[3,4] ITT essentially tests a treatment policy or strategy, and avoids overoptimistic estimates of the efficacy of an intervention resulting from the removal of non-compliers.

NHMRC Clinical Trial Centre, University of Sydney, Camperdown, NSW.

Stephane R Heritier, PhD, *Senior Lecturer in Statistics*
Val J Gebski, BA, MStat, *Principal Research Fellow*
Anthony C Keech, MScEpid FRACP, *Deputy Director*

Reprints will not be available from the authors.

Correspondence: Associate Professor Anthony C Keech, NHMRC Clinical Trial Centre, University of Sydney, Locked Bag 77, Camperdown, NSW 1450.
(email: enquiry@ctc.usyd.edu.au)

(*Received 3 Sep 2003, accepted 16 Sep 2003*)

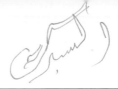

Ensuring ITT produces meaningful answers

The reality of conducting clinical trials means that the ITT principle is not usually fully met, especially when outcome data are missing for some participants. However, clinical trial researchers should consider this principle an ideal, and steps to achieve it should be considered in both the design and conduct of a trial.

Firstly, eligibility errors can be avoided by careful scrutiny before random allocation. Indeed, allocation of ineligible patients should be the exception, unless eligibility cannot be assessed quickly. Secondly, all efforts should be pursued to ensure minimal dropouts from treatment, crossover of participants between groups and losses to follow-up. An active run-in phase may be feasible to identify patients who are likely to drop out. A thorough consent process for participants and education of investigators will also minimise the number of dropouts. During the trial, adequate warning of the potential side effects of treatment, together with ongoing clinical support and reassurance, should be available to all participants. When a proportion of participants are expected to receive a treatment different from the assigned one, a dilution effect generally results. The subsequent potential loss of study power can be accounted for by increasing the planned sample size.[5]

Box 2 details the advantages and limitations of ITT analyses.

Alternatives to ITT analysis

Per-protocol (PP) analysis

There is a view that only patients who sufficiently complied with the trial's protocol should be considered in the analysis.[6] Compliance covers exposure to treatment, availability of measurements, and absence of major protocol violations. Such an analysis is often referred to as a "per-protocol" or "on treatment" analysis. The main issue arising from this approach is that it might introduce bias related to excluding participants from analysis. Therefore, the ITT analysis should always be considered as the ideal primary analysis, possibly supplemented by a secondary analysis using the PP approach. However, if investigators decide differently, their choice must be justified and should be subject to strict rules.[7–9]

Treatment-received (TR) analysis

Another approach is to analyse all participants according to the treatment they actually received, regardless of what treatment they were originally allocated. While this may have some initial appeal, once again the effect of random allocation is compromised, making the interpretation of the results difficult.

The impact of various approaches is illustrated in Box 3.

When ITT requirements are not fully met

A number of strategies can be adopted if the assumptions underpinning ITT are not satisfied.

If the crossover/non-compliance rates are small, then an ITT analysis should be the principal method of analysis.

There is still some debate about whether ineligible subjects can legitimately be omitted from the final analysis.[2] For instance, in a study involving a potentially life-threatening condition, such as severe acute respiratory syndrome, treatment may be routinely commenced before laboratory confirmation of the diagnosis. If the patients subsequently are not diagnosed with the condition, there may be a case for excluding them from the ITT population. In these instances, a "modified" or "quasi" ITT population may be defined, allowing for such exclusions. The following principles should be followed to allow participants to be excluded from such an analysis:

- the criteria for exclusion from the analysis should be pre-specified in the protocol, be objective and clearly defined;[7,8] and,
- to remain unbiased, decisions to exclude participants need to be made (i) by researchers blinded to treatment allocation, and (ii) on the basis of information not related to either the allocated treatment or to events or outcomes that occur after random allocation.

In all circumstances, all patients randomly allocated to a study arm should be followed up, as exposure to study treatment may still influence their safety and place them at risk of serious adverse events. All efforts must be made to ensure maximum compliance and that patients continue to take their allocated treatments, and that all patients are accounted for in the trial report.[9]

The modified or quasi ITT population may also be useful when outcomes are not assessed in all participants. For example, outcomes requiring colonoscopic follow-up can result in no information for patients who, for any reason, did not undergo colonoscopy during the study, requiring an analysis based on a subset of the patient population.[10] In such a case, modifying the ITT population allows some clinical interpretation of the results.

A more extreme example is a study evaluating hip protectors, in which only around 50% of those in the intervention arm were wearing a hip protector at the time of their fracture.[11] In this situation, neither an ITT or per-protocol analysis would necessarily provide reliable information about the value of hip protectors when actually worn.

There has been debate about the appropriateness of imputing missing values.[4] If missing data are imputed, it is recommended that some sensitivity analysis be performed to ensure that study conclusions are not misleading.[4,12]

Conclusion

ITT analysis gives unbiased and consistent estimates of a treatment policy, and should, wherever possible, be the analysis of choice. Deviations from this principle compromise the balance between groups that is achieved by random allocation, and are rarely justifiable as a principal analysis.

Competing interests

None identified.

Originally published in *Medical Journal of Australia* 2003; **179**: 438–40. Reproduced with permission.

3: Example illustrating the impact of intention-to-treat, per-protocol and treatment-received analyses in a placebo-controlled trial*

	Treatment group (n = 1000)		Control group (n = 1000)	
	Compliers	Non-compliers (drop-outs)	Compliers	Non-compliers (drop-ins)‡
Compliance 80%†‡	800†	200†	800‡	200‡
Untreated baseline risk	10%	10%	7.5%	20%
Number of events without any treatment	80	20	60	40
Overall event rate	100/1000 = 10%		100/1000 = 10%	

Expected number of events					Expected benefit (relative risk reduction)
Full compliance		80		100	20% benefit (1 – [80/100])
Intention-to-treat analysis	64	20	60	32	9% benefit (1 – [84/92])
Per-protocol analysis	64	—	60	—	7% detriment (1 – [64/60])
Treatment-received analysis	80	20	60	32	40% detriment (1 – [112/80]§)

Trial assumptions.

* The average risk of each group is 10% over the long term trial duration, and active treatment, when taken, reduces the risk by 20%.

† 20% of those allocated to receive the active drug do not take it because of early side-effects unrelated to the study outcome.

‡ 20% of those allocated to receive the matching placebo medication are prescribed the active therapy because of early clinical deterioration of their condition directly related to their risk of study outcome (these participants are a high-risk subset and have double the average risk [ie, 20%]).

§ This comprises expected events in those taking the active drug (treatment group compliers and control group non-compliers) divided by those not taking the active drug (control group compliers and treatment group non-compliers).

A simple adjustment factor to obtain a better estimate of what might happen with full compliance (100%) compared with observed compliance (80% for each group) can be applied to the ITT benefit (ie, 9% × 100/80 × 100/80 = 13% benefit).

References

1 Moher D, Schulz KF, Altman DG, et al, for the CONSORT group. The revised CONSORT statement for reporting randomized trials: explanation and elaboration. *Ann Intern Med* 2001; 134: 663–694.

2 Fisher L, Dixon D, Jerson J, et al. Intention to treat in clinical trials. In: Peace K, editor. Statistical issues in drug research and development. New York: Marcel Dekker, 1990.

3 Gillings D, Koch G. The application of the principle of intention-to-treat to the analysis of clinical trials. *Clinical Research Bulletin*. Basle: Santoz Pharma, September, 1990.

4 Hollis S, Campbell F. What is meant by intention to treat analysis? Survey of published randomized controlled trials. *BMJ* 1999; 319: 670–674.

5 Kirby A, Gebski VJ, Keech AC. Determining the sample size in a clinical trial. *Med J Aust* 2002; 177: 256–257.

6 Sackett D, Gent M. Controversy in counting and attributing events in clinical trials. *N Engl J Med* 1979; 301: 1410–1412.

7 Peto R, Pike MC, Armitage P, et al. Design and analysis of randomized clinical trials requiring prolonged observation of each patient. *Br J Cancer* 1976; 34: 585–612.

8 Armitage P. Exclusions, losses to follow-up and withdrawals in clinical trials. In: Shapiro SH, Louis TA, editors. Clinical trials. New York: Marcel Dekker, 1983.

9 Gail MH. Eligibility, exclusions, losses to follow-up, removal of randomised patients and uncounted events in cancer clinical trials. *Cancer Treat Rep* 1985; 69: 1107–1113.

10 Sandler R, Halabi S, Baron J, et al. A randomized trial of aspirin to prevent colorectal adenomas in patients with previous colorectal cancer. *N Engl J Med* 2003; 348: 883–890.

11 Cameron ID, Cumming RG, Kurrle SE, et al. A randomised trial of hip protector use by frail older women living in their own homes. *Injury Prevention* 2003; 9: 138–141.

12 Cakir B, Gebski V, Keech AC. Flow of participants in randomised studies. *Med J Aust* 2003; 718: 347–349.

Originally published in *Medical Journal of Australia* 2003; **179**: 438–40. Reproduced with permission.

UNIT 6
Comparing mean values

Aims

To understand the statistical methods used to compare the mean outcome values of two study groups, and to recognise features of the data analyses that may bias the summary statistics and therefore the interpretation of the results.

Learning objectives
On completion of this unit, participants will be able to:
- decide whether to use a parametric method (independent samples *t*-test or unpaired *z*-test) or a non-parametric method (Mann–Whitney *U* test) to compare an outcome measurement between two groups;
- calculate and interpret the results from an independent samples *t*-test;
- calculate effect sizes and 95% confidence intervals around differences between mean values;
- interpret figures which report mean values in graphical form.

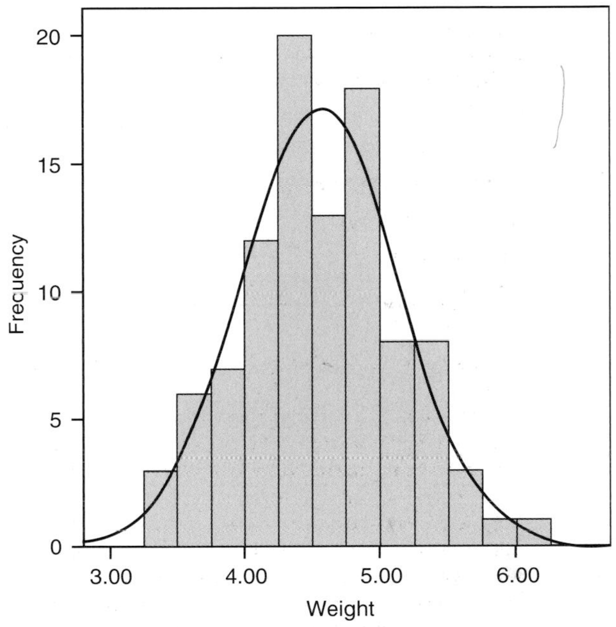

Figure 6.1 Distribution of weight at 1 month of age in 100 babies.

Background

In medical research, we often want to compare the mean value of an outcome measurement between two groups, say, between male and female, in an observational study or between a control group and an intervention group in an experimental study. For example, in a cross-sectional study, we may want to compare mean blood cholesterol levels between male and female or between people who are normal weight or overweight. In a clinical trial, we may want to compare mean fitness levels or mean body mass index in people who have been randomised to receive either an aerobic programme or a weight training schedule.

For applications such as this, parametric or non-parametric methods can be used to determine if a continuous outcome measurement is different between two groups. Parametric methods are used when the distribution

of the outcome measurement approximates to a normal distribution. When the frequency distribution of the outcome measurement follows a bell-shaped curve and is symmetrical about the central mean value, it is said to have a normal distribution.

Figure 6.1 shows the sample distribution of weight at one month of age in 100 babies who were born at term and who were selected randomly from the population. The distribution is approximately normal because it does not deviate in a large way from the shape of the bell curve that has been superimposed and is symmetrical around the mean value of 4.6 kg.

In comparing mean values when the explanatory (group) variable is binary and the outcome (group) variable has a normal distribution in each group, either an unpaired *z*-test or an independent samples *t*-test is the correct statistic

69

to use. A *z*-test is also known as a normal distribution test and an independent samples *t*-test is also known as a two-sample *t*-test, a Student's *t*-test or an unpaired *t*-test. These tests are parametric tests that are used to assess whether there is a significant difference between the mean values of two study groups. A *t*-test is provided by most statistical packages and is appropriate when the sample size has at least 30 participants. A *z*-test is appropriate when the sample size is very large, say, at least 100 participants in each group, but is rarely used in clinical research. When the sample size is large and the variability of both groups is equal, both tests return approximately the same *P* value. In this Unit, we focus on the use of an independent samples *t*-test because this is the most commonly reported test; however, the use of the *z*-test is included in the further reading.

Summary statistics for parametric tests

The summary statistics that are used to describe the central value of each group are the mean values of the outcome variable. Two statistical terms that are often confused in describing the variation of the data values around a mean value are the standard deviation (SD) and the standard error (SE).[1] A further term that is used to describe the dispersion of the data values is the variance.

The variance is used to describe the total variability in the sample. Individuals in the sample can be described in terms of their distance (deviation) from their mean value. When an outcome measurement is normally distributed, approximately half of the sample will have a negative deviation that is lower than the mean value and the other half will have a positive deviation that is higher than the mean value. Because the negative values will balance out the positive values, summing these deviations would result in a value close to zero. Therefore, to calculate the variance, the deviations from the mean are squared to obtain values which are all positive. The sum of the squared deviations is divided by the degrees of freedom to compute a measure of the total variation that is called the 'variance'. The degrees of freedom are equal to the sample size minus one ($n - 1$).

The standard deviation is a measure of how far the data spreads either side of the central mean value and, as such, is a measure of the variability in the population from which the sample was drawn.[1] The standard deviation is actually the square root of the variance and therefore is in the same units as the data values. If the distribution is normal, approximately 95% of the data values will lie within the range of 1.96 standard deviations below to 1.96 standard deviations above the mean. This range is called the 95% range. For the data shown in Figure 6.1, the mean value is 4.6 kg with a standard deviation of 0.6 kg. From this we can infer that 95% of babies in the sample have a weight that lies in the range of 4.6 ± (1.96 × 0.6) or between 3.4 and 5.8 kg. This seems reasonable given the range of values on the *x*-axis in Figure 6.1. The spread of the data values will remain similar

for random samples of the same population, and therefore the standard deviation does not change much if the sample size is larger or smaller.[1]

Glossary	
Term	**Definition**
Outcome variable	The outcome measurement in a study, that is the variable of interest such as the primary illness or disease status indicator.
Explanatory variable	A characteristic that is hypothesised to influence the outcome variable. In clinical studies the explanatory variable is often the group to which patients have been randomised. In cross-sectional and cohort studies, explanatory variables are often exposure variables.
Parametric statistics	Statistics used when the outcome measurement has a distribution that is approximately normal.
Variance	A squared term that describes the total variation in the sample.
Standard deviation (SD)	A measure of variability that describes how far the data spreads on either side of the central mean value. The standard deviation is the square root of the variance and therefore is in the same units as the data values.
Standard error (SE)	A measure of the precision with which the mean value has been measured.

The standard error has an entirely different meaning from the standard deviation in that it conveys the precision with which the mean value has been measured. The standard error is not an estimate of any quantity in the population from which the sample was drawn, but is an estimate that tells us how precisely the sample mean is an estimate of the true population mean. As such, the mean plus or minus 1.96 standard errors tells us the range in which we expect the true population mean to lie. If the sample size in a study is small, we are less certain of the accuracy with which the true mean value has been estimated and the standard error is wider than if the sample size is large, and we are more certain of the accuracy of the estimate. Unlike the standard deviation, which remains relatively constant with sample size, the standard error is inversely related to the sample size. Using the formula for standard error that is shown in Unit 1, the standard error for the data shown in Figure 6.1 is $0.6/\sqrt{100}$, or 0.06. If the sample size had been much smaller, at 25 babies, the standard error would be larger at $0.6/\sqrt{25}$, or 0.12, indicating less precision as a result of the smaller sample size.

Independent samples *t*-test

An independent samples *t*-test tells us how different two mean values are relative to the standard error of their difference. The *P* value from this test indicates whether there is a statistically significant difference between the mean values, that is, the probability that the mean values have come from two populations with the same distribution of the outcome measurement. As such, the *P* value tells us the probability that a difference between the groups has arisen by chance.

When comparing two groups, it is important to distinguish between clinical importance and statistical significance, particularly when the *P* value is on the margin of significance. The standard error that is used to compute a *t* value is influenced by the sample size. Thus, if the sample size is large enough, a small difference between mean values will be statistically significant. If the sample size is too small then a large difference will not be statistically significant. As discussed in Unit 1, a type I error occurs when a statistically significant difference between two mean values is found but no clinically important difference exists. A type II error occurs when no statistically significant difference between the mean values is found but a clinically important difference exists. When interpreting the results from an independent samples *t*-test, it is important to interpret the statistical significance of the *P* value in the light of whether the mean difference between the groups is clinically important and to remember that a type II error may occur – that is an important difference may not reach statistical significance when the sample size is small.

Assumptions

As with all statistical tests, some basic assumptions must be met for the results from an independent samples *t*-test to be valid. The assumptions are that each participant is represented in the analysis once only and that the outcome measurement is normally distributed in each group. Although the independent samples *t*-test is not sensitive to moderate departures from a normal distribution, it is probably best not to rely on this feature.[2] If the distribution of the outcome measurement is skewed, one option is to mathematically transform the measurement to a different scale, for example by using a logarithmic transformation so that the assumption of normality is reasonable.[3] If a measurement cannot be mathematically transformed to normality, a non-parametric test is preferred.

A third assumption for using an independent samples *t*-test is that the variance of the outcome measurement in each group should be approximately equal. When using a statistical package, a Levene's test of equality of variances is reported as an integral part of the independent samples *t*-test, and therefore this assumption does not need to be considered prior to conducting the test. If the Levene's test indicates that this assumption is not met, an adjustment is made to the calculation of the *t*-test statistic and its degrees of freedom and an adjusted *P* value is reported.

The fourth assumption is that the sample size is large enough. The sample size that is adequate for using an independent samples *t*-test is open to debate, but it is generally accepted that, if the other assumptions are met, there should be at least 30 participants in each of the study groups. If the assumptions of normality and equal variances are not properly met, then a larger sample of size of at least 50 participants in each group will provide an unbiased *t* value.[4]

In general, if there is a large imbalance in the group variances, if the distribution of the outcome in either group significantly departs from normality or if there are influential outliers in either group, that is, data points that are extreme and separated from the rest of the data, a non-parametric test should be used. The non-parametric equivalent to an independent samples *t*-test is the Mann–Whitney *U* test. This test should also be used when the sample size of one or both groups is small.

If the assumption of independence is violated, for example if a participant is included more than once in the analysis, such as when measurements have been taken from both kidneys or both eyes in the same participant, a paired *t*-test should be used. Paired *t*-tests, which are used to describe within-participant differences rather than between-group differences, are discussed in Unit 8. A paired *t*-test may also be more appropriate in other study designs such as matched case-control studies, in which the case-control pairs are related by their selection criteria.[5]

Effect size

When the outcome measurement has a continuous distribution, the term 'effect size' is used to describe the magnitude of the difference in mean values between the two study groups, relative to the size of their standard deviations. This is calculated as:

$$\text{Effect size} = (\text{Mean}_1 - \text{Mean}_2)/\text{SD}$$

where Mean_1 = mean of group 1, Mean_2 = mean of group 2 and SD = standard deviation.

When the standard deviations are approximately equal, the standard deviation of either group can be used to calculate the effect size. If one group is an experimental group and the other is a control group, the control group standard deviation is used. However, if the control group is small, its standard deviation may not be an accurate estimate of the population standard deviation. In this case, it is better to use the pooled standard deviation, which is calculated from the standard deviation of both groups. The pooled standard deviation is used when neither group is a control group or when the groups have unequal standard deviations and/or unequal sample sizes. The pooled standard deviation is calculated as follows:

$$\text{Pooled standard deviation} = \sqrt{\frac{(N_1-1) \times \text{SD}_1^2 + (N_2-1) \times \text{SD}_2^2}{N_1 + N_2 - 2}}$$

where N_1 and SD_1 are the sample size and standard deviation of group 1, and N_2 and SD_2 are the sample size and standard deviation of group 2.

Figure 6.2 shows the mean values in two groups that are one standard deviation apart, that is, there is an effect size of one standard deviation. When considering the difference between two mean values, it often helps to visualise them in this way.

Effect size can be used as a measure of the magnitude of a treatment or exposure effect. Calculating the effect size can be helpful because this allows treatment or exposure effects to be compared between different studies in which the standard deviation is different. Effect sizes estimated from a number of similar studies can be combined in a meta-analysis to provide an overall or average effect size for a treatment or exposure. In general, an effect size of 0.2 is considered to be small, 0.5 is considered medium and 0.8 is considered large.[6]

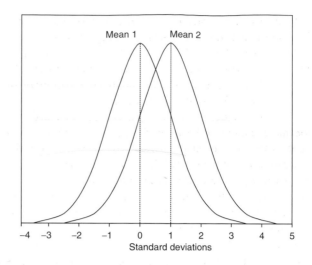

Figure 6.2 Effect size between two continuously distributed variables.

Table 6.1 Independent samples t-test statistics for male and female babies

Gender	N	Mean	SD	Levene's test F	Levene's test P value	t-test t value	t-test P value
Male	48	4.70	0.52	0.78	0.38	2.64	0.01
Female	52	4.41	0.60				

Calculating and interpreting results from an independent samples *t*-test

We can use an independent samples t-test to estimate whether the distribution of weight at one month of age as shown in Figure 6.1 is different between male and female babies. The results obtained from a statistics package are given in Table 6.1 and show that male babies have a mean weight of 4.70 kg, that is 0.29 kg higher than the mean weight of 4.41 kg for female babies, and a standard deviation of 0.52 that is slightly smaller than that of female babies which is 0.60.

The formulas to calculate the mean difference between groups, the standard error of the difference and its 95% confidence interval, and the t value, are shown below:

Mean difference = $\text{Mean}_1 - \text{Mean}_2$
SE (mean difference) = Pooled SD $\times \sqrt{1/N_1 + 1/N_2}$
95% confidence interval = Mean difference $\pm (1.96 \times \text{SE})$
t value = Mean difference/SE

In calculating a t value, the absolute value of t is used without regard to whether the sign is positive or negative. For example, the absolute value of -3 is equal to 3.

Glossary

Term	Definition
Outlier	Data points at the extremities of the range or separated from the normal range of the data values. Data points more than three standard deviations from the mean are usually considered to be outliers.
t value	A t value, which is calculated by dividing a mean value by its standard error, gives a number from which the probability of the event occurring is estimated from a t-distribution. A t-distribution is closely related to a normal distribution but depends on the number of cases in the sample.
Independent samples t-test	Test to measure whether a continuous outcome variable with a normal distribution is significantly different between two groups, e.g. between male and female or between an intervention and a control group.
Unpaired z-test	Test used to compare the mean values of two independent samples using a normal distribution. This test is only used when the sample size is very large or the mean and standard deviation of the population are known.
Effect size	The distance between two mean values, described in units of their standard deviations, that describes the relative magnitude of the difference between two groups.

In Table 6.1, the standard deviations of the groups are not largely different and the Levene's test of equal variance with a F statistic of 0.78 and a P value of 0.38 is not significant. This indicates that the variances in the two groups are not significantly different from one another and that the assumption of equal variances for using a t-test is met.

Using the values in Table 6.1, it can be calculated that the mean difference between the groups is calculated to be 0.29 kg, the pooled standard deviation is 0.56 and the standard error of the mean difference is 0.11. The t value is calculated by dividing the mean difference by its standard error, that is, 0.29/0.11 to give a t value of 2.64. When the variances are equal, the degrees of freedom are the sum of the number in each group minus the number of groups in this case, $48 + 52 - 2$ or 98. The t value can be converted into a P value by either using a t-distribution table in a statistics book or by using the Excel statistics function 'TDIST' which returns a P value when the t value, degrees of freedom and number of tails (in this case, two) is entered. For these data, the P value is 0.01, indicating it is very unlikely that the 0.29 kg weight difference between the gender groups has occurred by chance.

When documenting the results of an independent samples t-test, the mean value and standard deviation of each group as shown in Table 6.1 are usually reported. The 95% confidence interval around the mean of each group could also be reported because this conveys the precision with which each of the mean values has been estimated. In addition, the mean difference between groups is an important statistic that has its own confidence interval. A mean difference of zero would indicate that there is no difference between the mean values of the two groups. Thus, if the 95% confidence interval around the mean difference encompasses the value of zero, we can infer that the difference between the groups is not statistically significant.

For the data shown in Table 6.1, the mean difference between the groups has a standard error of 0.11, which can be converted into a 95% confidence interval of 0.07–0.51 kg. This interval does not cross the value of zero and thus confirms that we can be 95% certain that male babies have, on average, a birth weight that is 0.07–0.51 kg larger than that of female babies.

Presenting mean values in graphs

When presenting mean values in a figure, a dot plot is usually preferable to a bar chart, unless the y-axis begins at zero and the distance of the mean values from zero on the chart has an intuitive meaning. Figure 6.3 shows the mean birth weight in male and female babies as a dot plot. In this plot, the difference between the groups relative to their 95% confidence intervals is displayed correctly. Figures 6.4 and 6.5 shows how mean values are often presented as bar charts and

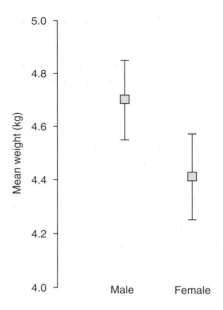

Figure 6.3 Mean values displayed as dot plots.

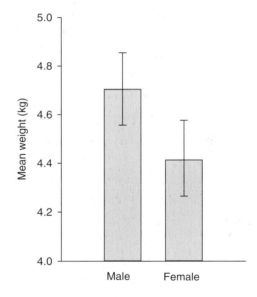

Figure 6.4 Mean values displayed as a bar chart with the y-axis beginning at 4.0 kg.

how, by selecting different starting points for the y-axis, it is possible to artificially change the perceived difference between the mean values. The size of the bars does not have a meaningful interpretation because the y-axis has been started at an arbitrary value in both plots. In general, mean values are better displayed using a dot plot so that the relative differences between the summary estimates are visually maintained and easily interpreted.

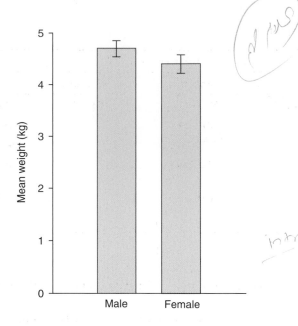

Figure 6.5 Mean values displayed as a bar chart with the *y*-axis beginning at 0 kg.

TAKE HOME LIST

- For measurements with a normal distribution, approximately 95% of the data points will fall within the range of two standard deviations above and below the mean value.

- Because the spread of the data remains approximately the same for random samples taken from a population, the standard deviation does not change much as the sample size increases.

- The standard error will become smaller as the sample size increases, indicating the greater precision with which the mean value has measured.

- The effect size is the difference between two mean values described in units of their standard deviations and is a measure of the relative magnitude of the difference between two groups.

- The statistical significance of a between-group difference is dependent on the sample size. If the sample size is small then a clinically important difference may not be statistically significant.

Reading and questions

Reprint

Driscoll P, Lecky F. Article 7. An introduction to hypothesis testing. Parametric comparison of two groups – 2. Emerg Med J 2001;18:214–221. (See p. 77.)

The reprint by Driscoll and Lecky (2001) shows how two groups can be compared using an unpaired *z*-test or an independent samples *t*-test. An unpaired *z*-test is used when the mean and the standard deviation of the population is known, or when the sample size is large and there is good reason to believe that the data have been drawn from a normal distribution. However, in health care research, population values are generally not known and sample sizes are not generally large, and therefore an independent samples *t*-test is the most frequently used statistic.

After reading the reprint, answer the following questions.

1 What does the 95% confidence interval around a mean difference between two groups actually show?
2 At what point in a study should you decide whether to use a one-tailed or a two-tailed significance test?
3 In the reprint, question 4 of the quiz, what would be the null hypothesis and the alternative hypothesis for the data from the study by Boyd *et al.*? Calculate the *t* value and the *P* value for the between-group difference. What conclusions would you make from these statistics? Then calculate the mean difference and its 95% confidence interval. Does this change your conclusions in any way?
4 For the data shown in Table 3 in the reprint, use an independent samples *t*-test to obtain a *P* value and also calculate the mean difference and its 95% confidence interval for the data as shown. Then, recalculate these values but change the sample size to 35 patients who were re-warmed by a blanket and 45 patients who were re-warmed by forced air. Compare the *P* values and confidence intervals calculated using the different sample sizes. What would you conclude about the likelihood of a type I or II error?
5 For Table 3, as it is shown in the reprint, would it be valid to use an independent samples *t*-test if you were using a statistical package to compare the mean values from the two groups? If you did, what effect would this have on your conclusion? What other statistical test could be used and why?

Worked example

Set article

Rivero-Arias O, Campbell H, Gray A, Fairbank J, Frost H, Wilson-MacDonald J for the Spine Stabilisation Trial Group. Surgical stabilisation of the spine compared with a programme of intensive rehabilitation for the management of patients with chronic low back pain: cost utility analysis based on a randomised controlled trial. BMJ, May 2005; 330: 1239. (See p. 85.)

The set article reports the results from a multi-centre study in which 349 patients were randomised to receive surgery (*N* = 176) or intensive rehabilitation (*N* = 173) as a treatment for chronic low back pain. Outcome measurements were collected at 24 months following enrolment.

Table 6.2 Other back pain-related NHS contacts for surgery and rehabilitation

	Surgery (N = 176)		Rehabilitation (N = 173)		
	Mean cost (SD)	95% range	Mean cost (SD)	95% range	P value
Surgery outpatient clinics	190 (159)	−122, 502	82 (119)	−151, 315	<0.001
Physiotherapy outpatient clinics	286 (523)		301 (584)		NS
Unplanned hospital admissions	451 (1881)		2128 (3522)		<0.001
Other back pain-related hospital admissions	130 (910)		73 (555)		NS
Other back pain-related NHS contact costs	1707 (2451)		3009 (4001)		<0.001

Table 6.2 is extracted from Table 3 in the set article: Other back pain-related costs to 24 months following randomisation. Figures are mean costs and standard deviations in pounds sterling.

Use the mean and standard deviations to calculate the 95% ranges in Table 6.1 and answer the following questions.

- Do you think that the SD describes the distribution of the data accurately?
- The authors say that skew in the cost data was modest and therefore that parametric confidence intervals were used. However, they do not say how the P values in the table were derived. Do you think that the distributions of cost in each group were approximately normal so that a t-test could be used to generate valid P values?
- Are the P values reported consistent with the 95% confidence intervals around the mean cost differences in Table 3 in the set article?

Figure 1 in the set article shows mean utility levels and their 95% confidence intervals at baseline and then at 6, 12 and 24 months. By comparing the confidence intervals what would you conclude about:

- the between-group differences;
- the change in mean utility levels over the period of the study.

Quick quiz

Tick the correct answer for each of the following questions.

1 An independent samples t-test is used when:
   (a) we want to decide if a mean value is different to zero;
   (b) the people in one group are not included in the other group;
   (c) the outcome measurement is not normally distributed;
   (d) people have two data points because they have returned for a follow-up study.

2 The results from an independent samples t value tells us whether:
   (a) the difference between two mean values is large relative to the standard error;
   (b) the two mean values are 1.96 standard deviations apart;
   (c) the group means are a good approximation of the population means;
   (d) one mean value is outside 1.96 standard deviations of the other mean.

3 When the 95% confidence interval around the difference between two mean values includes a zero value, this indicates that:
   (a) the estimate around the mean difference lacks precision;
   (b) one of the mean values is approximately equal to zero;
   (c) there is no evidence of a significant difference between the groups;
   (d) there is evidence that the between-group difference is statistically significant.

4 A non-parametric test is used in preference to an independent samples t-test when:
   (a) the participants have not been selected randomly;
   (b) the sample size is small;
   (c) the distribution of the measurement in the population is not known;
   (d) there are no outliers in either group.

Critical appraisal

Work through the critical appraisal checklist to review the paper by Rivero-Arias et al. (2005) and decide whether the results and the conclusions are valid and justified.

Critical appraisal checklist for an article that compares the mean values of two groups

A. Study design	
1. Are any cases included in a group more than once, for example, are any follow-up data treated as independent data?	
2. Are the two groups independent? Is there any matching or duplicate measurement involved?	
3. Are there sufficient cases in each group to warrant using an independent samples t-test?	
B. Statistical methods	
4. Is any evidence given that the outcome variable is normally distributed in each group?	
5. Are there likely to be any influential outliers that could have increased or decreased the difference in mean values between the groups?	
6. Is the variance of the two groups equal and, if not, has a P value for unequal variances been reported?	
C. Results	
7. Are bar charts used inappropriately for presenting mean values?	
8. Are mean values and/or the differences between groups presented with 95% confidence intervals?	
D. Interpretation	
9. Is the use of mean values and t values appropriate?	
10. Are any of the summary statistics biased? If yes, have any differences between the groups been under-estimated or over-estimated?	
11. Do any differences between groups represent type I or type II errors?	

References

1. Altman DG, Bland JM. Standard deviations and standard errors. BMJ 2005;331:903.
2. Altman DG, Bland JM. The normal distribution. BMJ 1995;310:298.
3. Bland JM, Altman DG. The use of transformation when comparing two means. BMJ 1996;312:1153.
4. Bland JM. Deviations from the assumptions of t methods. In: An introduction to medical statistics. Oxford: Oxford University Press, 1996; pp 165–166.
5. Bland JM, Altman DG. Matching. BMJ 1994;309:1128.
6. Cohen, J. A power primer. Psych Bull 1992;112:155–159.

Article 7. An introduction to hypothesis testing. Parametric comparison of two groups—2

P Driscoll, F Lecky

Objectives

- Dealing with unpaired (independent) parametric data
- Discuss common mistakes using the *t* test

In covering these objectives the following terms will be introduced:

- Unpaired *z* test
- Unpaired *t* test
- One and two tailed tests

In the previous article we discussed the comparison of paired (dependent) data.[1] These result when there is a relation between the groups, for example investigating the before and after effects of a drug on the same group of patients. The key measurement here is the difference between each pair. If this comes from a population that is normally distributed the mean difference can be calculated along with the standard error of the mean (SEM). The 95% confidence intervals for the true mean difference can then be derived along with the p value for the null hypothesis (table 1).

When there is no relation between the groups, the data are called "unpaired" or "independent". A common example of this is the controlled trial where the effect of an intervention on one group is compared with a control group without the intervention. Here the selection of the experimental group does not tell you which people will be in the control group. They are therefore independent of one another.

Table 1 Comparison of two groups using z and *t*-tests

Paired test	Unpaired test
Deals with the difference between the paired values	Deals with the difference between the means of both groups
Relies on the population of this difference being normally distributed	Relies on the population of this difference being normally distributed
It is not affected by the distribution of the before and after samples	Is affected by the inter and intra group distribution

Accident and Emergency Department, Hope Hospital, Salford M6 8HD, UK

Correspondence to: Mr Driscoll, Consultant in Accident and Emergency Medicine (email: pdriscoll@hope.srht.nwest.nhs.uk)

It is useful to note at this stage that when you compare groups you are taking into account two variations. One is due to the difference between subjects within the same group and is called the intra-group variation. The other results from the difference between the groups and so is known as the inter-group variation. With paired data the difference in subjects is removed because each subject acts as its own control. Consequently you are simply measuring the inter-group variation. In contrast, when using unpaired data, both these variations have an effect (table 1).

Unpaired z test

We have shown previously that a systematic approach is used to determine if the null hypothesis is valid (box 1).[1]

To see how this works when dealing with unpaired data consider the following example. Dr Egbert Everard has been working for just over a year in the emergency department of Deathstar General. During this time the department has dealt with 100 patients who have ingested a new rave drug "Hothead". He suspects these people may have an abnormal sodium concentration on presentation—how can he investigate this?

1 State the null hypothesis and alternative hypothesis of the study

Having considered the problem, Egbert writes down the null hypothesis as:

"There is no significant difference between the sodium concentration in the patient's ingesting "Hothead" and those of a similar age attending the emergency department". In other words they are part of the same population.

Box 1 System for statistical comparison of two groups

- State the null hypothesis and the alternative hypothesis of the study
- Select the level of significance
- Establish the critical values
- Select the groups and calculate their means and standard errors of the mean (SEM)*
- Choose and calculate the test statistic
- Compare the calculated test statistic with the critical values
- Express the chances of obtaining results at least this extreme if the null hypothesis is true

*or estimated standard error of the mean (ESEM) if using a sample size < 100.[2]

Originally published in *Emerg Med J* 2001; **18**: 214–21. Reproduced with permission.

This can be summarised to:

mean "Hothead" [Na$^+$] = mean control [Na$^+$]

The alternative hypothesis is the logical opposite of this, that is:

"There is a significant difference between the sodium concentration in the patient's ingesting "Hothead" and those of a similar age attending the emergency department".

This can be summarised to:

mean "Hothead" [Na$^+$] ≠ mean control [Na$^+$]

2 Select the level of significance

If the null hypothesis is correct, and the two groups are part of the same population, then their mean sodium concentrations should be the same. Therefore the difference between them would be zero. However, there is bound to be some small variation simply due to chance. Therefore how big a difference are we going to allow before we reject the idea that the two groups are all part of the same population?

In answering this question we rely on an interesting mathematical fact that the difference of the means represents a population that has a normal distribution. In other words, if you repeated the experiment many times, and plotted all the mean differences, the scatter diagram would take the form of a normal distribution. If the null hypothesis was correct this distribution would have a mean of zero. The standard deviation of this distribution is known as the standard error of the differences between the means (SE Diff). This is equivalent to the standard error of the mean (SEM) that has been discussed in previous articles (fig 1A).[1–3]

When comparing large groups of independent data we can determine the size of different areas under the distribution curve by using the z statistic:

z = [μ1– μ2]/SE Diff

Where:
μ1 = mean of group 1
μ2 = mean of group 2

You will note that this equation is slightly different from the one used to compare paired data.[1] The numerator has changed to reflect the fact that we are interested in the difference between the means of the two groups rather than the mean difference between paired readings. Furthermore, the standard error of the difference between the means (SE Diff) has replaced the SEM to take account of the errors in estimating the means in each group:

$$SE\ Diff = \sqrt{[(s_1^2/n_1) + (s_2^2/n_2)]}$$

Where:
s_1 = estimation of the population's standard deviation derived from group 1 with n_1 subjects
s_2 = estimation of the population's standard deviation derived from group 2 with n_2 subjects

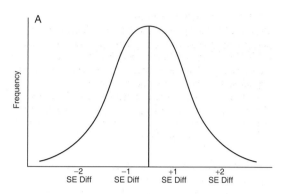

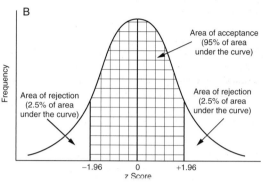

Figure 1 Normal distribution of the difference between the means of the two groups. (A) Shows the hypothetical population mean of this difference (central vertical line). The horizontal access is divided up into standard errors of the difference of the mean (SE Diff). (B) Displays the same data as a standard normal distribution and replaces the SE Diff with z scores. The areas of acceptance (0.95 of the total area under the curve) and rejection (0.05 of the total area under the curve) of the null hypothesis are demonstrated. The area of rejection is split into two tails of the distribution curve.

As discussed in article 4, s is used because in clinical practice we usually do not know the value of a population's standard deviation (σ). However, provided the sample size is large enough (that is, greater than or equal to 100) the z statistic can still be derived using s as an estimation of the population's standard deviation.[3]

By convention, the outer 0.025 probabilities (that is, the tips of the two tails representing 2.5% of the area under the curve) are considered to be sufficiently away from the population mean as to represent values that cannot be simply attributed to chance variation (fig 1B). Consequently, if the sample mean is found to lie in either of these two tails then the null hypothesis is rejected. Conversely, if the sample mean lies within these two extremes then the null hypothesis will be accepted (fig 1B).

Following convention, Egbert picks a significance level of 0.05 for his study. He now needs to determine the sodium concentration that demarcates these two tails.

Originally published in *Emerg Med J* 2001; **18**: 214–21. Reproduced with permission.

3 Establish the critical values

Using the z table Egbert finds that the critical value (z_{CRIT}) demarcating the middle 95% of the distribution curve is z = +/− 1.96 (fig 1B). In other words a z value of +/− 1.96 separates the middle 95% area of acceptance of the null hypothesis from two, 2.5% areas of rejection.

With the null and alternative hypotheses defined, and the critical values established (z_{CRIT}), the patients for the study can now be selected. The z statistic derived from the sample (z_{CALC}) can then be determined.

4 Select the groups and calculate their means

Egbert gathered the presenting sodium concentrations from a sample of 100 patients who have taken "Hothead". The mean ($\mu 1$) and estimation of the population's standard deviation (s_1) were calculated and found to be 131 mmol/l and 10 mmol/l respectively.

Egbert had arranged with Ivor Whitecoat, senior laboratory technician at Deathstar General, to measure the sodium concentration in a control group of patients who had not taken "Hothead". Ivor tells him that the mean sodium concentration in a 100 patients of a similar age presenting to the emergency department ($\mu 2$) is 134 mmol/l with as an s of 7 mmol/l (s_2).

5 Choose and calculates the test statistic

As explained before, the z statistic is equal to:

$$z = [\mu 1 - \mu 2]/\text{SE Diff}$$

Where:
$$\text{SE diff} = \sqrt{[(10^2/100) + (7^2/100)]} = \sqrt{[1 + 0.49]} = 1.2$$
(rounded down)

An interesting feature can be noted from the equation above. Supposed Ivor Whitecoat used several thousand patients to work out a mean. In this case s_2^2/n_2 would become so small as to be negligible. Consequently the SE Diff would simply be equal to the ESEM of Egbert's group.

The difference between the two means in this study is:

$$[\mu 1 - \mu 2] = 131 - 134 = -3$$

Therefore:
$$z = -3/1.2 = -2.5$$

Key point 1

When comparing a sample with a large group you only need to know the ESEM of the sample.

---

6 Compare the calculated test statistic with the critical values

The calculated value of −2.5 lies beyond the larger critical value of −1.96. It therefore falls outside the area of accepting the null hypothesis.

7 Express the chances that the null hypothesis is in keeping with the data

The p value is the probability of getting a difference equal to or greater than that found in the experiment (that is, −3), if the null hypothesis was correct.[4] As the z value can be negative or positive, there are two ways of getting a value with a magnitude of 2.5. Consequently the p value is represented by the area demarcated by −2.5 to the tip of the left tail plus the area demarcated by +2.5 to the tip of the right tail (fig 2).

From the tables of z statistics, it can be seen that the size of the tail from +2.5 to the right tip is 0.5−0.4938 = 0.0062. The equivalent value in the other half of the distribution curve is the same. The p value is therefore doubled to give a total value of 0.0124. Consequently there is a 1.2% chance that a difference with a magnitude of 3, or larger, could have resulted if the null hypothesis was true.

What is the estimated range for the true difference between the means?

In view of the importance of confidence intervals, Egbert also wants to determine the 95% CI for the difference. From the previous explanation, Egbert knows that 95% of all possible values of the difference between the means will lie within a range 1.96 SE Diff below his experimental difference to 1.96 SE Diff above it:

95% confidence intervals = mean ± [1.96 × SE Diff]

As described above, the difference between the means is 131 − 134 − −3 mmol/l. Therefore the 95% confidence intervals of the difference between the two groups are:

1.96 × 1.2 below −3 mmol/l = −5.4 (rounded up) mmol/l
to
1.96 × 1.2 above −3 mmol/l = −0.6 (rounded down) mmol/l

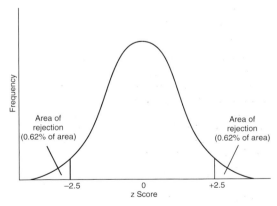

Figure 2 Standard normal distribution curve demonstrating two ways of getting a difference with a magnitude of 2.5. 0.0062 of the area under the curve lies between −2.5 to the tip of the left tail. A similar area lies between +2.5 to the tip of the right tail.

Originally published in *Emerg Med J* 2001; **18**: 214–21. Reproduced with permission.

As this range does not include zero, Egbert concludes that the data are not compatible with the null hypothesis being correct. The range is on the side of there being a lower sodium concentration in the patients taking "Hothead" but the differences are small. Therefore, rather than simply presenting a p value, it would be better if Egbert uses the 95% confidence intervals in discussing the clinical relevance of these data.

In summary, Egbert concludes that he can confidently reject the null hypothesis. Difference between the means of the two groups = –3 mmol/l (95% confidence intervals –5.4 to –0.6 mmol/l); p = 0.012.

Unpaired *t* test

When the sample size is less than 100, the effect of intra-group variation becomes greater. In these cases the normal distribution has to be replaced by the *t* distribution. Unlike the normal distribution, the shape of the *t* distribution is

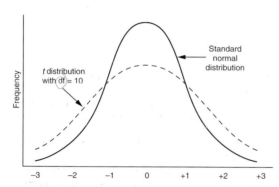

Figure 3 *t* distribution with 10 degrees of freedom and a standard normal distribution. As the degrees of freedom increase the *t* distribution becomes more like a normal distribution.

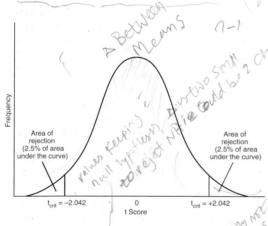

Figure 4 *t* distribution curve with 30 degrees of freedom demonstrating two tails. These are demarcated by $t_{(crit)}$ of –2.042 and 2.042. The area between these values represents those values that are in keeping with the null hypothesis and amount to 0.95 of the area under the curve.

dependent upon the size of the group (fig 3). It is always symmetrical but with small sample sizes the curve is flatter and has longer "tails". However, as the sample size increases, the curve becomes normally distributed.

Irrespective of which *t* distribution is chosen, the same principle applies regarding set areas under the curve representing particular probabilities. Consequently the p value for the null hypothesis is derived from the test statistic. However, tables of the *t* distribution are used rather than the z distribution ones. Likewise, the 95% confidence intervals for the true difference between the means are the experimental mean difference, (±) the appropriate *t* value, multiplied by the SE Diff.

To see how this works, consider the following example. Egbert by chance has a night off and discusses his findings over a romantic meal with Endora Lonely, an emergency physician at St Heartsinc. She is surprised by the topic of conversation but does wonder if the same applies to patients having taken an analogue of "Hothead" called "Brainboil". She tackles this using the previously described systematic approach but this time considers using an unpaired *t* test as her study and control groups have only 16 patients in each.

1 State the null hypothesis and the alternative hypothesis of the study

These remain unchanged from those used in the larger study. Consequently:

"There is no significant difference between the sodium concentration in the patient's ingesting "Brainboil" and those of a similar age attending the emergency department". In other words they are part of the same population.

This can be summarised to:

mean "Brainboil" [Na$^+$] = mean control [Na$^+$]

The alternative hypothesis is the logical opposite of this, that is:

"There is a significant difference between the sodium concentration in the patient's ingesting "Brainboil" and those of a similar age attending the emergency department".

This can be summarised to:

mean "Brainboil" [Na$^+$] ≠ mean control [Na$^+$]

2 Select the level of significance

Following convention, Endora picks a significance level of 0.05 for her study.

3 Establish the critical values

This is carried out in the same way as comparing larger groups but this time the *t* statistic is used because the group size is less than 100. The *t* table enables you to calculate the probability of lying within the middle 95% of the distribution where the null hypothesis is valid. The tables also take into account the changes in *t* with variation in sample size.

For mathematical reasons rather than use the absolute number in the group you use the degrees of freedom. In this type of comparison it is equal to the sum of the number in each group minus 1 (that is, $(n_1 - 1) + (n_2 - 1)$).

Originally published in *Emerg Med J* 2001; **18**: 214–21. Reproduced with permission.

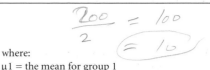

Consequently the degrees of freedom is [16 − 1] + [16 − 1] = 30.

Using the *t* distribution tables, Endora finds that the t value for a probability of 0.05 with 30 degrees of freedom is 2.042. This is known as the t_{crit} value. It means that for this study, a *t* value of ±2.042 divides the middle 95% of the population accepting the null hypothesis from the two, 2.5% tails of rejection (fig 4).

The *t* statistic from the study (t_{calc}) can now be determined.

4 Select the groups and calculate their means

After carrying out her study with "Brainboil" she finds the mean presenting sodium concentrations to be 130 mmol/l (s = 10 mmol/l). Dr Rooba Tube tells her the mean sodium concentration in a control group of patients at St Heartsinc is 135 mmol/l (s = 10).

5 Choose and calculate the test statistic

Unpaired t test

This test requires the data to have two properties:

(1) The two groups need to come from populations with normal distributions.

It is sometimes possible to determine if the distribution is skewed simply by checking the raw data or looking at a distribution curve. A more sophisticated way is to use a computer to develop a "normal plot" of the data. This programme manipulates normally distributed data so that they form a straight line. The closer the data comply with this line, the closer they are to being normally distributed. Altman gives a good description for those who are interested to getting further information about this type of manipulation.[5] It is possible to also prove the same thing mathematically using various probability tests. However, these are of little additional benefit when populations are less than 30 and the normal probability plot gives a reasonably straight line.

(2) The groups should be from populations with the same standard deviation.

It is not possible to know the standard deviations of the populations but an estimation comes from using the s value calculated from each group. The closer these values are, the more likely they have similar standard deviations. As with distributions, it is possible to formally assess the difference in group variance by carrying out an *F* test (see appendix).

Endora checks her datasets for both groups and is satisfied that these pre-conditions are met. She therefore proceeds with the analysis.

Key points 2 Requirements for unpaired *t* tests
- The groups need to have normal distributions
- The groups need to have similar standard deviations

Calculate the t statistic

The *t* statistic for comparing two unpaired groups is:

$$t = [\mu1 - \mu2] / \text{SE Diff}$$

where:
$\mu1$ = the mean for group 1
$\mu2$ = the mean for group 2

When using the *t* test for comparing unpaired means the SE diff is derived from the following formula:

$$\text{SE diff} = \sqrt{[(s^2/n_1) + (s^2/n_2)]}$$

Where:
n_1 and n_2 are the number of subjects in the two groups.
s represents the pooled variance of the two groups:

$$s^2 = [(n_1 - 1)s_1^2 + (n_2 - 1)s_2^2]/[n_1 + n_2 - 2]$$

From the data Endora calculates:

$$s^2 = [(16 - 1)\,100 + (16 - 1)\,100]/30 = [3000]/30 = 100$$

Therefore:

$$\text{SE diff} = \sqrt{[(100/16) + (100/16)]} = \sqrt{12.5} = 3.5$$

Therefore:

$$t = [130 - 135]/3.5 = -1.43$$

6 Compare the calculated test statistic with the critical values

The calculated value of −1.43 lies inside the area of accepting the null hypothesis (that is, a *t* value of ± 2.042).

7 Express the chances that the null hypothesis is in keeping with the data

As the *t* value can be negative or positive, there are two ways of getting a difference with a magnitude of 1.43. Consequently the p value is represented by the area demarcated by −1.43 to the tip of the left tail plus the area demarcated by +1.43 to the tip of the right tail.

To determine this p value, Endora needs to consult the *t* distribution table using the appropriate degrees of freedom (table 2). In this case the degrees of freedom equals two less than the total number of subjects in both groups (that is, 30). The table indicates that the size of these two tails is greater

Table 2 Extract of the table of the *t*-statistic values. The first column lists the degrees of freedom (df). The headings of the other columns give probabilities for t to lie within the two tails of the distribution.

df	0.1	0.05	0.01	0.001
1	6.314	12.706	63.657	636.619
5	2.015	2.571	4.032	6.869
10	1.812	2.228	3.169	4.587
15	1.753	2.131	2.947	4.073
20	1.725	2.086	2.845	3.850
30	1.697	2.042	2.750	3.646
43	1.681	2.017	2.695	3.532

Originally published in *Emerg Med J* 2001; **18**: 214–21. Reproduced with permission.

than 0.1. Consequently there is over a 10% chance that a difference of 5 mmol/l, or larger could have resulted if the null hypothesis was true.

The null hypothesis is therefore accepted and Endora can conclude that the sodium concentrations in patients taking "Brainboil" are not significantly different from the general population.

What is the estimated range for the true difference between the means?

Similar to Egbert, Endora would also like to know the 95% confidence intervals for the difference. The SE Diff is used in the usual way to determine this:

$$95\% \text{ CI} = \text{difference between the means} \pm [t_o \times \text{SE Diff}]$$

Where t_o is the t statistic appropriate for the required CI for the true difference between the means.

To find the t value representing the middle 95% of the distribution curve, Endora needs to look down the column representing the outer 5% (0.05 probability) of the curve because this identifies the extreme point of the middle section. The t value in the column representing p = 0.05 at 30 degree of freedom is 2.042. This is the number of SE Diff above and below the mean that cover the middle 95% of the distribution curve.

Therefore:

95% CI = −5 ± [2.042 × 3.5] = −12 to 2 mmol/l (to the nearest whole numbers)

As this includes zero, the null hypothesis is valid at the 5% level. The confidence intervals are wide indicating that the study lacks precision, possibly due to the small sample size.[1]

Common mistakes made in using the z and t test

One and two tailed test

When using the null hypothesis in comparing two groups, you are determining what is the probability that they are from the same population. p Values of less than 0.05 are usually taken as the point where the null hypothesis can be rejected. However, this result does not tell you how they are different. Indeed when you set up your initial study you commonly do not know which group will produce the biggest result.

To demonstrate this consider a trial comparing the analgesic effect of a new non-steroidal anti-inflammatory drug (NSAID) with ibrufen. Before carrying out this trial you may hope that the new drug is better than the old one but you cannot be sure—it could be worse. Your study, and statistical analysis, should therefore be able to detect three possibilities:

- The new NSAID is no different then ibrufen (that is, supporting the null hypothesis)
- The new NSAID is a better then ibrufen (that is, rejects the null hypothesis)
- The new NSAID is worse then ibrufen (that is, rejects the null hypothesis)

The latter two displacements are referred to as the "tails" or "sides". Consequently the tests measuring the probability of

the null hypothesis being valid in one or both situations are called "one" and "two" tailed (sided) tests respectively.

When using a "one tailed test" there is only one area of rejection on the random sampling distribution of the means. Consequently the area of rejection is concentrated on one of the tails. This reduces the critical value for t and so makes the p value smaller and more impressive for any given difference between means.

For example, if Endora used a one tail test for a t statistic of −1.43 she would find it to lie in an area of rejection of the null hypothesis (p < 0.05, shaded area). This is because the t_{crit} for this degree of freedom is −1.31. In contrast, as we have seen, using a two tailed test leads to acceptance of the null hypothesis (p > 0.05, checkered area) (fig 5).

You may therefore be tempted to use a one tailed test in an analysis. Beware though; it is rare that the direction of displacement can be predicted before the study. Furthermore, in comparison to the standard treatment a worse result by the new treatment is also clinically important. Consequently two tailed tests should be routinely used when comparing two groups. If a decision is made to carry out a one tailed test then the rationale must be clearly described. An example of such a case is in public health work when you want to determine if a product does not fall below a particular standard (for example, water purity). Here you are not concerned with how pure the water is, just as long as it is better than a preset level.

Key points 3
- The decision to use a one tailed test must depend upon the nature of the hypothesis being tested and should therefore be decided upon before the data are collected.
- As a rule of thumb, when comparing two groups always use a two tailed test for the null hypothesis.
- The concept of one tailed and two tailed tests does not apply when more than two groups are being compared.

Using a computer without considering the data and the question being asked

Obviously using computer software can greatly help you in working out the long calculations described above. This leads to the temptation of doing the analysis on your own and not seeking statistical help when necessary. However, be aware in doing this that you make sure the appropriate test is carried out so that the correct calculations and distribution tables are used. Applying the wrong test will still produce an answer, but it will be meaningless!

Assumptions of normality and similar variance

The t test is able to deal with all but major deviations from normality or uniform variance between the groups. The main problems occur when dealing with small data with a skewed

---

Originally published in *Emerg Med J* 2001; **18**: 214–21. Reproduced with permission.

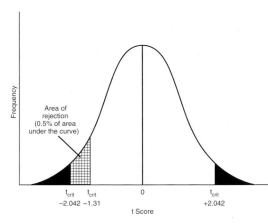

Figure 5 t distribution curve with 30 degrees of freedom demonstrating one and two areas of rejection. A t statistic to be −1.43 lies in an area of acceptance of the null hypothesis using the two tailed test $[t_{(crit)} = -2.042]$ or rejection using the one tailed test $[t_{(crit)} = -1.31]$.

Table 3 Comparison of age and admission temperatures in two groups of patients selected for Steele et al's study[9]

Characteristic	Blanket rewarming (7 patients)	Forced-air rewarming (9 patients)
Mean age (s)	54 yr. (14 yr.)	58 yr. (19 yr.)
Mean admission temperature (s)	29.8°C (1.5°C)	28.8°C (2.5°C)

distribution. In these cases the *t* statistic does not comply with the *t* distribution curve. A possible solution in these cases is to see if transforming the data can make them have a normal distribution and uniform variance.[6] Data that still fail to be achieve these prerequisites cannot be analysed using the *t* test. Instead a non-parametric method will have to be used.

Multiple comparisons

This article has concentrated on comparing two groups. In medical research however we may be faced with having to compare three or more groups. If this problem is tackled using two group comparisons for every possible pair of combinations then we run the risk of finding some "significant" differences simply by chance. This probability gets bigger as the number of pairs increase. Therefore for multiple comparisons, *t* tests should not be used. Instead a different test, known as an analysis of variance, is required.

Summary

When carrying out medical studies we often have to compare two unpaired (independent) groups. This is best carried out using a systematic approach in which the null hypothesis, the levels of significance and the critical levels are decided upon before the experiment is started. Once the data have been collected the appropriate statistic test is chosen and calculated. The likelihood of the null hypothesis being valid can then be determined along with the confidence intervals for the difference between the means of the two groups.

When comparing large samples (a 100 or greater), the z statistic can be used. However, with smaller groups the assumptions made in its calculation are no longer valid. In these

circumstances the *t* statistic should be calculated, provided the data are normally distributed and the two groups have similar standard deviations.

Quiz

1 Why are the confidence intervals for unpaired comparisons usually greater than the paired variety?
2 What are the requirements of the data if an unpaired *t* test is to be carried out?
3 Allison *et al.* carried out an experiment to compare the capillary leakage in trauma victims resuscitated with either hydroxyethyl starch (n = 24) or gelatine (n = 21).[7] State the null hypothesis and alternative hypothesis of the study? Assuming a level of significance of 0.05, what would be the critical values (t_{crit}) of the study if an unpaired *t* test was carried out?
4 The following question is adapted from Boyd *et al.* study comparing two activated charcoal preparations.[8] They found the mean (s) amount of charcoal drunk was 26.5 (13.3) g for Carbomix and 19.5 (13.7) g for Actidose-Aqua. The sample size for the Carbomix group was 47 and 50 for Actidose-Aqua. Assuming the prerequisites for carrying out an unpaired, two tailed *t* test are valid, calculate the *t* statistic.
5 One for you to try on your own. Steele *et al.* carried out a study comparing two types of rewarming of hypothermic patients.[9] Part of the data are adapted and shown in table 3.

Carry out an unpaired, two tailed *t* test comparing these datasets in the two groups. Is there a significant difference between the groups for the two variables?

Answers

1 When using paired data the confidence interval is smaller because you have removed the variability between the subjects and are solely comparing the inter-groups difference.
2 The groups need to have normal distributions and similar standard deviations.
3 The null hypothesis is:
"There is no significant difference in the capillary leakage of trauma victims resuscitated with hydroxyethyl starch or gelatine.

Originally published in *Emerg Med J* 2001; **18**: 214–21. Reproduced with permission.

The alternative hypothesis is:

"There is a significant difference in the capillary leakage of trauma victims resuscitated with hydroxyethyl starch or gelatine.

To determine the critical value the degrees of freedom need to be calculated first. In this study this is equal to $[24 - 1] + [21 - 1] = 43$.

Using the t distribution tables, the t_{crit} value for a probability of 0.05 with 43 degrees of freedom is ± 2.017 if a two tailed test is being used.

4 The t statistic for comparing two unpaired groups is:

$$t = [\mu 1 - \mu 2] / SE\ Diff$$

where:

$\mu 1$ = the mean for Carbomix
$\mu 2$ = the mean for Actidose-Aqua
$SE\ diff = \sqrt{[s^2 / n_1 + s^2 / n_2]}$

and:

$$s^2 = [(n_1 - 1)s_1^2 + (n_2 - 1)s_2^2]/[n_1 + n_2 - 2]$$

From the data of Boyd *et al.*:

$$s^2 = [(46 \times 176.89) + (49 \times 187.69)]/95 = 182.46$$

Therefore:

$$SE\ diff = \sqrt{[182.46/47 + 182.46/50]} = 2.74$$

Therefore:

$$t = [26.5 - 19.5]/2.74 = 2.6\ (rounded\ up)$$

The authors would like to thank Jim Wardrope and Iram Butt for their invaluable suggestions.

Appendix

The F test is the ratio of the larger variance/smaller variance. The resulting F value is then used to determine the probability that the two variances are from the same population (that is, that the null hypothesis is correct). This is done by reading the F tables using the F value and the appropriate degrees of freedom. The latter is equal to the sum of $(n_1 - 1)$ and $(n_2 - 1)$ where n_1 and n_2 are the number in both groups.

If the null hypothesis is not consistent with the data (that is, the "F" statistic is significant), the t test should not be used.

References

1 Driscoll P, Lecky F. An introduction to hypothesis testing. Parametric comparison of two groups—1. *Emerg Med J* 2001;**18**:124–30.
2 Driscoll P, Lecky F, Crosby M. An introduction to estimation—1. Starting from z. *J Accid Emerg Med* 2000;**17**:409–15.
3 Driscoll P, Lecky F. An introduction to estimation—2. From z to t. *Emerg Med J* 2001;**18**:65–70.
4 Driscoll P, Lecky F, Crosby M. An introduction to statistical inference. *J Accid Emerg Med* 2000;**17**:357–63.
5 Altman D. Normal plot. In: *Practical statistics for medical research*. London: Chapman and Hall, 1997:133–43.
6 Driscoll P, Lecky F, Crosby M. *An introduction to everyday statistics—1*. *J Accid Emerg Med* 2000;**17**:205–11.
7 Allison K, Gosling P, Jones S, *et al*. Randomised trial of hydroxyethyl starch versus gelatine for trauma resuscitation. *J Trauma* 1999;**47**:1114–21.
8 Boyd R, Hanson J. Prospective single blinded randomised controlled trial of two orally administered activated charcoal preparations. *J Accid Emerg Med* 1999;**16**:24–5.
9 Steele M, Nelson M, Sessier D, *et al*. Forced air speeds rewarming in accidental hypothermia. *J Trauma* 1996;**27**:479–84.

Further reading

Altman D. Theoretical distributions. In: *Practical statistics for medical research*. London: Chapman and Hall, 1991:48–73.
Bland M. *An introduction to medical statistics*. Oxford: Oxford University Press, 1987.
Gaddis G, Gaddis M. Introduction to biostatistics: Part 4, statistical inference techniques in hypothesis testing. *Ann Emerg Med* 1990;**19**:820–5.
Gardner M, Altman D. Calculating confidence intervals for means and their differences. In: *Statistics with confidence*. London: BMJ Publications, 1989:20–7.
Glaser A. Hypothesis testing In: *High yield biostatistics*. Baltimore: Williams and Wilkins, 1995:31–46.
Koosis D. Difference between means. In: *Statistics—a self teaching guide*. 4th ed. New York: Wiley, 1997:127–52.
Swincow T. The t test. In: *Statistics from square one*. London: BMJ Publications, 1983:33–42.

Originally published in *Emerg Med J* 2001; **18**: 214–21. Reproduced with permission.

Surgical stabilisation of the spine compared with a programme of intensive rehabilitation for the management of patients with chronic low back pain: cost utility analysis based on a randomised controlled trial

Oliver Rivero-Arias, Helen Campbell, Alastair Gray, Jeremy Fairbank, Helen Frost, James Wilson-MacDonald for the Spine Stabilisation Trial Group

Abstract

Objective   To determine whether, from a health provider and patient perspective, surgical stabilisation of the spine is cost effective when compared with an intensive programme of rehabilitation in patients with chronic low back pain.

Design   Economic evaluation alongside a pragmatic randomised controlled trial.

Setting   Secondary care.

Participants   349 patients randomised to surgery (n = 176) or to an intensive rehabilitation programme (n = 173) from 15 centres across the United Kingdom between June 1996 and February 2002.

Main outcome measures   Costs related to back pain and incurred by the NHS and patients up to 24 months after randomisation. Return to paid employment and total hours worked. Patient utility as estimated by using the EuroQol EQ-5D questionnaire at several time points and used to calculate quality adjusted life years (QALYs). Cost effectiveness was expressed as an incremental cost per QALY.

Results   At two years, 38 patients randomised to rehabilitation had received rehabilitation and surgery whereas just seven surgery patients had received both treatments. The mean total cost per patient was estimated to be £7830 (SD £5202) in the surgery group and £4526 (SD £4155) in the intensive rehabilitation arm, a significant difference of £3304 (95% confidence interval £2317 to £4291). Mean QALYs over the trial period were 1.004 (SD 0.405) in the surgery group and 0.936 (SD 0.431) in the intensive rehabilitation group, giving a non-significant difference of 0.068 (−0.020 to 0.156). The incremental cost effectiveness ratio was estimated to be £48 588 per QALY gained (− £279 883 to £372 406).

Conclusion   Two year follow-up data show that surgical stabilisation of the spine may not be a cost effective use of scarce health care resources. However, sensitivity analyses show that this could change—for example, if the proportion of rehabilitation patients requiring subsequent surgery continues to increase.

Introduction

Chronic low back pain, defined as pain lasting for more than three months, is common and places a major economic burden on individuals, the health care system, and society as a whole. Direct costs associated with the disability were estimated to be around £1.6bn in the United Kingdom in 1998,[1] and the condition is estimated to be responsible for close to 120 million UK work days lost per year.[2]

doi 10.1136/bmj.38441.429618.8F

Health Economics Research Centre, Department of Public Health, University of Oxford, Oxford OX3 7LF

Oliver Rivero-Arias *research officer*
Helen Campbell *research officer*
Alastair Gray *professor of health economics*

Nuffield Orthopaedic Centre, Oxford OX3 7LD

Jeremy Fairbank *consultant orthopaedic surgeon*
James Wilson-MacDonald *consultant orthopaedic surgeon*

Division of Health in the Community, University of Warwick, Warwick CV4 7AL

Helen Frost *research fellow*

Correspondence to: H Campbell
(email: helen.campbell@dphpc.ox.ac.uk)

(Accepted 29 March 2005)

Originally published in *BMJ* 2005; **300**. Reproduced with permission.

The optimal treatment strategy for patients with chronic low back pain in whom conservative therapy has failed remains uncertain. For three trials, the results of randomised comparisons between surgical and conservative management techniques have been published.[3-5] Evidence from these trials shows that surgery may have some clinical benefit, but it is not clear whether intensive rehabilitation in conjunction with cognitive educational programmes can generate similar benefits for patients. Results from the first UK based trial, the spine stabilisation trial, show a significant difference in the Oswestry disability index at two years in patients randomised to spinal fusion surgery compared with intensive rehabilitation, which is arguably of clinical importance.[6] This statistical difference between treatment groups in only one of the two primary outcome measures was marginal and only just reached the predefined minimal clinical difference. The potential risk and additional cost of surgery also need to be considered. No clear evidence emerged that primary fusion was any more beneficial than intensive rehabilitation. We report an economic evaluation conducted prospectively alongside the UK spine stabilisation trial. We employ a cost utility framework to determine whether any net health gain from using surgery would be sufficient to justify a likely increase in the costs of treatment. The chosen form of analysis will facilitate comparisons between the cost effectiveness of surgery and that of other health care interventions competing for health care resources.

Methods

Full details of the randomised controlled trial are published in parallel with this paper.[6] Briefly, the trial was powered to detect a four point difference on the Oswestry disability index (a questionnaire designed to assess limitations of various activities of daily living[7,8]) between surgery and intensive rehabilitation at 24 months. We recruited 349 patients who met trial eligibility criteria from 15 centres around the UK between June 1996 and February 2002. Of these patients, 176 were randomised to spinal fusion surgery and 173 to intensive rehabilitation.

For surgery patients, the local operating surgeon decided the type of spinal stabilisation used. Rehabilitation patients attended a paced exercise and education programme based on principles of cognitive behaviour therapy totalling about 75 hours. We followed patients and collected back pain related NHS data and data on use of resources by patients to 24 months after randomisation. Patients who considered that their allocated treatment for chronic low back pain had failed could have further treatment including surgery. At baseline, six, 12, and 24 months, patients completed the EuroQol EQ-5D questionnaire, a generic health outcome instrument used to estimate utility scores[9] and quality adjusted life years (QALYs).

Resource use

Patient specific data on the use of NHS resources included initial treatments, other back pain related hospital inpatient and outpatient visits, primary care contacts, and prescribed items of medication. We also collected data on over the counter medications purchased and visits made to private practitioners. The number of centres participating in the trial and constraints on resources precluded the collection of centre specific unit costs. Unless otherwise indicated, we used national average unit costs. All costs calculated are expressed in 2002–3 pounds sterling, inflated to this base year where appropriate.[10]

Spinal fusion surgery

A "micro" approach to the costing of surgery used patient specific data itemised by use of resources. We costed duration spent by each patient in the operating theatre to allow for the time of staff involved and use of the theatre.[10,11] We used unit costs obtained from the lead investigating centre to value types and numbers of surgical implants and intraoperative spinal x rays.

We calculated costs for anaesthetic agents and blood products administered during each patient's surgery.[12] We assumed that the costs of any surgical complications were reflected in the time spent by the patient in theatre. Finally, we costed each patient's surgery related inpatient stay in hospital.[13]

Intensive rehabilitation

For each patient, we collected information on the number of half day rehabilitation sessions attended and applied staff costs per session.[10] Patients had one hydrotherapy session per day, valued by using a unit cost from the lead investigating centre. We costed exercise equipment and use of the hospital gym and a meeting room, by adding 15% (the overhead rate employed by the lead investigating centre) to staff, hydrotherapy, and equipment costs. Finally, we costed overnight accommodation at either a private bed and breakfast (paid for by the NHS) or on a hospital ward.[14]

Other back pain related NHS contacts

Patients reported attendances at hospital outpatient clinics for spinal surgery, physiotherapy, and other back pain related care at six, 12, and 24 months, which we then costed.[10,13,15,16] We used the mean cost of the initial fusion procedures (calculated as described above) to cost hospital admissions for unplanned spinal fusion surgeries. Admissions for investigations included the cost of the evaluative procedure (provided by the lead investigating centre) plus overnight hotel costs on a general medical ward.[14] We costed visits to and home visits from general practitioners and practice nurses.[10] We used the average cost of a rehabilitation programme (calculated as described above) to cost any additional intensive rehabilitation.

Patients' costs

Patients reported contacts with private complementary practitioners, for which we obtained costs from relevant national organisations. Patients also documented items of medication prescribed, and the cost of over the counter

Originally published in *BMJ* 2005; **300**. Reproduced with permission.

medication purchased for back pain (see bmj.com for more details of costing methods).

Paid employment

Patients reported their employment status, occupation, and hours worked at baseline, six, 12, and 24 months. We calculated and costed total hours worked by each patient.[17]

Health related quality of life and quality adjusted life years

We used the EuroQol EQ-5D social tariff, estimated from a representative sample of the UK population, to convert patients' responses to the EuroQol EQ-5D questionnaire at baseline, six, 12, and 24 months into single utility levels.[18] We then constructed patient specific utility profiles, assuming a straight line relation between each of the patient's utility levels. We calculated the number of QALYs experienced by each patient from baseline to 24 months as the area beneath this profile.

Discounting

We discounted costs and effects at an annual rate of 3.5%.[19]

Statistical analysis

A small amount of trial data (12% of follow-up resource use items, 10% of utility scores, and 14% of work status data) were missing between baseline and 24 months. We used multiple imputation,[20] which replaces each missing value with a set of m plausible values, to generate three replacement values (m = 3) for each of the missing cells in these datasets, using multiple linear regression models containing the covariates intervention group, age, and sex. Arithmetic means presented for resource use, costs, and QALYs in each trial arm are an average of the means from the three datasets created. Associated standard deviations include a variance correction factor to account for variability as a result of the imputation process.

Arithmetic means and 95% confidence intervals are presented when making cost and QALY comparisons between the two arms of the trial. Skewness in cost data was modest, and we therefore report conventional parametric confidence intervals.

We carried out incremental analysis, with the mean cost difference between surgery and rehabilitation divided by the mean QALY difference to give the incremental cost effectiveness ratio (ICER). The non-parametric percentile method[21] for calculating the confidence interval around this ratio used 1000 bootstrap estimates of the mean cost and QALY differences. We used the cost effectiveness acceptability curve to show the probability that surgery is cost effective at two years for different values of the NHS's willingness to pay for an additional QALY.[22]

Results

Baseline patient characteristics are summarised in table 1 and reported in detail in the companion paper.[6]

Table 1 Patients' demographics at baseline. Values are numbers (percentages) of patients unless otherwise indicated

Characteristic	Surgery group (n = 176)	Rehabilitation group (n = 173)
Male	79 (44.9)	93 (53.8)
Female	97 (55.1)	80 (46.2)
Age:		
<30 years	24 (13.6)	20 (11.6)
30–39 years	63 (35.8)	67 (38.7)
40–49 years	56 (31.8)	66 (38.1)
≥50 years	33 (18.8)	20 (11.6)
Median (range) duration of back pain in years	8 (1–35)	8 (1–35)

Resource use and costs: initial interventions

Surgery—Spinal stabilisation was carried out for 139/176 (79%) patients randomised to surgery. Procedures were divided into three different groups: posterolateral fusion (n = 57), 360° fusion (n = 57), and Graf stabilisation (n = 25). Table 2 presents data on use of surgical resources and cost, averaged across all 139 patients who had surgery. The mean total cost of a spinal operation was estimated at £7610 (SD £2643). Zero surgery costs were assigned to the 37 patients who did not have spinal fusion and an average treatment cost of £6011 (SD £3896) calculated across all surgery patients.

Intensive rehabilitation—151/173 (87%) of the patients randomised to intensive rehabilitation attended some proportion of their programme. Table 2 shows a breakdown of the mean total cost of intensive rehabilitation among the 151 patients who attended rehabilitation. The total cost was estimated to be £1615 (SD £644). Including zero rehabilitation programme costs for the 22 patients who did not attend, averaging across all 173 patients generated a cost estimate of £1410 (SD £808).

Intensive rehabilitation was substantially less costly than surgery (cost difference £4601, 95% confidence interval £4013 to £5189, P < 0.001).

Other back pain related NHS costs

Forty eight patients randomised to rehabilitation underwent surgical stabilisation of the spine—10 instead of rehabilitation, 38 in addition to rehabilitation. Table 3 shows that these unplanned surgery costs averaged £2128 per patient across the rehabilitation group. This was greater than the corresponding cost of £451 in the surgery group, which was primarily attributable to 11 patients who required spinal re-operations.

Fourteen surgery patients underwent unplanned intensive rehabilitation (seven instead of surgery, seven as well as surgery). These costs amounted to £162 per patient. The overall mean cost per patient of follow-up back pain related NHS contacts was £1302 lower in the surgery group (95% confidence interval −£1999 to −£605, P < 0.001).

Originally published in *BMJ* 2005; **300**. Reproduced with permission.

Table 2 Breakdown of resource use and costs associated with initial treatments (in 2002–3 pounds sterling)

Resource use item	Mean (SD) resource use per patient*		Mean (SD) cost per patient*	
	Surgery (n = 139)	Rehabilitation (n = 151)	Surgery (n = 139)	Rehabilitation (n = 151)
Surgical stabilization				
Duration in theatre in minutes	182 (76)	N/A		
Costs related to theatre duration:				
Cost of theatre per se			£204 (£85)	N/A
Cost of theatre personnel			£2635 (£1409)	N/A
Cost of anaesthetics†			£24.07 (£29.55)	N/A
Radiography‡	0.69 (1.06)	N/A	£18.39 (£24.48)	N/A
Surgical implants used	96%§	N/A	£1703 (£1589)	N/A
Blood products used	18%§	N/A	£77.79 (£241)	N/A
Surgery related inpatient hospital stay in days	7.70 (3.13)	N/A	£2933 (£1192)	N/A
Mean total cost of a surgical stabilisation operation¶			£7610 (£2643)	N/A
Intensive rehabilitation				
Number of half day rehabilitation sessions attended	N/A	26.32 (6.94)		
Costs related to session attendance:				
Cost of programme personnel			N/A	£513.79 (£135.51)
Cost of hospital gym or exercise rooms			N/A	£223.70 (£59)
Cost of hydrotherapy sessions			N/A	£526.36 (£138.82)
Accommodation required	N/A	36.5%§	N/A	£350.81 (£506.99)
Mean total cost of a course of intensive rehabilitation**			N/A	£1615 (£644)
Mean total cost of interventions			£6011 (£3896)††	£1410 (£808)††

N/A = Not applicable.

*Calculated for 139/176 surgery patients and 151/173 rehabilitation patients receiving allocated therapy.

†Includes cost of administering and monitoring anaesthetics.

‡Includes cost of radiography plus a 30 minute allocation of radiographer time.

§Proportion of patients consuming resource.

¶Includes low cost items not shown in the table—that is, use of image intensifier and post-operative pain control costing £0.20 and £14.82 per patient, respectively.

**Includes low cost item not shown in table—that is, exercise equipment (chair and mat) at £0.74 per patient.

††Calculated across all 176 surgery patients and all 173 rehabilitation patients.

Patient costs

Table 3 shows that patient costs related to back pain were similar in both arms.

Overall costs

Table 4 shows that at two years, spinal fusion costs £7830 (SD £5202), and intensive rehabilitation £4526 (SD £4155). The cost difference of £3304 favoured intensive rehabilitation (£2317 to £4291, P < 0.001).

Return to work

At baseline, 88/176 (50%) of the surgery group and 79/173 (46%) of the rehabilitation group were not in paid employment. By 24 months, 18 of these 88 in the surgery group (20%) and 19 of the 79 in the rehabilitation group (24%) had started some form of employment, a non-significant difference of 4% (−8% to 12%, P = 0.71). The mean number of days to obtaining paid employment was 326 (SD 167) days and 323 (SD 278) days, respectively.

The mean total number of hours worked from baseline to 24 months in the surgery group was 1678 (SD 1847) hours and in the rehabilitation group 1707 (SD 1870) hours (difference −29, 95% confidence interval −419 hours to 361 hours, P = 0.89). Corresponding gross earnings were £19 648 (SD £22 256) and £20 034 (SD £22 564), respectively—a non-significant difference of −£386 (−£5088 to £4317, P = 0.87).

Originally published in *BMJ* 2005; **300**. Reproduced with permission.

Table 3 Other back pain related NHS contacts and patient costs to 24 months after randomisation (2002–3 pounds sterling)

Resource use item	Mean (SD) No per patient		Mean (SD) cost per patient		Mean cost difference (95% parametric CI)
	Surgery (n = 176)	Rehabilitation (n = 173)	Surgery (n = 176)	Rehabilitation (n = 173)	
Other back pain related NHS contacts					
Surgery related follow-up outpatient clinics	2.87 (2.41)	1.21 (1.77)	£190 (£159)	£82 (£119)	£108 (£78 to £137)*
Physiotherapy outpatient clinics	3.88 (7.09)	3.91 (7.60)	£286 (£523)	£301 (£584)	−£15 (−£131 to £101)
Other back pain related outpatient clinics	2.06 (4.33)	2.51 (6.41)	£124 (£241)	£121 (£224)	£3 (−£46 to £52)
Unplanned hospital admissions for spinal surgery	0.07 (0.27)	0.31 (0.50)	£451 (£1881)	£2128 (£3522)	−£1677 (−£2271 to −£1083)*
Other back pain related hospital admissions.	0.18 (0.49)	0.07 (0.25)	£130 (£910)	£73 (£555)	£57 (−£101 to £215)
General practitioner consultations	7.38 (9.23)	6.81 (8.49)	£198 (£232)	£185 (£212)	£13 (−£33 to £60)
Practice nurse consultations	0.86 (2.09)	0.62 (1.84)	£15 (£35)	£11 (£31)	£4 (−£3 to £11)
General practitioner home visits	0.69 (1.81)	0.31 (1.03)	£44 (£113)	£19 (£62)	£24 (£5 to £43)†
Practice nurse home visits	0.61 (2.07)	0.24 (1.15)	£12 (£41)	£4 (£18)	£8 (£2 to £15)†
Patients attending unplanned intensive rehabilitation	14	0	£162 (£453)	£0	£162 (£94 to £229)*
Prescriptions received	14.23 (27.05)	13.43 (20.26)	£95 (£200)	£84 (£141)	£11 (−£25 to £46)
Total other back pain related NHS contact costs			£1707 (£2451)	£3009 (£4001)	−£1302 (−£1999 to −£605)*
Back pain related costs to patients					
Visits to complementary practitioners	4.00 (13.19)	2.77 (11.70)	£89 (£325)	£92 (£501)	−£3 (−£92 to £86)
Home visits from complementary practitioners	0.19 (2.26)	0.03 (0.17)	£6 (£71)	£1 (£5)	£5 (−£6 to £15)
Items of over the counter medication purchased	N/A	N/A	£17 (£34)	£14 (£36)	£3 (−£4 to £11)
Total back pain related patient costs			£112 (£350)	£107 (£502)	£5 (−£86 to £96)
Total back pain related follow-up costs			£1819 (£2511)	£3116 (£4120)	−£1297 (−£2014 to −£580)*

N/A = Not available.

*P ≤ 0.001.
†P < 0.05.

Table 4 Summary of initial treatment and 24 month follow-up costs (2002–03 pounds sterling)

Cost category	Surgery group (n = 176) Mean (SD) cost per patient	Rehabilitation group (n = 173) Mean (SD) cost per patient	Mean cost difference (95% parametric CI)
Initial treatment cost	£6011 (£3896)	£1410 (£808)	£4601 (£4013 to £5189)*
Other back pain related NHS contacts at 24 months	£1707 (£2451)	£3009 (£4001)	−£1302 (−£1999 to −£605)*
Total NHS cost	£7718 (£5138)	£4419 (£4026)	£3299 (£2322 to £4267)*
Back pain related patient costs at 24 months	£112 (£350)	£107 (£502)	£5 (−£86 to £96)
Total cost of care	£7830 (£5202)	£4526 (£4155)	£3304 (£2317 to £4291)*

*P ≤ 0.001.

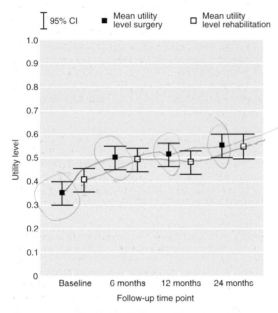

Figure 1 Mean utility levels (with 95% confidence intervals) generated by applying the EuroQol EQ-5D social tariff to patients' self reported health state descriptions.

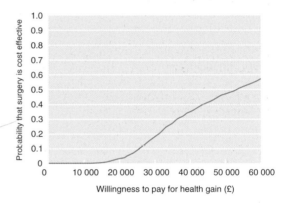

Figure 2 Cost effectiveness acceptability curve showing the probability that surgery is cost effective for different ceilings of willingness to pay.

Utility

Figure 1 shows utility levels at baseline, six, 12, and 24 months. We found no significant differences in utility at any of the follow-up points. A notable difference in utility existed at baseline (0.35 for surgery, 0.41 for rehabilitation). Adjusting for such a difference (using a regression based approach with trial arm and baseline score as explanatory variables) and recalculating the area under utility frontiers specific to patients produced a mean QALY difference in favour of surgery of 0.068 (−0.02 to 0.156, P = 0.13; mean 1.004 (SD 0.405) for surgery and 0.936 (SD 0.431) for rehabilitation).

Cost utility

The incremental cost per QALY of using a policy of immediate surgery was estimated to be £48 588 (−£279 883 to £372 406). Figure 2 shows the cost effectiveness acceptability curve. Reading off from the curve shows that if decision makers are willing to pay £30 000 for a QALY (the value above which the National Institute for Clinical Excellence is less likely to accept a technology as cost effective[23]), at two years, the chance that surgery will be cost effective is less than 20%.

Sensitivity analysis

Although uncertainty surrounds several trial variables, alternative assumptions for some would not affect the baseline conclusion. For example, replacing unit costs provided by the lead investigating centre with national averages had they been available would make little difference. Similarly, alternative discount rates will have little effect over a two year time horizon.

Originally published in *BMJ* 2005; **300**. Reproduced with permission.

We used sensitivity analysis to examine uncertainty surrounding the use of different surgical techniques for spinal stabilisation. Assuming any patient in the trial receiving surgery underwent posterolateral fusion, the least costly technique at £6170 (£5638 to £6803), reduced the total cost in the surgery group to £6655 and in the rehabilitation group to £4252. The incremental cost per QALY fell to £35 338 (−£188 876 to £410 404). Alternatively had all patients undergone 360° fusion, the most costly technique at £9279 (£8632 to £9917), then the mean cost difference would have increased to £4132 (£3065 to £5199) and the incremental cost per QALY to £60 765 (−£420 210 to £617 081).

If the difference in utility observed at 24 months (0.566 for surgery and 0.532 for rehabilitation after adjustments for baseline) was maintained for a further two years, the incremental cost per QALY at four years would fall to £25 398 (£13 121 to £75 916).

We also examined the impact of patients receiving other treatments subsequent to their allocated therapy. At two years, 45 patients (38 in the rehabilitation group and seven in the surgery group) had received both treatments under comparison. Holding all else constant and assuming patients in each arm would continue to receive both treatments in years three, four, and five at the rates observed in years one and two, the cost difference is reduced to £1144 (−£312 to £2600) and the cost per QALY to £16 824 (−£156 358 to £138 911). If the trend continued but at half the rate observed in years one and two, the excess cost of the surgery arm at five years would fall to £2165 (£904 to £3425) and the cost per QALY to £31 838 (−£407 056 to £283 783).

Discussion

A policy in which patients receive spinal fusion surgery as first line therapy for their chronic low back pain seems not to be a cost effective use of health care resources at two year follow-up.

Strengths of the study

The main strength of this study lies in the pragmatic approach adopted by the randomised controlled trial. Patients were not denied alternative health care interventions for chronic pain of the low back, and consequently the treatment patterns observed are likely to reflect those prevailing in routine practice.

At 24 months, the numbers of patients receiving both trial interventions differed significantly between the two arms. It is possible that this difference will increase beyond the two year follow-up point, and sensitivity analyses have shown that this could substantially affect the cost effectiveness of surgery.

Our study found no significant differences in work status measures. Employment data were available from two of the three previously published randomised trials comparing surgical and conservative intervention for chronic pain of the low back.[3,5] The number of patients returning to work differed between arms (in favour of surgery) in one of these

trials, but the same trial found no significant differences in the mean number of sick days per patient and resulting productivity costs at 24 months.[5,24]

This paper presents a cost utility analysis of surgery compared with intensive rehabilitation by using principles of cognitive behaviour therapy in the management of chronic pain of the low back. Although other economic evaluations of interventions for chronic low back pain have been published,[24–26] only one compared operative and conservative treatment.[24] Rehabilitation included in that study focused primarily on routine physiotherapy: comparison of cost effectiveness results between these two trials would not therefore be useful.

Conclusion

Although a policy of spinal fusion surgery as first line therapy for chronic low back pain seems not to be a cost effective use of health care resources at two year follow-up, our analyses have shown that this conclusion could alter if the number of rehabilitation patients subsequently receiving surgery continues to increase in the future. Only with further follow-up of patients can a robust and reliable estimate of the long term cost effectiveness of surgery compared with intensive rehabilitation in the management of chronic low back pain be obtained.

We thank the patients who permitted a difficult decision to be made for them, physiotherapists and surgeons both inside and outside the trial who helped develop the protocol and made the study possible, Anthony Morton for provision of unit costs, the Medical Research Council for supporting the study, and the NHS R&D programme (especially Richard Lilford) for supporting and promoting the study.

Contributors: OR-A collected unit cost data, analysed resource use data, produced cost effectiveness estimates, and revised the paper. HEC supervised the collection of unit costs, analysed HRQoL data, wrote and revised the paper. AG designed and supervised the economic evaluation and revised the paper, and is guarantor of the economic analysis. JF was responsible for the overall trial design, the organisation of the trial, recruitment, surgical intervention, provision of unit costs, and revision of the paper. HF was responsible for overall trial design, the organisation of the trial, the design and implementation of the rehabilitation programme, and revising the paper. JW-M was responsible for overall trial design, the organisation of the study, recruitment, operating on trial participants, and editing the paper. Patricia Carver, Nuffield Orthopaedic Centre, was responsible for data collection, maintenance, and cleaning. Ly-Mee Yu, Centre for Statistics in Medicine, provided statistical advice and commented on the paper. Karen Barker, Nuffield Orthopaedic Centre NHS Trust, assisted with the collection of unit costs and provided valuable comments on the paper. Rory Collins, Clinical Trial Service Unit, Nuffield Department of Clinical Medicine, University of Oxford, was involved in the overall trial design and revising the manuscript. Douglas Altman, Centre for Statistics in Medicine, was responsible for statistical analysis and sat on the data monitoring committee. Nikolaos Maniadakis, Patras General University Hospital, assisted with the design of the economic evaluation. Katharine Johnston, Economics and Statistics Division, Scottish Executive, monitored progression of the study and produced power

Originally published in *BMJ* 2005; **300**. Reproduced with permission.

What is already known on this topic

An economic evaluation of surgery for chronic low back pain that used unspecified physical therapy as the comparator indicated that surgery may be cost effective

A small trial reported that an intensive rehabilitation programme including cognitive behaviour therapy produced similar clinical benefits to spinal fusion surgery0

The cost effectiveness of surgery compared with such a programme has not been assessed

What this study adds

In the short term, compared with intensive rehabilitation, surgical stabilisation of the spine as first line treatment for chronic low back pain patients who have already failed standard non-operative care seems not be cost effective

If the number of rehabilitation patients observed having surgery continues to increase beyond two years, or the small treatment benefit at two years continues, this conclusion may change

calculations. Lesley Morgan, Nuffield Department of Anaesthetics, John Radcliffe Hospital, was responsible for helping to set up the study, data collection, and database design. Kate Stevens, Victoria Erlanger, and Rebecca Bale (previous trial managers) collected and entered data. Peter Smith, X-I Interactive Database and Internet Solutions, developed and maintained the database.

Funding: This study was supported by the UK Medical Research Council. The NHS (326) or private patient insurance (23) funded the treatment of patients. The Health Economics Research Centre is partly funded by the National Coordinating Centre for Research Capacity Development. JF and JW-M receive funding from Synthes for a spinal fellow.

Competing interests: None declared.

Ethical approval: Granted by 15 local research ethics committees and one multicentre research ethics committee.

References

1 Maniadakis N, Gray A. The economic burden of back pain in the UK. *Pain* 2000;84:95–103.
2 BUPA. *Health information, ABC of health, back pain.* http://hcd2.bupa.co.uk/fact_sheets/mosby_factsheets/backpain.html (accessed 8 Apr 2005).
3 Fritzell P, Hägg P, Wessburg P, Nordwall A. 2001 Volvo award winner in clinical studies: lumbar fusion versus nonsurgical treatment for chronic low back pain. A multicenter randomized controlled trial from the Swedish lumbar spine group. *Spine* 2001; 26:2521–34.
4 Moller H, Hedlund R. Surgery versus conservative management in adult isthmic spondylolisthesis—a prospective randomized study: part 1. *Spine* 2000;25:1711–5.
5 Brox JI, Sorensen R, Friis A, Nygaard O, Indahl A, Keller A, et al. Randomized clinical trial of lumbar instrumented fusion and cognitive intervention and exercises in patients with chronic low back pain and disc degeneration. *Spine* 2003;28:1913–21.
6 Fairbank J, Frost H, Wilson-MacDonald J, Yu L, Barker K, Collins R, for the Spine Stabilisation Trial Group. The MRC spine stabilisation trial: a randomised controlled trial to compare surgical stabilisation of the lumbar spine versus an intensive rehabilitation programme for patients with chronic low back pain. *BMJ* 2005;330: (in press, May 28 issue).
7 Fairbank JC, Couper J, Davies JB, O'Brien JP. The Oswestry low back pain disability questionnaire. *Physiotherapy* 1980;66:271–3.
8 Fairbank JC, Pynsent PB. The Oswestry disability index. *Spine* 2000;25:2940–52.
9 EuroQol Group. EuroQol – a new facility for the measurement of health-related quality of life. *Health Policy* 1990;16:199–208.
10 Netten A, Curtis L. *Unit costs of health and social care.* Canterbury: Personal Social Services Research Unit, University of Kent, 2003.
11 MASS Group. Multicentre aneurysm screening study (MASS): cost-effectiveness analysis of screening for abdominal aortic aneurysms based on four year results from a randomized controlled trial. *BMJ* 2002;325:1135–41.
12 Dion P. The cost of anaesthetic vapours. *Can J Anaesthesia* 1992;39:633.
13 Chartered Institute of Public Finance and Accountancy. *The health service financial database and comparative tool.* Croydon: Institute of Public Finance, 2000.
14 Mallender Hancock Associates (MHA). *National average specialty treatment and hotel costs.* London: Department of Health, 1998.
15 Information Services Division NHS Scotland. *The cost book 2003.* www.isdscotland.org/isd/info3.jsp?p_service=Content.show&pContentID=360&p_applic=CCC& (accessed 1 Jul 2004).
16 Department of Health. *NHS reference costs 2003.* Wetherby: DoH, 2004
17 Bulman J. Patterns of pay: results of the 2003 new earnings survey. In: *Labour Market Trends.* Newport, Wales: Office for National Statistics, 2003:601–12.
18 Dolan P, Gudex C, Kind P, Williams A. The time trade-off method: results from a general population study. *Health Econ* 1996;5:141–54.
19 Great Britain H.M. Treasury. *Green book, appraisal and evaluation in central government.* London: Stationery Office, 2003.
20 Van Buuren S, Boshuizen H, Knook D. Multiple imputation of missing blood pressure covariates in survival analysis. *Stat Med* 2000;18:681–94.
21 Briggs AH, Wonderling DE, Mooney CZ. Pulling cost-effectiveness analysis up by its bootstraps: a non-parametric approach to confidence interval estimation. *Health Econ* 1997;6:327–40.
22 Van Hout BA, Al MJ, Gordon GS, Rutten FF. Costs, effects and the C/E ratios alongside a clinical trial. *Health Econ* 1994;3:309–19.
23 Rawlins MD, Culyer AJ. National Institute for Clinical Excellence and its value judgments. *BMJ* 2004;329:224–7.
24 Fritzell P, Hagg O, Jonsson D, Nordwall A. Cost-effectiveness of lumbar fusion and nonsurgical treatment for chronic low back pain in the Swedish lumbar spine study: a multicenter, randomized, controlled trial from the Swedish Lumbar Spine Study Group. *Spine* 2004;29:421–34.
25 Skouen JS, Gradsal AL, Haldorsen EM, Ursin H. Relative cost-effectiveness of extensive and light multidisciplinary treatment programs versus treatment as usual for patients with chronic low back pain on long term sick leave: randomized controlled study. *Spine* 2002;27:901–9.
26 Kuntz KM, Snider RK, Weinstein JN, Pope MH, Katz JN. Cost-effectiveness of fusion with and without instrumentation for patients with degenerative spondylolisthesis and spinal stenosis. *Spine* 2000;25:1132–9.

UNIT 7

Correlation and regression

Aims

To understand and interpret correlation coefficients and regression models and to decide whether these statistics can be generalised to other populations or used to estimate 'normal or reference' values.

Learning objectives

On completion of this unit, participants will be able to:
- interpret a correlation coefficient;
- recognise the limitations of correlation coefficients;
- interpret the meaning of linear and multiple regression coefficients;
- describe the characteristics of reliable explanatory variables;
- decide whether a regression model is valid;
- explain the requirements for calculating normal or reference population values.

Background

In research, we often want to know how closely two continuously distributed measurements are related. For example, we may want to know how closely weight is related to height in a sample of school children. To measure the strength of association between two continuously distributed variables, a correlation coefficient is used. We may also want to know how well one continuously distributed measurement predicts the value of another measurement. For example, we may want to know how well height predicts 'normal' values of lung capacity in a community of adults. To use one measurement to predict the value of another measurement, a regression model is required. Although both a correlation coefficient and a regression model can be used to describe the degree of association between two variables, the two methods provide very different statistical information.

Correlation coefficients

Correlation coefficients describe how closely two variables are related, that is, the extent to which the variation in one measurement is explained by another measurement. Pearson's correlation coefficient (r) is a parametric statistic that is used to measure the strength of a linear association between two continuous variables that are both normally distributed. A linear association indicates that as the value of one variable changes, so does the value of the other variable.

The range of the correlation coefficient, r, is from -1 to $+1$. A correlation coefficient of $+1$ indicates a perfect positive linear association, that is, as the value of one variable increases the value of the other variable also increases. A correlation coefficient of -1 indicates a perfect negative linear association, that is, as the value of one variable increases the value of the other variable decreases. In practice, it is rare to have a perfect linear association between two variables because, even if they are measurements of the same characteristic, measurement error results in 'noise' around them. A correlation coefficient of zero indicates that there is no linear association between the two variables. Suggested guidelines for interpreting the size of the correlation coefficient in psychological research are that values between 0.1 and 0.3 are regarded as small correlations, between 0.3 and 0.5 are moderate correlations, and above 0.5 are large correlations.[1] In clinical medicine 0.2 is considered weak, 0.5 moderate and 0.8 a strong association.[2] However, these guidelines will not apply to all types of data. Large correlations may look unimpressive when the data are plotted and therefore each study must be judged on its merits given that a small correlation that is important in an epidemiological study may not be clinically important.[3]

The P value associated with a correlation coefficient is simply a test of whether the slope of the line through the plotted data points is significantly different from zero, that is, a horizontal line. The P value is heavily reliant on the sample size and thus a small correlation of no clinical importance will become statistically significant when the sample size is large enough.

A perfect positive linear relationship with the correlation coefficient $r = 1$ is shown by the dotted lines connecting

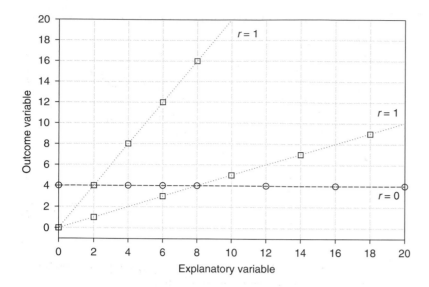

Figure 7.1 Linear relationship between two variables.

the data points in Figure 7.1. For the upper dotted line, the outcome variable increases by 2 units for every 1 unit increase in the explanatory variable. For the lower dotted line, the outcome variable increases by 0.5 units for every 1 unit increase in the explanatory variable. Thus, the r value does not distinguish between different slopes and a high r value does not necessary imply that the two variables are equal to one other. The dashed line in Figure 7.1 has an r value of zero because the outcome variable has the same value for all values of the explanatory variable, and therefore the slope is zero.

It is important to remember that the absence of a linear association does not mean that there is no association between the variables because the relationship could be more complex, such as a cyclical or curved relationship. Moreover, a high correlation coefficient between two variables does not imply that the variables have a causal relationship.

The correlation coefficient (r) can be squared to give the coefficient of determination (r^2). The coefficient of determination is useful because it provides an estimate of the per cent of variation in one variable that is explained by the other variable. For example, a correlation coefficient of 0.6 has a coefficient of determination equal to 0.36, which indicates that 36% of the variation in one variable is explained by the other variable.

The assumptions that must be satisfied to use a Pearson's correlation coefficient are that:

- the sample has been selected randomly from the general population;
- both variables are normally distributed;
- the observations are independent, that is, each person is included once only;
- the relationship between the two variables is linear.

The assumption that both variables are approximately normally distributed is important, and if either variable departs from normality in a significant way, a non-parametric correlation coefficient, such as Spearman's rho or Kendall's tau, should be used. In the following example, the association between weight and length in 100 babies of one month of age who were born at full term is examined. The distribution of weight was shown in Figure 6.1 in Unit 6. Figure 7.2 shows the distribution of length. Both weight and length are both approximately normally distributed in the sample. Although neither distribution is perfectly normal, the distributions are approximately bell-shaped and there

Glossary	
Term	**Definition**
r value	Pearson's correlation coefficient that measures the strength of a linear relationship between two continuous normally distributed variables.
r^2	The coefficient of determination is equal to the squared correlation coefficient and provides an estimate of the per cent of variation in one variable that is explained by the other variable.
Random selection	Sample taken from a population in which all people have an equal chance of being selected.

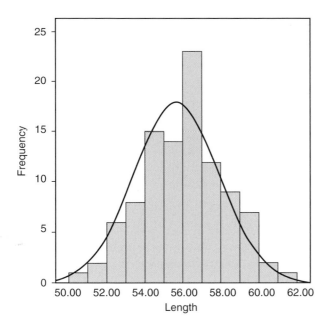

Figure 7.2 Distribution of length at 1 month of age in a population sample of 100 babies who were born at term.

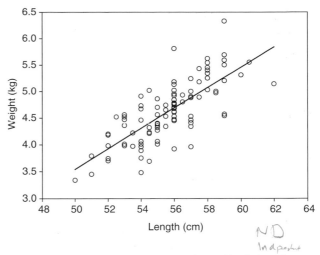

Figure 7.3 Relationship between weight and body length at 1 month of age in 100 term babies.

are no outliers, that is, extreme data points that would bias the estimate of a correlation coefficient.

It is always important to obtain a scatter plot of the data to provide a visual image of the relationship, otherwise known as the 'look-and-see' test. A scatter plot is a visual representation of the data points that provides information about the strength of the relationship between two variables, the degree of linearity, whether the association is positive or negative and if any outliers are present. In a scatter plot, the values of one variable are plotted along the horizontal or x-axis with the corresponding values of the other variable plotted along the vertical or y-axis. Either variable can be plotted along either axis, because the correlation coefficient will be identical whichever axes are used. However, best practice is to plot the outcome variable along the y-axis and the explanatory variable along the x-axis. Scatter plots are invaluable for helping to interpret both the correlation coefficient and the regression model correctly.

Figure 7.3 is a scatter plot showing how length and weight are related to one another in babies at 1 month of age. The plot indicates that weight increases linearly with an increase in body length, with a moderate amount of scatter around the line through the data points. The Pearson's correlation coefficient (r) for this relationship is 0.74, indicating that in this sample, 55% (0.74 × 0.74 multiplied by 100 to obtain a percentage) of the variation in weight is explained by body length. The r value of 0.74 is positive because weight increases as body length increases. The P value of <0.0001 indicates that the slope of the line through the data points is significantly different from zero.

Limitations

Correlation coefficients are rarely used as statistics in their own right because they do not discriminate between different types of relationships in the data. Figure 7.1 shows how an r value can be +1 for two very different lines. In addition, correlation coefficients can be over-valued and misinterpreted when used without regard for their assumptions and limitations. The size of a correlation coefficient depends on many factors, such as the relationship between the two variables.[4] A major limitation is that the range of values on either axis influences the size of the correlation coefficient. For the same relationship between two variables, the correlation coefficient becomes larger, and therefore more significant, as the range

TAKE HOME LIST

- An r value of +1 or −1 indicates a perfect linear relationship and an r value of 0 indicates no linear relationship.

- In general, an r value below 0.3 indicates a poor association and an r value above 0.8 indicates a strong association.

- An r value does not give an indication of the slope or the shape of the relationship between the variables.

- An r value is highly influenced by the range of the data points and the P value is highly influenced by the sample size.

- Only data from a random sample of the population can be used to describe the true relationship between two variables.

- Valid comparisons of r values can only be made between random population samples.

of a variable increases. For this reason, correlation coefficients cannot be compared between studies in which the range of values is different. The only correlation coefficients that describe the true relationship between two variables are those measured in random samples of the population in which the range of values represents the true range in the population.

If the assumption of random selection is not met, the correlation coefficient may be a biased estimate of the true association between two variables. Thus, it would not be valid to generalise the association from a small selected sample to other populations, or to compare r values from studies in which the selection criteria and therefore the characteristics of the sample are different.

Linear regression

A linear regression model generally conveys more useful information than a correlation coefficient because the model provides a mathematical equation that explains the association between two or more variables. Regression models are sometimes used for hypothesis testing, but their main value lies in building predictive equations. For example, regression equations can be used to predict 'normal' population values for variable characteristics such as weight, blood pressure, lung function etc. from other characteristics such as height, age or gender. In general, a regression equation is used to predict the range of values that are expected to occur naturally in the general population given the value of the predictive variable. In this case, the usual emphasis is on building an accurate predictive model that only contains variables that have important statistical and biologically plausible roles.

When using linear regression, it is essential that the research question is framed so that the explanatory and outcome variables are classified correctly. In a scatter plot, the data to be used in a linear regression are displayed with the explanatory variable on the x-axis and the outcome variable on the y-axis, as shown in Figure 7.3. An important concept is that the regression equation predicts the mean y' value for any observed x value. In regression, the measurement error around the explanatory variable on the x-axis is not taken into account. For this reason, measurements that can be taken accurately, such as age and height, make good explanatory variables. Measurements that are difficult to measure accurately or are subject to bias, such as birth weight recalled by parents when their child has reached school age, should be avoided as explanatory variables because measurement error, in this example as a result of recall bias, will compromise the accuracy of the predictive equation.

For a simple linear regression the 'line of best fit', that is the regression line through the data points, is described by the following equation:

$$y = a + bx$$

where 'y' is the outcome variable, 'x' is the explanatory variable, 'a' is the intercept of the line on the y-axis and 'b' is

the regression coefficient. The intercept value 'a' is the point at which the regression line intersects with the y-axis when the value of 'x' is zero. The intercept rarely has a clinical interpretation. On the other hand, the slope of the line, estimated by 'b', does have a clinical interpretation in that it represents the unit change in the outcome variable 'y' with each unit change in the explanatory variable 'x'. From the lower dotted line shown in Figure 7.1, the intercept (a) is zero and the slope of the line (b) is 0.5 because the outcome variable increases by 0.5 units for every increase of 1 unit in the explanatory variable. For this line, the equation would be:

Outcome variable = 0 + (0.5 × explanatory variable)

The regression coefficients for a line of best fit through a scatter plot can be obtained by using a statistics program. The equation of the regression line through the data shown in Figure 7.3 is:

$y = -6.28 + 0.19 \times x$, that is
Weight = $-6.28 + 0.19 \times$ Length

The sign for the coefficient for length is positive, indicating that weight increases with increasing length. In addition, R and R square (R^2) values are given for the regression model. In simple linear regression with only one explanatory variable, the R value is the absolute value of the correlation coefficient (r) and R^2 is the coefficient of determination (r^2). In regression, the capital letter 'R' rather than lower case 'r' is generally used – this helps to distinguish Pearson's correlation coefficients from multiple correlation coefficients that are obtained when there is more than one explanatory variable in the regression model. The R square value for the above model is 0.55, the same value as r^2, and indicates that at 1 month of age, length explains 55% of the variation in weight. The P value for length in the model is <0.0001, indicating that length is a highly significant predictor of weight. The regression coefficient for length indicates that, on average, weight increases by 0.19 kg for each centimetre increase in the length of the baby. The length of a baby can be substituted into the equation to obtain a predicted value for weight. From the equation, the predicted weight for a 1 month old baby of 56 cm would be $-6.28 + (0.19 \times 56)$, or 4.4 kg.

Glossary	
Term	**Definition**
Normal values	Range of values in which the majority of people in a population are expected to lie.
Residuals	Distance between an observed value and its predicted value, in this case the value predicted by the regression line.
Line of best fit	Regression line through a set of data points calculated to minimise the sums of the squared residuals.

Assumptions for regression

To avoid bias in a regression model, or a lack of precision around the estimates, there are several statistical assumptions that must be met. For hypothesis testing, the sample does not have to be a random population sample because, unlike a correlation coefficient, the range of the data values does not influence the regression equation. However, the final prediction equation should only be applied to populations with the same sampling criteria, and therefore the same characteristics, as the study sample.

The assumptions for using linear regression are discussed in detail in the attached reprint by Garnett et al. (2005) and are summarised below.

The assumptions that must be satisfied to use a regression model are that:

- the observations are independent of one another;
- the data have been collected in a period when the relationship between the variables remains constant;
- all important explanatory variables are included in the model;
- the explanatory variables must not be strongly related to one another;
- the relationship between each explanatory variable and the outcome is linear;
- the residuals are normally distributed;
- the variance is constant over the model;
- there are no influential outliers.

Regression models are robust to moderate degrees of non-normality in the distribution of the outcome and explanatory variables, provided that the sample size is large and there are no influential outliers. In general, it is the 'residuals' and not the variables that have to be normally distributed. The residual for each data point is its distance from the regression line. Regression models are often described as 'best fit' or 'least squares' models because calculating the equation is based on the mathematics of minimising the sum of squared residuals relative to the total variation.[5] As for most statistics, the residuals are squared to remove negative values. Most statistical programs provide options for examining whether the distribution of the residuals is normal and whether the variance is constant across the model.

Normal or reference values

A common use of regression equations is to calculate 'normal values', which are often called 'reference values'. Normal values represent the range in which the values for the majority of people in the population lie.[4] The region in which most people are expected to lie is usually described by the area that is 1.96 standard deviations above and below

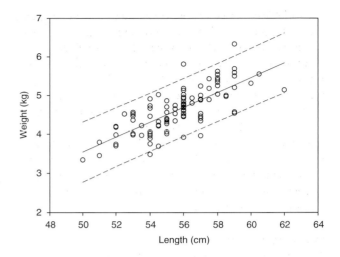

Figure 7.4 Relationship between weight and body length shown with reference range.

the line of best fit, that is, the region between the 2.5 and 97.5 percentiles. Thus, by definition, 2.5% of people will lie below the reference range and 2.5% of people will lie above the reference range. The reference intervals for the scatter plot shown in Figure 7.3 have been added as shown in Figure 7.4. As expected, only 5% of the sample, that is, 5 of the sample of 100 babies, are outside the reference range.

Reference intervals are often used in health care settings and clinics in which diagnostic testing is important. For example, psychologists use reference values to predict whether a patient is within the range for normal cognitive functioning, and respiratory specialists use reference values to decide whether a patient's lung function is within the normal range. Reference intervals are also used to provide a range of normal values against which to assess the results of biochemical blood tests. Obviously, for calculating normal population values, it is essential that a random population sample is selected and, if precision around the estimates is required, then a large sample needs to be enrolled. To build equations to predict accurate reference ranges, a sample size of at least 200 people is recommended.[6]

Multiple regression

Regression models can be built using more than one explanatory variable. The term multiple regression is used to describe models in which there are multiple predictive variables. For a regression equation with two or more explanatory variables, the equation is as follows:

$$y = a + b_1 x_1 + b_2 x_2 + b_3 x_3 \ldots$$

Adding further predictors into the model has the potential to increase the R square value and therefore the amount of variation that can be explained. For example, instead of predicting weight from body length as in Figure 7.3, other predictors such as maternal height, number of siblings, gender etc. could be examined to assess whether they improve the predictive value of the model by explaining more of the variation in weight. In the data set, gender is a binary variable and coded as 0 = male and 1 = female. When gender is added to the model, the regression equation for the data is:

Weight = −5.93 + (0.19 × Length) − (0.22 × Gender)

The P value for length in the model remains significant at <0.0001 and the P value for gender is 0.01, indicating that it is also a significant predictor of weight. The addition of gender to the model increases the R square value from 0.55 to 0.59, and thus gender explains a further 4% of the variation in weight. The regression equation still indicates that weight increases by 0.19 kg for each centimetre increase in the length of the baby. The negative sign for the coefficient for gender indicates that weight decreases as the coding for gender increases, that is, female babies have a lower weight than male babies. This is shown when the regression lines for male and female babies are plotted, as shown in Figure 7.5.

The regression equation indicates that female babies are, on average, 0.22 kg lighter than male babies because for gender = 0, that is, male, the last term in the model is zero, and for gender = 1, that is, female, the last term in the model is −0.22. Thus, the predicted weight for a one-month-old male baby of 56 cm would be −5.93 + (0.19 × 56) or 4.7 kg, and for a one-month-old female baby would be 0.22 kg less at 4.5 kg.

Predictor variables that do not have a significant P value and/or that explain only a small amount of additional variation are usually excluded from regression models. It is important to avoid creating a model that includes more variables than can be supported by the sample size or many variables that explain little of the variation. Such models are described as being 'over-fitted' and the coefficients may be unreliable predictors of the outcome so that their signs (positive or negative) and slopes have no meaningful interpretation.

In building a multiple regression model, it is essential that explanatory variables that are highly correlated with one another should not be included in the model. Explanatory variables that are related to one another in an important way share the same amount of variation in the model, and for this reason tend to distort the regression coefficients and lead to a loss of precision in estimating reference intervals. For example, parental height should not be included as a predictor of babies' weight because it correlates significantly with babies' length with an r value of 0.7. A high correlation between two explanatory variables suggests that they are both slightly different estimates of the same characteristic and that only one variable is needed. It is always preferable to use the variable that has the most biological plausibility and that can be measured with the most accuracy, although other factors such as cost, invasiveness, and ease of measurement are also important factors.

TAKE HOME LIST

- Regression models provide a mathematical equation that can be used to predict expected values of the outcome variable using one or more explanatory variables.

- When a large random sample of the population is enrolled, 'normal or reference' population values can be calculated.

- Explanatory variables should be measurements that can be made accurately.

- Outcome and explanatory variables must be correctly classified.

- In multiple regression, the explanatory variables must not be significantly related to one another.

Reading and questions
Reprint
Garnett S, Hayen A, Peat JK. The art and science of regression modelling; methods for building valid models to explore hormone and body composition interactions. Ped Endocrinol Rev 2005;3:40–44. (See p. 102.)

The reprint by Garnett *et al.* (2005) discusses the assumptions of regression models and explores how spurious associations can be generated through unsound modelling techniques.

After reading the reprint answer the following questions:
1 What are the two major uses of regression models in health research?

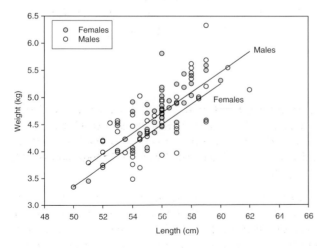

Figure 7.5 Regression lines of best fit shown for male and female babies.

Table 7.1 Predicted FVC and per cent predicted FVC

Height (m)	Age (years)	Gender	Measured FVC (L)	Predicted FVC (L)	Per cent predicted FVC
1.50	20	Female	3.8	3.19	119.0%
1.74	20	Female	3.8		
1.50	60	Female	3.8		
1.74	60	Female	3.8		
1.58	20	Male	3.8		
1.82	20	Male	3.8		
1.58	60	Male	3.8		
1.82	60	Male	3.8		

2 What criteria need to be met in order to compare correlation coefficients with one another?

3 If regression assumptions are violated, what influence does this have on the model?

4 If two explanatory variables are highly related to one another, what is the effect when they are both included in the model?

Worked example

The equations for predicting normal values for adult lung volume measured as forced vital capacity (FVC) were reported by Belousova *et al.* in 1997.[7] The values were derived from a large random sample of adults aged between 18 and 73 years. In the paper, the multiple regression equation for predicting FVC with rounding to two decimal places is:

$$FVC = 1.70 + (0.62 \times Height^3)$$
$$- (0.03 \times Age) + (0.59 \times Male)$$

In this equation, FVC is expressed in units of litres, height in units of metres, age in units of years, and 'male' is a binary variable coded as 1 = male and 0 = female. The R^2 value for the model is moderately high at 0.76 and all variables are significant predictors with $P < 0.0001$.

Using this regression equation, calculate predicted values for FVC for adults with the height, age and gender characteristics shown in Table 7.1. Also, calculate the per cent predicted FVC for each value, assuming that the measured FVC for each line was 3.8 L. Per cent predicted values are calculated as:

Per cent predicted value = (Measured value/Predicted value) × 100

After calculating FVC values, answer the following questions:
- How would you interpret the coefficient for the binary variable 'gender'?
- Are your calculations of predicted FVC in accordance with the signs and sizes of the regression coefficients?

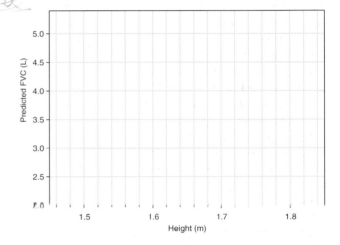

Figure 7.6 Regression lines for predicted FVC values for male and female.

- What do the estimates of per cent predicted FVC indicate?
- What clinical importance would you attach to these estimates of per cent predicted FVC?

Plot the separate regression lines for male age 20, male age 60, female age 20 and female age 60 in Figure 7.6.

Exercise

Campeotto F, Kapel N, Kalach N, Razafimahefa H, Castela F, Barbot F, Soulaines P, Dehan M, Gobert JG, Dupont C. Low levels of pancreatic elastase 1 in stools of preterm infants. Arch Dis Child Fetal Neonatal Ed 2002; 86:198–199. (See p. 107.)

Read the short report by Campeotto *et al.* (2002). In the report, the authors explore whether the amount of faecal pancreatic enzyme elastase 1 (E1), which is a marker of pancreatic function, is related to nutrient intake in pre-term and term babies. In the report, Figure 2 shows the relation of faecal E1 to four measures of nutrient intake.

The *r* values and their corresponding *P* values are shown in Figure 2.

- What populations can these results be generalised to?
- Can the *r* values be compared across the four figures to assess which measure of nutrient intake is the 'best' predictor of faecal E1?

  The line of best fit is also shown in Figure 2.
- Are the measurements displayed correctly on the *x*- and *y*-axis, that is, are the outcome and explanatory variables correctly classified?
- Are the lines of best fit that are shown on the figures valid assessments of the relationships given the presentation of the explanatory and outcome variable on the *x*- and *y*-axis?
- Do you think that each line meets the assumptions for using regression?

Critical appraisal

Work through this critical appraisal checklist to review the paper by Campeotto *et al.* (2002), and other papers that report regression models, to decide whether the results and the conclusions are valid and justified.

Quiz

Tick the correct answer for each of the following questions:

1 A correlation coefficient tells us:
  (a) the slope of the equation through the data;
  (b) how well one variable predicts another;
  (c) how closely two variables are linearly related;
  (d) whether the relationship is linear or non-linear.

Critical appraisal checklist for an article that reports correlation and/or regression analyses

A. Study design	
1. What is the design of the study?	
2. Was the sample selected randomly?	
3. Is the sample size adequate to justify the statistics used?	
B. Statistical methods	
4. Have the assumptions for correlation been met?	
5. Have the assumptions for regression been met?	
6. Are any repeated measures treated as independent observations?	
7. Are there any outliers that could influence the regression estimates?	
8. Has the model been tested for relationships between explanatory variables, normality of residuals and constant variance?	
C. Results	
9. Are the outcome and explanatory variables correctly classified?	
10. Have the explanatory variables been measured reliably?	
11. If a line of best fit is used, is the full regression equation reported?	
12. Are there sufficient data at the extremities of the model or should the prediction range be shortened?	
D. Interpretation	
13. Which patient or population group do the results generalise to?	
14. Have the results been interpreted appropriately?	
15. Are the conclusions valid?	

2 A correlation coefficient is a reliable estimate of association if:
(a) a large sample size has been enrolled;
(b) the sample is randomly selected from the population;
(c) extra cases are enrolled to ensure a wide range of y values;
(d) there is a positive association between two variables.

3 A regression model is more reliable if:
(a) it has been created using a statistical package;
(b) there is only one explanatory variable;
(c) one of the explanatory variables is a binary characteristic;
(d) the explanatory variables are not related to one another.

4 Normal or reference values show:
(a) the mean +1.96 standard deviations of a measurement in a population;
(b) the range of values for 95% of people without an illness;
(c) the range of values for all of the normal people in the population;
(d) the range in which 95% of values lie in a random population sample.

References

1. Cohen J. Statistical power analysis for the behavioral sciences (2nd ed.) Hillsdale, NJ: Lawrence Erlbaum Associates, 1988; pp 75–108.
2. Zou KH, Tuncali K, Silverman SG. Correlation and simple linear regression. Radiology 2003; 227:617–628.
3. Altman DG. Interpretation of correlation. In: Practical statistics for medical research. London: Chapman & Hall, 1991; pp 296–299.
4. Bland JM, Altman DG. Measurement error and correlation coefficients. BMJ 1996;313:41–42.
5. Bland JM. Regression and correlation. In: An introduction to medical statistics. Oxford: Oxford University Press, 1996; pp 180–504.
6. Altman DG. Reference intervals. In: Practical statistics for medical research. London: Chapman & Hall, 1996; pp 419–426.
7. Belousova EG, Haby MM, Xuan W, Peat JK. Factors that affect normal lung function in white Australian adults. Chest 1997;112: 1539–1546.

The Art and Science of Regression Modelling; Methods for Building Valid Models to Explore Hormone and Body Composition Interactions

Sarah P Garnett, BSc, M Nutr and Diet[1], *Andrew Hayen: BA (Hons), PhD, M Biostat*[2], *Jennifer Peat, BSc (Hons), PhD*[3]

Abstract

Multiple linear regression modelling is commonly used to investigate how hormones and body composition interact, but for valid interpretation a sound methodological approach must be used. It is particularly important that the assumptions for regression are met so that spurious associations are not generated. In this article we show how different approaches to building a multiple linear regression model can influence perceived associations, using examples from the literature and our own data related to predicting fasting insulin and leptin levels from total body fat and fat distribution in children.

Ref: Ped. Endocrinol. Rev. 2005;1:40–44

Key words: Regression modelling, Body composition, fat distribution, Insulin, leptin

Introduction

Multiple linear regression modelling, often referred to as multiple regression, is commonly used to investigate how hormones and body composition interact. However, perceived associations can be misleading if the regression model is invalid. The assumptions for regression models which must be met in order to avoid biased coefficients are shown in Table 1. If an assumption is violated, both the reliability and stability of the model may be influenced leading to inaccurate or biased results.

In this article, we outline the problems in interpretation that can occur if regression assumptions are not met. In our examples, from the literature and our own data, we show how invalid regression models can influence the prediction of fasting insulin and leptin levels from total body fat and fat distribution in children.

Purposes of multiple regression modelling

There are two principal uses of multiple regression models that affect the way a model is built and the variables that are

included. One use is for hypothesis testing in which the effect of an explanatory variable (or an exposure) on the outcome of interest is examined while adjusting for the effects of other known explanatory variables (or confounders). This type of model is used, for example, to explore the effect of physical activity on total body fat after adjusting for age and gender. With this type of model, it is important to specify before building the model and preferably before collecting the data, which variables will be considered for inclusion in the final regression model.

The second use of multiple regression is to predict the value of an outcome using a set of explanatory or predictive variables, for example to predict normal values for characteristics such as total body fat, fat free mass and bone mass. An ideal model enables accurate predictions to be made for a wide sector of the community but should be parsimonious, that is only contain variables that have an important statistical and theoretical role.

Model Building

Many strategies are used to build multiple regression models. Although automatic software facilities such as forward or backward stepwise regression are available, a more rigorous approach is to carefully build models using expert knowledge at each step. The best predictive variables are explanatory variables that have a high correlation with the outcome variable and a low correlation with other explanatory variables. Ordering explanatory variables by their strength of association (correlation coefficient) with the dependent variable is central to the art of building reliable predictive models. Associations can be obtained with a correlation matrix. Modelling should begin by

[1]Research Officer, Institute of Endocrinology and Diabetes, the Children's Hospital at Westmead, Australia

[2]Biostatistical Officer, Centre for Epidemiology and Research, NSW Department of Health, Australia

[3]Senior Statistician, Research and Development Office, The Children's Hospital at Westmead, Australia

Corresponding Author:
Sarah Garnett, Institute of Endocrinology and Diabetes, The Children's Hospital at Westmead, Locked Bag 4001, Westmead, NSW 2145, Australia, Telephone: +61 2 98453152, Fax: +61 2 98453170 (e-mail: sarahg@chw.edu.au)

Originally published in *PER*; 3: 40–44. Reproduced with permission.

Table 1 Regression assumptions that must be met for a model to be valid

Study design
1 The sample is representative of the population to which inference will be made
2 All important explanatory variables (confounders) and interactions between explanatory variables are included in the model
3 The data have been collected in a period when the relationship between the variables remains constant
4 The sample size is sufficient to support the model

Independence
5 All observations must be independent of each other
6 The explanatory variables should not be highly linearly related to one another, ie should not have a high degree of collinearity

Model building
7 The relation between the dependent variable and each explanatory variable is approximately linear
8 The residuals are normally distributed
9 The variance is constant over the length of the regression model (homoscedacity)
10 There are no multi-variate outliers that have an undue influence on the regression model

adding the predictor with the highest correlation coefficient (R value) first and noting the size of the regression coefficient, its standard error and the P value. Then other explanatory variables are added one at a time in order of their correlation. After the addition of each variable, it is important to inspect changes in each coefficient and its standard error. A coefficient that changes substantially or a standard error that inflates by more than 10% when another variable is added to the model is a sign of possible collinearity and an indication that one variable should be omitted from the model.

Multiple regression models are dynamic and the changes that occur when new variables are added provide important information. A final model in which all of the important predictors are included and in which all assumptions have been met has the highest validity for testing a hypothesis or providing a prediction equation.

Study Design
Assumptions 1–4 (Table 1) are determined by the study design. For multiple regression, the sample does not have to be selected randomly. However, the final prediction equation applies only to a group with the same characteristics as the study sample.

It is important to recognise that correlation coefficients cannot be compared between different multiple regression models when the sampling criteria are different or when the range of measurements in one data set is wider than in the other. Correlation coefficients are highly dependent on these factors in addition to the true relationship between the variables (1). For example, the correlation between two variables such as fat free mass and total body fat is higher at $R^2 = 0.57$ in children age 3 to 18 years than at $R^2 = 0.36$ in children age 7 to 8 years largely because the range of values is wider in the older age group and not because the relationship is different.

Sample Size
Sample size (assumption 4) is an important issue because a multivariate model with a small number of cases and

several explanatory variables will lack precision and will be unreliable. Imprecise estimates may have no sensible interpretation. While there is no clear consensus for estimating the minimum sample size, recommendations tend to range from 15 to 40 times the number of variables included in the model (2).

The larger the sample size, the more likely the model will generalise beyond the sample. With a very large sample size, variables that predict only a negligible amount of variance in the outcome variable may become statistically significant even though they may not be clinically important.

Independence
All observations must be independent of each other (assumption 5), so that the effect of one explanatory variable on the outcome variable is the same regardless of the values of the other explanatory variables in the model. Variables are said to interact if the effect of one explanatory variable on the outcome variable depends upon the level of the second variable. Interaction between two variables can be examined by creating a new variable which is their product and adding the variable in the model.

Collinearity, which is addressed in assumption 6, occurs when two explanatory variables are strongly and linearly related to one another. In practice, collinearity indicates that two variables are both measures of the same entity and therefore, the theory behind the model should be examined.

In published equations, it is common to find two variables that measure a similar entity have been included, for example total body fat and sum of skinfolds. In other models, two variables of which one is a component of the other, for example weight and total body fat, or total body fat and subcutaneous abdominal adipose tissue (SAAT), are included as explanatory variables. In these situations, collinearity is likely to distort the measurements of associations. Only one of the variables needs to be included and ideally, the variable to include should be the one that can be measured with least error and/or most easily depending on the situation.

When building a model, the extent of collinearity between variables can be assessed using the variance inflation factor (VIF). Most commonly used statistical packages, including SPSS, SAS and STATA, will calculate VIF. In regression models, the P values and confidence intervals are computed from an estimate of variance around the regression coefficients which is proportional to the VIF. The reliability of a regression coefficient decreases as the VIF increases. When the VIF is large, the regression coefficients, their variances and the P values will have no reliable interpretation. In extreme cases, the standard error will be significantly inflated and the direction of effect of the regression coefficient may change.

The magnitude of VIF that leads to an unreliable model depends on sample size and application. A VIF value above 2.0, which corresponds with a correlation coefficient above 0.7, should be a cause for concern and further investigation. However, smaller correlations can be problematic if the sample size is small or a large number of variables are included. Collinearity must be resolved in the model building process because, in published results, it is impossible to judge the extent to which the inclusion of collinear variables destabilises a model.

Interactions and Polynomials

Collinearity naturally arises when a quadratic term is included in a model, for example in a model such as $Y = a + b_1 X + b_2 X^2$ in which a variable that is the square of another variable is linearly related to it. However, subtracting a constant from the explanatory variable, reduces the collinearity between X and X^2. The constant that minimises collinearity is the mean of the explanatory variable and subtracting this value is called centering (2). Centering is crucial for removing collinearity when higher order terms are used to improve fit.

Linearity

In regression modelling, the relation between the dependent and explanatory variables should be linear (assumption 7). A dependent variable that is not normally distributed may also lead to violations of assumptions 8. The explanatory variables do not have to be normally distributed but the residuals of the model must be. Violations of assumption 7 may be overcome by transforming either the explanatory or dependent variable and violations of assumption 8 by transforming the dependent variable.

In medical research, often variables take only positive values and are right-skewed which may result in some multivariate outliers. For this type of data, logarithmic transformation can be helpful. This transformation also has the important property that it converts multiplicative relations into additive relations. However, when variables are logarithmically transformed, the regression coefficients must be interpreted in terms of the transformed variable, or the model can be back-transformed.

The concept of linearity between an outcome and explanatory variable also applies to any categorical variable such as Tanner staging of pubertal status, which is an ordered variable that is ranked from 1 to 5. If there is no linear trend across categories or if variables are used in which the categories are not ordered, for example ethnicity, then dummy variables need to be created in order to describe the effects accurately.

Regression Diagnostics

When a regression model meets assumptions 1 to 8 and stable estimates have been fitted, it is then important to check assumption 9 by examining whether the spread of the residuals is the same for all predicted scores. This can be done by plotting residuals against the explanatory variable. A plot that is funnel shaped can indicate that the dependent variable requires transformation or that there is an interaction with an unmeasured effect. If the problem cannot be easily resolved, a weighted least squares model that gives more weight to smaller residuals may be appropriate.

Finally, assumption 10 can be tested by using standard diagnostics. A high number of large standardised residuals, that is those greater than 2 in absolute value, should be a cause of concern. Another diagnostic is to examine points of leverage to detect any data points that have an undue influence on the fitted regression line. The leverage of points range from 1/n to 1, where n is the number of observations in the model. Values close to zero indicate that a value has little influence and values close to 1 indicate that the value may have a large influence on the model. Leverage values above 0.2 are problematic and leverage values above 0.5 may indicate an undue influence on the model.

Describing the Relation between Body Composition and Leptin Levels

Multiple regression has been used to explore associations between body composition and leptin levels. It has been reported that when leptin levels are adjusted for differences in body composition and body fat distribution, a sex difference is no longer apparent (3). The regression coefficients from this study are shown in Table 2. In the first model, the negative sign for fat free mass is in contrast to the positive relation shown in bi-variate analysis. Given that the variables fat free mass and total body fat are likely to be related, this indicates instability resulting from collinearity.

Although the final model contains six variables, the sample size was only 74 children. This could explain why sex, which is significant in smaller models, becomes non-significant in the final model. The instability of the final model would also be increased by the addition of two further variables, SAAT and intra-abdominal adipose tissue (IAAT), which are presumably related not only to one another but also to total body fat and fat free mass. When SAAT and IAAT are added the coefficient for total body fat changes from 1.26 to 0.98 (a 22% reduction) and the standard error inflates from 0.09 to 0.16 (a 77% increase), which indicates collinearity. Moreover, the sign of the coefficient for IAAT is reversed when compared with the bi-variate analyses, which indicated a strong, positive relation between IAAT and leptin level.

Originally published in *PER*; 3: 40–44. Reproduced with permission.

These changes in the regression coefficients and their standard errors should alert researchers to question the way in which the model can be interpreted.

It has also been reported that serum leptin and IGF-I do not have a significant effect on fasting insulin level after adjusting for other factors, including sex, anthropometry, total body fat and fat distribution (4). Again, this was a relatively small study with 61 children but 10 variables were included in the final model. The main conclusion that leptin and IGF-I levels, the final two variables added to a model containing sex, pubertal stage, height, weight, total body fat, muscle fat, IAAT and sum of skinfolds, were not significant predictors of fasting insulin level could well be a type II error because of small sample size. Unfortunately, no details of the coefficients, their signs or standard errors are reported to allow us to judge whether collinearity between variables may have been a cause of instability. Given the nature of the variables and the signs of their regression coefficients, which indicate a changed direction of effect, it is likely that the final model was destabilised.

Neither of these papers includes information that verifies the assumptions of regression modelling were met. Although both papers discuss possible interactions between variables as an explanation of effects, no formal interactive terms were included in either model. It seems more likely that collinearity and instability rather than interactions will have influenced the perceived relation between the variables.

Effects of Removing Collinear Terms

We used data from 60 children randomly selected from a larger sample [Garnett unpublished data] to explore how sample size and collinearity may have produced the problems discussed above. Regression coefficients for predicting fasting insulin level are shown in Table 3. Fasting insulin level was logarithmically transformed to meet the assumptions of normality. The columns on the left hand side of the table show the regression coefficients that would be reported from univariate analysis and the columns on the right hand side show the coefficients for the same variables after they have all been entered into the model. The changes in signs from the univariate analysis to the model, the inflation of standard errors, the radically different P values and large VIF values in the final model show clear collinearity. We could not conclude that after taking sex, height and weight into consideration, no other variable reliably increased the prediction of fasting insulin.

If we wanted to test the hypothesis that there was a relation between fasting insulin, total body fat, abdominal fat, leptin and IGF-I levels, then weight and sum of skinfolds would not be included in the same model because both are surrogate measures of total body fat. If good model building strategies

Table 2 Multiple linear regression to predict leptin (3)

Independent variable	Beta[a]	SE (beta)	Model R square	P value
Model 1				
Sex	0.10	0.04	0.81	0.02
Ethnicity	−0.04	0.04		0.33
Total body fat (kg)	1.26	0.09		<0.001
Fat free mass (kg)	−0.74	0.26		<0.01
Final Model				
Sex	0.06	0.04	0.84	0.12
Ethnicity	−0.001	0.04		0.99
Total body fat (kg)	0.98	0.16		<0.001
Fat free mass (kg)	−0.75	0.25		<0.01
SAAT (cm²)	0.37	0.12		<0.01
IAAT (cm²)	−0.22	0.14		0.12

[a] Beta: correlation coefficient.

Table 3 Univariate analysis and regression for predicting insulin level (logarithmically transformed)

	Univariate analysis			Model: all variables entered			
	Beta[a]	SE	P	Beta[a]	SE	P	VIF
Sex	0.23	0.14	0.10	−0.09	0.14	0.52	1.3
Height (cm)	0.04	0.01	<0.001	0.04	0.02	0.04	3.7
Weight (kg)	0.05	0.01	<0.001	−0.01	0.04	0.81	14.1
Fat mass (kg)	0.07	0.02	<0.001	−0.08	0.08	0.33	23.1
Abdominal fat (kg)	0.10	0.02	<0.001	0.45	1.0	0.66	20.7
Sum skinfolds (cm)	0.007	0.002	<0.001	0.04	0.04	0.35	7.6
IGF-I	0.03	0.01	0.007	0.002	0.01	0.82	1.5
Leptin	0.09	0.02	<0.001	0.07	0.04	0.12	4.9

[a] Beta: correlation coefficient.

Originally published in *PER*; 3: 40–44. Reproduced with permission.

are used, the best predictive equation for insulin level from our data would include only leptin and height. Both variables have positive beta coefficients that are consistent with univariate analyses and together the two variables explain 35% of the variation in fasting insulin level. Other variables including total body fat, abdominal fat and IGF-I levels were excluded on the basis of their non-significant P values.

Recommendations

For a sound understanding of how hormones and body composition interact, it is important that data are analysed carefully. Researchers often invest large resources in conducting invasive tests of children. In such situations, it is especially important that multiple regression models are built with great care and that all of the assumptions are met in order to prevent errors that lead to misconceptions in understanding. In small, multivariate models with instability and collinearity, neither the directions of effect of the coefficients or the size of the P values have a logical interpretation. Science is a search for the truth and until a rigorous approach to building multivariate models becomes standard practice, it is unlikely that we will come to understand the true relationship between hormones and body composition in children.

References

1 Bland JM and Altman DG. Measurement error and correlation coefficients. BMJ 1996;313:41–42.
2 Kleinbaum DJ, Kupper LL, Muller KE, Nizam A. Applied regression analysis and other multivariable methods. Duxbury Press., 1998.
3 Nagy TR, Gower BA, Trowbridge CA, Dezenberg C, Shewchuk RM, Goran MI. Effects of gender, ethnicity, body composition, and fat distribution on serum leptin concentrations in children. J Clin Endo Met 1997;82:2148–2152.
4 Roemmich JN, Clark PA, Lusk M, Friel A, Weltman A, Epstein LH, Rogol AD. Pubertal alterations in growth and body composition. VI. Pubertal insulin resistance: relation to adiposity, body fat distribution and hormone release. Int J Obes 2002; 26: 701–709.

Originally published in *PER*; 3: 40–44. Reproduced with permission.

Low levels of pancreatic elastase 1 in stools of preterm infants

F Campeotto, N Kapel, N Kalach, H Razafimahefa, F Castela, L Barbot, P Soulaines, M Dehan, J G Gobert, C Dupont

The amount of faecal pancreatic enzyme elastase 1 was significantly lower in 42 preterm newborns than in 12 full term babies at day 2 (89 (3–539) *v* 354 (52–600) µg/g, p<0.0007) and day 5 (164 (3–600) *v* 600 (158–600) µg/g, p<0.05) and correlated positively with total nutrient intake during the first week of life in preterm infants. This should probably be taken into account during early feeding.

Pancreatic elastase 1 (E1) is considered to be a highly sensitive and specific marker for exocrine pancreatic function, allowing the diagnosis of pancreatic insufficiency at all ages.[1] After two weeks of life, whatever the gestational age, 96.8% of infants without pancreatic disorders exhibit faecal E1 levels comparable to those of adults.[2] A preliminary study suggested decreased faecal E1 levels in infants below 2 weeks of age,[3] and this prospective study measured faecal E1 in preterm and full term newborn infants during the first week of life.

Methods and results

A bicentric prospective study enrolled 42 preterm infants (18 girls and 24 boys) born at 28 weeks gestation (median, range 25–35 weeks) and weighing 1140 g (range 640–1890), including 13 extreme premature infants (<28 weeks gestation). Controls were 12 full term infants (eight girls and four boys) born at term (38–41 weeks) and weighing 3455 g (range 2840–4160).

For each child, one to three stool samples (about 5 g) were obtained during the first two weeks of life and stored at −20°C before analysis. The first sample was obtained between days 0 and 7 (median 2), the second between days 3 and 9 (median 5), and the third between days 7 and 11 (median 9). Owing to monitoring difficulties, two stool samples were collected for 29 of the 42 premature infants and three for the remaining 12. Three stool samples were not collected for any of the term infants, as they were discharged at 5 days of age.

Pancreatic E1 levels were determined using a "sandwich" type enzyme immunoassay (Schebo-Biotech, Guiessen, Germany), using two monoclonal antibodies binding to two distinct epitopes specific to human pancreatic E1. Results were expressed as µg/g of stool; 200 µg/g was the lower normal limit.[1] All quantitative results are given as median (range).

Statistical comparisons were performed using the non-parametric Mann-Whitney U test. Single regression analysis was used to calculate correlation coefficients for parametric data.

In all newborns, faecal E1 levels increased significantly (p<0.0001) from the first to the third sample: 113 (3–600), 242 (3–600), and 459 (559–600) µg/g respectively. E1 levels were significantly lower in preterm infants than in full term infants at day 2 (89 (3–539) *v* 354 (52–600) µg/g, p<0.0007) and day 5 (164 (3–600) *v* 600 (158–600) µg/g, p<0.05) (fig 1). No difference was found between extremely premature (74 (3–228) µg/g) and premature infants (102 (3–539) µg/g) (p = 0.58), within the first week of life. All preterm infants displayed normal E1 levels from the second week onwards.

F Campeotto, N Kalach, F Castela, P Soulaines, C Dupont, Service de Néonatologie, Hôpital Cochin-Saint Vincent de Paul, 82 Avenue Denfert Rochereau, 75674 Paris Cedex 14, France and Université René Descartes, Paris V, France

N Kapel, L Barbot, J G Gobert, Service de Coprologie Fonctionnelle, Groupe Hospitalier Pitié-Salpetrière, 47 Boulevard de l'Hôpital, 75651 Paris Cedex 13, France

H Razafimahefa, M Dehan, Service de Réanimation Néonatale, Hôpital Antoine Béclère, 157 rue de la Porte-de-Trivaux, 92141 Clamart, France

Correspondence to: Dr Campeotto, Service de Néonatologie, Hôpital Saint Vincent de Paul, 82 Avenue Denfert Rochereau, 75674 Paris cedex 14, France (email: florence.campeotto@noos.fr)

(*Accepted 11 December 2001*)

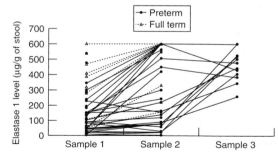

Figure 1 Pancreatic elastase (E1) levels in the two groups of newborn infants. Samples 1, 2, and 3 were collected on median day 2, median day 5, and median day 9 respectively. Reference concentrations for pancreatic E1 in adult stools are: normal, ≥200 µg/g; moderate to light exocrine pancreatic insufficiency, 100 to < 200 µg/g; severe pancreatic insufficiency, ≤100 µg/g.

Originally published in *Arch Dis Child Fetal Neonatal Ed* 2002; **86**: 198–99. Reproduced with permission.

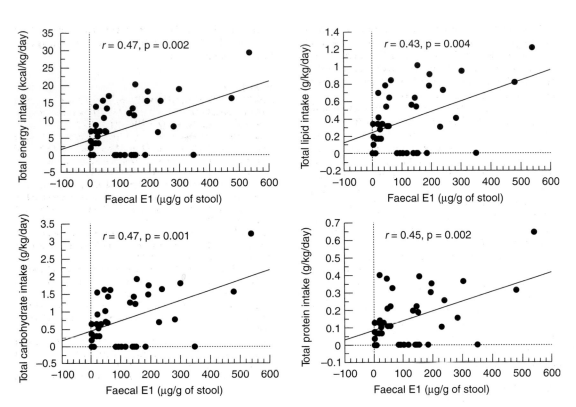

Figure 2 Correlation between faecal elastase 1 (E1) level and nutritional intake in preterm infants in the first sample.

Considering all infants, a positive correlation was observed between E1 levels and gestational age in both first week samples: $r = 0.5$, $p = 0.0001$ and $r = 0.3$, $p = 0.03$. A positive correlation was also observed between E1 levels in the first sample and birth weight: $r = 0.5$, $p = 0.0001$.

In preterms, a positive correlation was observed between E1 levels in the first sample and total energy ($r = 0.47$, $p = 0.002$), lipid ($r = 0.43$, $p = 0.004$), protein ($r = 0.45$, $p = 0.002$), and carbohydrate ($r = 0.47$, $p = 0.001$) intake (fig 2).

No correlation was found between faecal E1 and any of the other clinical parameters of the studied population: sex, maternal treatment with steroids, maternal blood hypertension, acute fetal distress, infection, respiratory distress, intrauterine growth retardation, necrotising enterocolitis, treatment, the day of stool sampling (table 1).

Discussion

Preterm infants have low levels of faecal E1 during the first week of life, whereas full term infants do not, suggesting exocrine pancreatic immaturity in the former. The beneficial effect of early enteral feeding on pancreatic exocrine function is supported by the correlation between faecal E1 increase and nutrient intake.

Table 1 Clinical features of the 42 preterm infants

	Preterm infants
Sex (F:M)	18:24
Gestational age (weeks)	28 (25–35)*
Birth weight (g)	1140 (640–1890)*
Maternal steroids	33 (78%)
Maternal hypertension	11 (26%)
Acute fetal distress	12 (28%)
Infection	8 (19%)
Respiratory distress	39 (93%)
Intrauterine growth retardation	7 (17%)
Necrotising enterocolitis	1 (2.4%)
Steroids	17 (40%)
Sedation	24 (57%)
Inotropes	5 (12%)
Volume expansion	9 (21%)
Insulin	2 (5%)
Feeding	29 (70%)

* Values are median (range).

Originally published in *Arch Dis Child Fetal Neonatal Ed* 2002; **86**: 198–99. Reproduced with permission.

Considerable variations in faecal E1 between stool samples and from day to day have been described by Hamwi *et al.*[4] The first sample was obtained close to birth, according to the availability of stools during this period of intensive care. This collection may have involved either stool or meconium, which is known to contain low E1 levels.[2,5]

More than half (52%) of preterm infants still had low pancreatic E1 (<200 µg/g of stool) at the end of the first week, independent of gestational age. Maturation occurs in preterm infants as well as in full term babies after the first week of life, as described by Terbrack *et al*[5] and Von Seebach and Henker[2]: after one week of life, 97.4% of term infants (but only 85% of preterm babies) had reached adult levels of E1 of > 200 µg/g faeces. After the first week of life, E1 concentrations remained within the normal adult range. The levels observed during the first week of life remained above values currently observed in cystic fibrosis (<50 µg/g of stool).[6]

The positive correlation between energy and nutrient intakes during the first week of life in preterm infants supports "minimal enteral feeding" as a strategy for accelerating the maturation of gastrointestinal function.[7] Digestion of nutrients in preterm infants may not be optimal in the first week of life, despite increased needs. Therefore, the trend to sustain "early aggressive enteral feeding"[8] has probably to be dealt with taking into account pancreatic immaturity: an adaptation of nutrients during the first week seems desirable.

Conclusion

A pancreatic maturation deficit exists in the first week of life in preterm infants, depending on gestational age. E1 levels normalise within the first days, more rapidly with enteral nutrition. This should be taken into account during early feeding of preterm infants.

References

1 Soldan W, Henker J, Sprossig C. Sensitivity and specificity of quantitative determination of pancreatic elastase 1 in feces of children. *J Pediatr Gastroenterol Nutr* 1997;24:53–5.

2 Von Seebach K, Henker J. Pancreatic Elastase 1 in feces of preterm and term born infants up to 12 months without insufficiancy of exocrine pancreatic function [abstract]. *21st European Cystic Fibrosis Conference, Davos (Switzerland), June 1–6, 1997.*

3 Campeotto F, Kapel N, Kalach N, *et al.* Evaluation de la fonction pancréatique exocrine du nouveau-né à terme et du prématuré au cours de la première semaine de vie par le dosage de l'élastase 1 fécale. *Arch Pediatr* 2001;8:445–6.

4 Hamwi A, Veitl M, Maenner G, *et al.* Pancreatic elastase 1 in stool: variations within one stool passage and individual changes from day to day. *Wien Klin Wochenschr* 2000;112:32–5.

5 Terbrack HG, Gurtler KH, Klor HU, *et al.* Human pancreatic elastase 1 concentrations in faeces of healthy children and children with cystic fibrosis. *Gut* 1995;37:(suppl 2):A253.

6 Walkowiak J. Faecal elastase-1: clinical value in the assessment of exocrine pancreatic function in children. *Eur J Pediatr* 2000;159: 869–70.

7 Burrin DG, Stoll B, Jiang R, *et al.* Minimal enteral nutrient requirements for intestinal growth in neonatal piglets: how much is enough? *Am J Clin Nutr* 2000;71:1603–10.

8 Thureen PJ. Early aggressive nutrition in the neonate. *Pediatrics in Review* 1999;20:e45–55.

Originally published in *Arch Dis Child Fetal Neonatal Ed* 2002; **86**: 198–99. Reproduced with permission.

Follow-up studies

Aims

To understand how to make within-subject and between-group comparisons of outcome measurements which have been collected from participants at baseline and at the end of a study.

Learning objectives

On completion of this unit, participants will be able to understand how to analyse data from clinical trials and longitudinal studies, and:

- identify the situations in which an independent samples *t*-test or a paired *t*-test is used;
- explain the consequences of excessive drop-out rates;
- interpret analyses in which adjustments are made for unbalanced baseline characteristics;
- understand why different P values are obtained for the same data set when different types of analyses are used.

Background

Follow-up studies are used to find out what happens to a group of participants over a defined period of time. These studies may be observational, such as cohort, prospective or longitudinal studies, or experimental, such as randomised controlled trials or cross-over trials. In such studies, measurements are taken from participants at baseline and at a later date to assess the significance of any changes that have occurred over time.

In this Unit, we refer to the outcome measurement at the end of a study as a 'follow-up score', and the within-participant difference between baseline and follow-up measures as a 'change score'. The analyses described in this Unit apply to continuously distributed measurements only, but the same principles can be applied to the analysis of categorical data. For categorical data, chi-square tests can be used for independent between-group comparisons,

as discussed in Unit 3, and a paired categorical analysis called McNemar's test can be used when the outcome measurement is binary.

Glossary

Term	Definition
Observational study	A study which is conducted to measure rates of disease in a population or to measure associations between exposures (risk factors) and disease.
Experimental study	A study which is conducted to test the effect of a treatment or intervention.
Randomised controlled trial	A study which is conducted to measure whether a new treatment is superior or equivalent to no treatment or an existing treatment, and in which participants are randomly allocated to the study groups.
Cross-over trial	A study in which participants receive two or more treatments given consecutively, usually in a random order. The response to the first treatment can be contrasted with the response to the second treatment in the same participants.
Paired *t*-test	A test to measure whether the means of two related continuous measurements are different from one other, typically measurements taken from the same participants on two occasions.

Follow-up studies with no between-group comparison

In studies without a between-group comparison, a paired *t*-test is used to estimate whether the baseline and follow-up measurements, which are expected to be related because they are collected from the same participant, are significantly different from one another. Paired *t*-tests are used in observational cohort studies and in experimental cross-over trials in which participants are randomised to receive active and control treatments in random order. In cohort studies, the outcome of interest is how much change occurs in the study group over time. In cross-over trials, the outcome of interest is whether the participants improve more when taking the experimental treatment than when taking the control treatment. In both types of studies, we are interested in the mean within-subject difference, unlike comparisons of independent samples (see Unit 6) in which we are interested in the mean between-group difference. In critically appraising the literature, it is important to identify what the term 'mean difference' actually describes.

In follow-up studies in which no comparison is being made between two groups, the outcome of interest is whether participants change significantly over time. In such studies, patients form their own control group. Thus, the mean within-subject difference between the baseline and follow-up measurements, that is, the mean change score, is the summary statistic of interest. For this, a paired t-test is the appropriate statistic to use.

When using a paired t-test, the within-subject variation for the participants is of most interest and the between-subject variation, which is considered when using an independent samples t-test, is of little interest. In effect, a paired t-test is used to assess whether the mean change score between the two related measurements is significantly different from zero – the value that indicates no change. The assumption for using a paired t-test is that the differences between the pairs of measurements (the change scores) rather than the measurements themselves are normally distributed. This assumption should be tested using a histogram or other summary statistics before the t-test is performed.

Paired t-tests are used in cross-over trials in which the outcome of interest is within-participant improvement for the new treatment period compared to the control or standard treatment period. For example, a paired t-test was used in a cross-over trial in which 48 people with chronic obstructive pulmonary disease were enrolled to test the efficacy of sustained release morphine compared to placebo for treating symptoms of dyspnoea (breathlessness).[1] During the study, the participants made twice daily ratings of their dyspnoea severity on a visual analogue scale, with the range of scores from zero (no breathlessness) to 100 (worst possible breathlessness). The design of the study involved participants receiving four days of the treatment and also four days of the placebo, the order of which was randomised. The authors report that a washout period (a period when the treatment is withdrawn so that any effects of the treatment are no longer present) between treatment arms was not required because a steady treatment state was reached in each arm by 60 hours. Thus, the authors made an *a priori* decision to compare follow-up scores at the end of each treatment period rather than change scores between the beginning and end of each treatment period. This method is recommended as an alternative to using a washout period to reduce the carry

Table 8.1 Effect of morphine versus placebo on ratings of dyspnoea at the end of each treatment period in 38 participants with chronic obstructive pulmonary disease

	Morphine mean (SD)	Placebo mean (SD)	Mean difference (95% CI)	P value
Morning	40.1 (24)	46.7 (26)	6.6 (1.6, 11.6)	0.011
Evening	40.3 (23)	49.8 (24)	9.5 (3.0, 16.1)	0.006

over effect, that is, the effect of the first treatment carrying over into the second treatment period.[2] To evaluate treatment effects, paired t-tests were used in an intention to treat analysis to evaluate between-treatment differences for each of the morning and evening dyspnoea scores. A summary of the study results with corrected mean values are shown in Table 8.1.

In both time periods, the mean follow-up dyspnoea score when participants were receiving morphine was approximately 7–9 points lower than when participants were receiving the placebo treatment. The mean change score was 6.6 for the morning period and 9.5 for the evening period. The P values shown in Table 8.1 are derived from paired t-tests. Both differences were statistically significant and this is reflected by the 95% confidence intervals around the mean differences which do not cross the value of zero. Thus, both the P values and confidence intervals indicate a difference between treatment phases, that is, that morphine was more effective than the placebo for reducing breathlessness.

Independent sample t-tests cannot be used for analysing paired data such as this, because the assumption that the observations are independent would be violated. In addition, treating paired measurements as independent samples would artificially inflate the sample size and lead to an inaccurate estimate of P values. In Table 8.1, the effective sample size is the number of participants, that is $N = 38$, and not the number of outcome measurements, that is $N = 76$, because the outcome in each participant was measured twice.

Although paired t-tests are an effective way to analyse follow-up data, drop-outs can be a major problem because participants with missing values cannot be included in the analysis. In practice, missing data reduce both the study power and the generalisability of results, and therefore it is important to have methods in place to ensure that drop-out rates are minimised in clinical trials and observational follow-up studies.

Follow-up studies with a between-group comparison

In many longitudinal studies we are interested in how much one group changes compared to another group. Randomised controlled trials are often longitudinal in nature in that

Table 8.2 Baseline and follow-up measures of enjoyment in a randomised controlled trial in 41 overweight primary school children

Time	Group	Mean (SD)	Mean difference (95% CI)	t value	P value
Baseline	Control	47.2 (11.1)	—	—	—
	Intervention	48.3 (11.7)			
Follow-up	Control	49.6 (10.4)	5.1 (−0.9, 11.2)	1.69	0.10
	Intervention	54.7 (8.9)			

both baseline and follow-up outcome measurements are collected from participants allocated to either an intervention or control treatment. In this type of study, we are interested in whether participants in the intervention group do better than participants in the control group after a set period of time. For this, an independent samples t-test can be used to assess the significance of the between-group difference in mean follow-up scores at the end of the trial. Alternatively, follow-up scores can be compared using regression to adjust for baseline values. Another method to take account of the longitudinal nature of the data is to calculate change scores (the difference between baseline and follow-up scores) and use an independent samples t-test to assess whether the within-subject change over time is significantly different between the two groups.

In studies with a follow-up component, the between-group comparison can be assessed in three different ways. Below, we use an example of a randomised controlled trial in which a control and an intervention group was enrolled to show how the three different methods can be applied. However, the principles can be extended to observational studies or to studies in which three or more groups are compared.

TAKE HOME LIST

The three different methods to analyse data from studies in which follow-up measurements are collected and a between-group comparison is being made are:

- to compare the mean follow-up scores between groups;

- to compare the mean change scores between groups;

- to compare the follow-up scores between groups after adjusting for baseline scores.

Comparing follow-up scores

The simplest type of analysis is to compare the mean follow-up scores between groups. For example, in an unpublished randomised controlled trial, overweight primary school children were randomised to a control group who received a walking programme ($N = 21$) or to an intervention group who received an active skills teaching programme ($N = 20$). Both groups received their programme twice weekly for a period of eight weeks. The aim of the trial was to measure

whether enjoyment of exercise could be improved with taught sporting skills. Thus, the primary outcome measurement was enjoyment of exercise as measured using a standardised questionnaire at baseline and at follow-up, which was three months later. The possible range of the scores was from zero (no enjoyment) to eighty (total enjoyment).

Table 8.2 shows the mean baseline and follow-up enjoyment scores. The intervention group had a mean enjoyment score that was 1.1 points higher than the control group at baseline. This type of baseline imbalance is more common in trials with a small number of participants in each group than in larger trials in which chance tends to balance groups more evenly.

Because the participants were randomised to their study group, it does not make sense to use a statistical test to assess whether the baseline enjoyment scores are different between the groups. Running this type of statistical test would equate to testing a null hypothesis that there is no difference in baseline characteristics between groups, and would merely be testing whether the randomisation procedure was effective.[3] However, the hypothesis that there is no difference between the groups at follow-up can be tested using an independent samples t-test. Table 8.2 shows that the active intervention group had a mean follow-up score which was, on average, 5.1 points higher than in the control group, with a 95% confidence interval of −0.9 to 11.2 points. This confidence interval just crosses the zero line as shown in the bottom plot of Figure 8.1. The P value is low but is not significant at 0.10.

Comparing change scores

A second way to analyse the data from this trial would be to compare change scores, that is, the difference between follow-up and baseline measurements in each participant. Again, these scores can be compared using an independent samples t-test as shown in Table 8.3.

Table 8.3 shows that enjoyment increased from baseline to follow-up in both groups as indicated by a positive mean change score. Enjoyment increased by an average of 2.4 points in the control group and 6.4 points in the intervention group. The mean between-group difference shows that the change scores increased, on average, by 4.0 points more in the intervention group than in the control group with a 95% confidence interval of −1.4 to 9.4. As shown in Figure 8.1, this confidence interval crosses the zero line of no difference to a slightly greater extent than the confidence

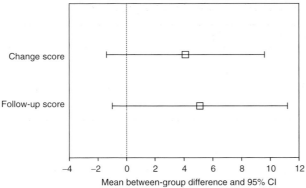

Figure 8.1 Mean within-group differences in enjoyment scores.

Table 8.3 Mean change scores and mean within-subject difference in enjoyment in a randomised controlled trial in overweight primary school children

Control group Mean (SD)	Intervention group Mean (SD)	Mean difference (95% CI)	P value
2.4 (7.7)	6.4 (9.6)	4.0 (−1.4, 9.4)	0.14

interval for the follow-up scores. As a result the *P* value is higher, and slightly less significant, with a value of 0.14.

It is problematic when two different statistical tests from the same data provide different estimates of effect and different *P* values. The difference in *P* values between the analyses occurs because of the difference in baseline scores between the two groups.[4]

If baseline scores are lower in the control group, as they are in Table 8.2, comparing follow-up scores may lead to an under-estimation of the treatment effect.[4] In practice, participants who have extremely low or high scores will have less extreme scores the next time they are measured. Therefore, the mean of these participants at follow-up will be reduced. This is known as regression to the mean and is a statistical occurrence.[5] Regression to the mean occurs because the first and second measurement will not be perfectly correlated.[5] If baseline scores are lower in the control group and regression to the mean occurs, both the mean follow-up and change scores between the groups will seem more alike and the treatment effect will be under-estimated compared to when the baseline scores are balanced.

In general, less variability in each group decreases the standard deviation and increases the effect size between groups for the same mean difference and conversely, more variability in each group increases the standard deviation and decreases the effect size. If the correlation between the baseline and follow-up scores is low, say less than 0.4, the change score will have more variability than the follow-up score and the *P* value is less likely to be statistically significant than if the follow-up score is used. On the other

hand, if the correlation between baseline and follow-up scores is high, say over 0.80, then the change score will reduce variability and the *P* value is more likely to be significant than if the follow-up score is used.[4] For the results shown in Tables 8.2 and 8.3, the correlation between baseline and follow-up scores was moderate at 0.7 and therefore the significance for the between-group differences in follow up and change scores was similar at *P* = 0.10 and 0.14 respectively, with neither being statistically significant.

Adjusting for baseline differences

The third method of analysing the data is to adjust for baseline differences using a regression model. In a randomised controlled trial, baseline differences are a bias that has occurred by chance. By using regression, the effect of the baseline differences can be minimised. However, the decision of whether to adjust for baseline differences in the analyses needs to be made before the data are analysed. Neither hypothesis testing nor visually inspecting the baseline statistics after the study is completed is a good method to decide whether to use regression. Ideally, a decision about the method of data analysis should be made before the study is conducted. In making decisions about what factors to adjust for, baseline values that might have prognostic value should be identified on the basis of available evidence from other sources at the beginning of the study or while the study is in progress.[6] Once decided *a priori*, regression can then be used to remove the influence of the baseline imbalance on the study result.

In Figure 8.2, follow-up enjoyment scores from the example are plotted against the baseline scores and the line of identity. The figure shows that all of the children with a baseline score of less than approximately 44 improved in that their follow-up score is above the line of identity.

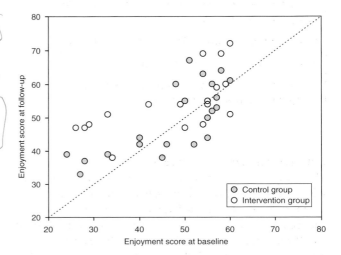

Figure 8.2 Follow-up scores for enjoyment plotted against baseline scores and shown with the line of identity.

On the other hand, in children who had a baseline score above 44, approximately 50% improved their score and 50% decreased their score –although the improvements are generally larger than the decreases.

The method of using regression to adjust for a continuous explanatory variable, in this case baseline score, and to test for a group difference, was discussed in Unit 7. In this analysis, the follow-up score is the outcome and the baseline score and the group are the explanatory variables. This method is also called analysis of covariance (ANCOVA) – the mathematics of ANCOVA and of regression, with one continuous explanatory variable and one binary group variable, are identical. By using regression, the follow-up scores of participants are adjusted for their baseline score and then an independent *t*-test is conducted to assess whether there is a significant between-group difference in the adjusted follow-up score. This method has the advantage that if the correlation between the baseline and follow-up scores is less than 0.8, it maximises statistical power to show a treatment effect. However, as with all multivariate analyses, the model should be built carefully, especially if further covariates are added, and all of the assumptions for regression that were discussed in Unit 7 need to be met.

For the data shown in Figure 8.2, the regression equation is:

Enjoyment at follow-up
    = 22.7 + 0.7 × Enjoyment at baseline
    + 4.5 for intervention group

This indicates that, after adjusting for baseline differences, the intervention group had a follow-up score that was, on average, 4.5 units higher than the control group. The 95% confidence interval around this mean value is −0.1 to 9.1, which now only marginally crosses the zero line of no difference. Reflecting this, the *P* value is on the margin of significance at 0.05. This *P* value is more significant than the independent samples *t*-tests used to compare follow-up scores ($P = 0.10$) and change scores ($P = 0.14$) showing the additional statistical power that this method of analysis may provide.

When the regression lines are plotted against the line of identity as shown in Figure 8.3, they convey the finding that children in the intervention group have, on average, follow-up scores that are 4.5 units higher than children in the control group. The slopes of the lines also confirm the observation that children with lower baseline scores improved more than children with higher baseline scores. That is, regression to the mean has occurred and the size of improvement is larger for participants with lower baseline scores. The control group line crosses the line of identity at an enjoyment score of just over 50, showing no mean improvement above this score in this group. This type of figure is a nice way to convey the estimate of effect in graphical form and to demonstrate when regression to the mean occurs.

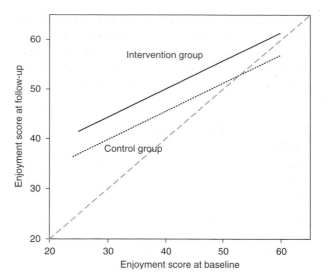

Figure 8.3 Regression lines for predicting enjoyment at follow-up compared against the line of identity.

Table 8.4 Results obtained using three different methods of data analysis for follow-up studies

Method	Mean difference	P value
1. Follow-up scores	5.1 (−0.9, 11.2)	0.10
2. Change scores	4.0 (−1.4, 9.4)	0.14
3. Regression	4.5 (−0.1, 9.1)	0.05

Comparison of methods

The mean difference between the groups and the *P* values obtained from the three different methods of analysis are summarised in Table 8.4. In essence, the three methods provide slightly different results because they are addressing slightly different questions.[7]

The first analysis with follow-up scores answers the question of whether the two groups are different at the end of the study, without adjusting for any initial differences at the beginning of the study. In both the second and third analyses, an adjustment for initial baseline scores is made. The second analysis with change scores answers the question of whether there is any difference between groups in the average change over the course of the study. The third analysis answers a slightly different question of whether there is any difference in the expected change between two groups who have the same baseline scores.

Obviously, framing the research question in a way that is congruent with the aims of the study is important and the most appropriate analysis should be decided when the study is designed, that is, *a priori*. The difference in *P* values results from the correlation between the baseline and follow-up scores and the number of people with higher or lower values in each group who may regress to the mean.

When there is a reasonable correlation between the baseline and follow-up scores, regression provides more statistical power to show a between-group difference. However, the scientific question of interest, and not issues of statistical precision, should be used to decide which type of analysis will be used.[7]

Reading and questions
Reprint
Vickers AJ, Altman DG. Analysing controlled trials with baseline and follow up measurements. BMJ 2001;323: 1123–1124. (See p. 118.)

The reprint by Vickers and Altman (2001) discusses some important issues in the analysis of follow-up data from randomised controlled trials. After reading the reprint answer the following questions:

1 If baseline and follow-up data are collected from an intervention and control group in a clinical trial, what statistics can be used to decide if the intervention was effective at follow-up?
2 In what situations are change scores poor at controlling for baseline imbalance?
3 If the follow-up measurement is highly correlated with the baseline measurement, how will the result of the t-test to compare follow-up scores be different from that of the t-test to compare change scores?
4 If there is a low correlation between the baseline measurement and the follow-up measurement, will the P value for the change scores be more significant or less significant than the P value for the follow-up scores and why?
5 If the mean baseline measurement in the intervention group is higher than in the control group, will the P value for the change scores be higher or lower than if the baseline measurements were balanced between groups?

Worked example
Set article
Fairbank J, Frost H, Wilson-MacDonald J, Yu L, Barker K, Collins R and for the Spine Stabilisation Trial Group.

Randomised controlled trial to compare surgical stabilisation of the lumbar spine with an intensive rehabilitation programme for patients with chronic low back pain: the MRC spine stabilisation trial. BMJ 2005;330. (See p. 120.)

In the set article, Fairbank et al. (2005) compare differences in the disability index and other indices of back pain in patients with chronic low back pain who underwent a surgical lumbar spine fusion ($N = 176$) or who attended an intensive rehabilitation programme ($N = 173$). At baseline and 24 months following the intervention, outcome data on the disability index, walking tests and quality of life were collected from patients. The primary and secondary study outcomes are shown in Table 4 in the set article.

In Table 4, the authors present mean follow-up scores, a mean change score and a P value based on analysis of covariance. The means and standard deviations of the follow-up scores for four outcomes are summarised in Table 8.5. If we wanted to interpret the data based on the follow-up scores, the means and their standard deviations can be used to calculate the mean between-group difference, effect size, 95% confidence interval, independent samples t value and P value. Using the formulas provided in Unit 6, complete Table 8.5, using the pooled standard deviation in the calculations.

After completing Table 8.5, answer the following questions:
• What does a negative effect size mean?
• Do the P values reflect the effect size between the groups?
• Do any of the P values suggest that a type II error has occurred?
• How do the P values that you have computed compare with the P values in Table 4 of Fairbank et al. (2005)? Can you explain why they are higher or lower?
• Do you agree with the authors' interpretation of their data?

Table 8.5 Mean outcome values at follow-up, effect size and mean difference

Outcome	Surgery group Mean (SD) ($n = 176$)	Rehabilitation group Mean (SD) ($n = 173$)	Effect size (SDs)	Mean difference (95% CI)	t-value	P value
Disability index	($n = 138$) 34.0 (21.1)	($n = 146$) 36.1 (20.6)	−0.1	−2.1 (−7.0, 2.8, 4.4)	0.85	0.40
Shuttle walk	($n = 118$) 352 (244)	($n = 126$) 310 (202)				
SF-36 physical	($n = 115$) 28.8 (14.9)	($n = 131$) 27.6 (14.6)				
SF-36 mental	47.4 (12.2)	48.1 (12.6)				

Critical appraisal checklist for an article that reports follow-up data	
A. Study design	
1. Is the follow-up rate sufficient to warrant making conclusions about long-term effects?	
2. If two groups are involved are the groups independent, that is, each person is in one group only?	
3. Are there sufficient participants to warrant using an independent samples *t*-test or a paired *t*-test?	
B. Statistical methods	
4. If a paired *t*-test is used, is there evidence that the change scores are normally distributed?	
5. Do the baseline data suggest that within-subject change scores need to be standardised for baseline differences?	
6. If the change scores are not normally distributed, has a non-parametric test been used?	
C. Results	
7. Is it clear whether the mean differences and 95% confidence intervals reported are within-subject or between-group estimates?	
8. Are mean within-subject change scores reported if a paired *t*-test is used?	
D. Interpretation	
9. Is the drop out rate low enough so that both the generalisability of results and the statistical power are maintained?	
10. Is there any evidence that the *P* values reported may be biased?	
11. If there is bias, is it likely that any differences within-subjects or between-groups have been under-estimated or over-estimated?	
12. Can any of the results be described as type I or type II errors?	

Critical appraisal

Work through the critical appraisal checklist to review the paper by Fairbank *et al.* (2005) and other reported follow-up studies to decide whether the results and the conclusions are valid and justified.

Quick quiz

Tick the correct answer for each of the following questions.

1 The mean within-subject difference is a term used to describe:
   (a) the mean change score in the participants;
   (b) the difference in mean values between the two study groups;
   (c) the mean of the difference in the outcome value between study groups;
   (d) the mean difference in follow-up scores.

2 A low correlation between baseline and follow-up scores indicates that an independent samples *t*-test using change scores is likely to be:
   (a) influenced by unequal variances;
   (b) more significant than for a test using follow-up scores;
   (c) less significant than for a test using follow-up scores;
   (d) an incorrect test to use.

3 A high correlation between baseline and follow-up scores indicates that an independent samples *t*-test using change scores is likely to be:
(a) biased;
(b) more significant than for a test using follow-up scores;
(c) less significant than for a test using follow-up scores;
(d) an incorrect test to use.

4 Regression to the mean indicates that participants outcome scores:
(a) can be predicted from a regression equation;
(b) are likely to get worse than expected;
(c) are likely to improve more than expected;
(d) are likely to change towards the mean value.

References

1. Abernethy AP, Currow DC, Frith P, Fazekas BS, McHugh A, Bui C. Randomised, double blind, placebo controlled crossover trial of sustained release morphine for the management of refractory dyspnoea. BMJ 2003;327:523–528.
2. Sibbald B, Roberts C. Understanding controlled trials: Crossover trials. BMJ 1998;316:1719–1720.
3. Altman DG, Dore CJ. Randomisation and baseline comparisons in clinical trials. Lancet 1990;335:149–153.
4. Vickers AJ, Altman DG. Analysing controlled trials with baseline and follow up measurements. BMJ 2001;323:1123–1124.
5. Bland JM, Altman DG. Regression towards the mean. BMJ 1994; 308:1499.
6. Roberts C, Torgerson DJ. Understanding controlled trials: Baseline imbalance in randomised controlled trials. BMJ 1999;319:185.
7. Fitzmaurice G. A conundrum in the analysis of change. Nutrition 2001;17:360–361.

Analysing controlled trials with baseline and follow up measurements

Andrew J Vickers, Douglas G Altman

In many randomised trials researchers measure a continuous variable at baseline and again as an outcome assessed at follow up. Baseline measurements are common in trials of chronic conditions where researchers want to see whether a treatment can reduce pre-existing levels of pain, anxiety, hypertension, and the like.

Statistical comparisons in such trials can be made in several ways. Comparison of follow up (post-treatment) scores will give a result such as "at the end of the trial, mean pain scores were 15 mm (95% confidence interval 10 to 20 mm) lower in the treatment group." Alternatively a change score can be calculated by subtracting the follow up score from the baseline score, leading to a statement such as "pain reductions were 20 mm (16 to 24 mm) greater on treatment than control." If the average baseline scores are the same in each group the estimated treatment effect will be the same using these two simple approaches. If the treatment is effective the statistical significance of the treatment effect by the two methods will depend on the correlation between baseline and follow up scores. If the correlation is low using the change score will add variation and the follow up score is more likely to show a significant result. Conversely, if the correlation is high using only the follow up score will lose information and the change score is more likely to be significant. It is incorrect, however, to choose whichever analysis gives a more significant finding. The method of analysis should be specified in the trial protocol.

Some use change scores to take account of chance imbalances at baseline between the treatment groups. However, analysing change does not control for baseline imbalance because of regression to the mean[1,2]: baseline values are negatively correlated with change because patients with low scores at baseline generally improve more than those with high scores. A better approach is to use analysis of covariance (ANCOVA), which, despite its name, is a regression

Integrative Medicine Service, Biostatistics Service, Memorial Sloan-Kettering Cancer Center, New York, New York 10021, USA

Andrew J Vickers *assistant attending research methodologist*

ICRF Medical Statistics Group, Centre for Statistics in Medicine, Institute of Health Sciences, Oxford OX3 7LF

Douglas G Altman *professor of statistics in medicine*

Correspondence to: Dr Vickers
(email: vickersa@mskcc.org)

method.[3] In effect two parallel straight lines (linear regression) are obtained relating outcome score to baseline score in each group. They can be summarised as a single regression equation:

follow up score = constant + a × baseline score + b × group

where a and b are estimated coefficients and group is a binary variable coded 1 for treatment and 0 for control. The coefficient b is the effect of interest—the estimated difference between the two treatment groups. In effect an analysis of covariance adjusts each patient's follow up score for his or her baseline score, but has the advantage of being unaffected by baseline differences. If, by chance, baseline scores are worse in the treatment group, the treatment effect will be underestimated by a follow up score analysis and overestimated by looking at change scores (because of regression to the mean). By contrast, analysis of covariance gives the same answer whether or not there is baseline imbalance.

As an illustration, Kleinhenz et al randomised 52 patients with shoulder pain to either true or sham acupuncture.[4] Patients were assessed before and after treatment using a 100 point rating scale of pain and function, with lower scores indicating poorer outcome. There was an imbalance between groups at baseline, with better scores in the acupuncture group (see table). Analysis of post-treatment scores is therefore biased. The authors analysed change scores, but as baseline and change scores are negatively correlated (about r = −0.25 within groups) this analysis underestimates the effect of acupuncture. From analysis of covariance we get:

follow up score = 24 + 0.71 × baseline score + 12.7 × group

(see figure). The coefficient for group (*b*) has a useful interpretation: it is the difference between the mean change scores of each group. In the above example it can be interpreted as "pain and function score improved by an estimated 12.7 points more on average in the treatment group than in the control group." A 95% confidence interval and P value can also be calculated for *b* (see table).[5] The regression equation provides a means of prediction: a patient with a baseline score of 50, for example, would be predicted to have a follow up score of 72.2 on treatment and 59.5 on control.

An additional advantage of analysis of covariance is that it generally has greater statistical power to detect a treatment effect than the other methods.[6] For example, a trial with a correlation between baseline and follow up scores of 0.6 that

Originally published in *BMJ* 2001; **323**: 1123–24. Reproduced with permission.

Results of trial of acupuncture for shoulder pain[4]

	Pain scores (mean and SD)		Difference between means (95% CI)	P value
	Placebo group (n = 27)	Acupuncture group (n = 25)		
Baseline	53.9 (14)	60.4 (12.3)	6.5	
Analysis				
Follow up	62.3 (17.9)	79.6 (17.1)	17.3 (7.5 to 27.1)	0.0008
Change score*	8.4 (14.6)	19.2 (16.1)	10.8 (2.3 to 19.4)	0.014
ANCOVA			12.7 (4.1 to 21.3)	0.005

*Analysis reported by authors.[4]

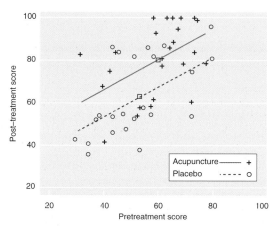

Pretreatment and post-treatment scores in each group showing fitted lines. Squares show mean values for the two groups. The estimated difference between the groups from analysis of covariance is the vertical distance between the two lines.

required 85 patients for analysis of follow up scores, would require 68 for a change score analysis but only 54 for analysis of covariance.

The efficiency gains of analysis of covariance compared with a change score are low when there is a high correlation (say r > 0.8) between baseline and follow up measurements. This will often be the case, particularly in stable chronic conditions such as obesity. In these situations, analysis of change scores can be a reasonable alternative, particularly if restricted randomisation is used to ensure baseline comparability between groups.[7] Analysis of covariance is the preferred general approach, however.

As with all analyses of continuous data, the use of analysis of covariance depends on some assumptions that need to be tested. In particular, data transformation, such as taking logarithms, may be indicated.[8] Lastly, analysis of covariance is a type of multiple regression and can be seen as a special type of adjusted analysis. The analysis can thus be expanded to include additional prognostic variables (not necessarily continuous), such as age and diagnostic group

We thank Dr J Kleinhenz for supplying the raw data from his study.

References

1 Bland JM, Altman DG. Regression towards the mean. *BMJ* 1994;308:1499.
2 Bland JM, Altman DG. Some examples of regression towards the mean. *BMJ* 1994;309:780.
3 Senn S. Baseline comparisons in randomized clinical trials. *Stat Med* 1991;10:1157–9.
4 Kleinhenz J, Streitberger K, Windeler J, Gussbacher A, Mavridis G, Martin E. Randomised clinical trial comparing the effects of acupuncture and a newly designed placebo needle in rotator cuff tendonitis. *Pain* 1999;83:235–41.
5 Altman DG, Gardner MJ. Regression and correlation. In: Altman DG, Machin D, Bryant TN, Gardner MJ, eds. *Statistics with confidence*. 2nd ed. London: BMJ Books, 2000:73–92.
6 Vickers AJ. The use of percentage change from baseline as an outcome in a controlled trial is statistically inefficient: a simulation study. *BMC Med Res Methodol* 2001;1:16.
7 Altman DG, Bland JM. How to randomise. *BMJ* 1999;319:703–4.
8 Bland JM, Altman DG. The use of transformation when comparing two means. *BMJ* 1996;312:1153.

Originally published in *BMJ* 2001; **323**: 1123–24. Reproduced with permission.

Randomised controlled trial to compare surgical stabilisation of the lumbar spine with an intensive rehabilitation programme for patients with chronic low back pain: the MRC spine stabilisation trial

Jeremy Fairbank, Helen Frost, James Wilson-MacDonald, Ly-Mee Yu, Karen Barker, Rory Collins for the Spine Stabilisation Trial Group

Abstract

Objectives   To assess the clinical effectiveness of surgical stabilisation (spinal fusion) compared with intensive rehabilitation for patients with chronic low back pain.

Design   Multicentre randomised controlled trial.

Setting   15 secondary care orthopaedic and rehabilitation centres across the United Kingdom.

Participants   349 participants aged 18–55 with chronic low back pain of at least one year's duration who were considered candidates for spinal fusion.

Intervention   Lumbar spine fusion or an intensive rehabilitation programme based on principles of cognitive behaviour therapy.

Main outcome measure   The primary outcomes were the Oswestry disability index and the shuttle walking test measured at baseline and two years after randomisation. The SF-36 instrument was used as a secondary outcome measure.

Results   176 participants were assigned to surgery and 173 to rehabilitation. 284 (81%) provided follow-up data at 24 months. The mean Oswestry disability index changed favourably from 46.5 (SD 14.6) to 34.0 (SD 21.1) in the surgery group and from 44.8 (SD14.8) to 36.1 (SD 20.6) in the rehabilitation group. The estimated mean difference between the groups was –4.1(95% confidence interval –8.1 to –0.1, P = 0.045) in favour of surgery. No significant differences between the treatment groups were observed in the shuttle walking test or any of the other outcome measures.

Conclusions   Both groups reported reductions in disability during two years of follow-up, possibly unrelated to the interventions. The statistical difference between treatment groups in one of the two primary outcome measures was marginal and only just reached the predefined minimal clinical difference, and the potential risk and additional cost of surgery also need to be considered. No clear evidence emerged that primary spinal fusion surgery was any more beneficial than intensive rehabilitation.

Introduction

Chronic low back pain is a common cause of distress and results in considerable personal and public financial consequences. Management is mostly non-operative, but spinal fusion has been used for nearly 90 years. Spinal fusion rates vary between and within countries.[1] In England about 1000 lumbar fusions are performed per year.[2] An almost direct relation exists between the numbers of operations

doi 10.1136/bmj.38441.620417.8F

Nuffield Orthopaedic Centre, Oxford OX3 7LD

Jeremy Fairbank *consultant orthopaedic surgeon*
James Wilson-MacDonald *consultant orthopaedic surgeon*
Karen Barker *director of physiotherapy research*

University of Warwick, Division of Health in the Community, Coventry CV4 7AL

Helen Frost *research fellow*

Centre for Statistics in Medicine, Oxford OX3 7LF

Ly-Mee Yu *statistician*

Clinical Trial Service Unit and Epidemiological Studies Unit, Radcliffe Infirmary, Oxford OX2 6HE

Rory Collins *professor*

Correspondence to: J Fairbank
(email: jeremy.fairbank@ndos.ox.ac.uk)

(*Accepted 24 March 2005*)

Originally published in *BMJ* 2005; **330**. Reproduced with permission.

performed each year and of orthopaedic and neurosurgeons per head of population.[3] In the United States, spinal fusions for "degenerative changes" rose sharply from around 11 000 operations per year in 1996 to 37 000/year in 2001 (a 336% increase).[4] Both the rationale and the techniques used to fuse the spine have been questioned.[5] Multi-disciplinary rehabilitation programmes that focus on physical, psychological, social, and occupational factors have been advocated for patients with chronic pain of the low back.[6–8]

This trial was conceived in response to the identification of weak evidence for surgery as a priority by the NHS standing group on health technology in 1994.[9,10] The pragmatic trial was designed to compare two treatment strategies (spinal stabilisation surgery or intensive rehabilitation) for patients considered by surgeons to be candidates for surgical stabilisation of the lumbar spine.

Methods

This multicentre, randomised trial was set in 15 hospitals in the United Kingdom. Only consultant surgeons with training and expertise in performing spinal fusions participated. We approached an additional 39 centres where either the surgeon was unwilling to recruit patients or implementation of the intensive rehabilitation programme was impossible.

Eligibility criteria

We used the uncertainty of outcome principle to define our entry criteria and therefore depended on the current practice of many experienced spine surgeons and their patients.[11] Patients who were candidates for surgical stabilisation of the spine were eligible if the clinician and patient were uncertain which of the study treatment strategies was best. Patients had to be aged between 18 and 55, with more than a 12 month history of chronic low back pain (with or without referred pain) and irrespective of whether they had had previous root decompression or discectomy.

Patients were ineligible if the surgeon considered that any medical or other reasons made one of the trial interventions unsuitable. These included infection or other comorbidities (inflammatory disease, tumours, fractures), psychiatric disease, inability or unwillingness to complete the trial questionnaires, or pregnancy. If patients had had previous surgical stabilisation surgery of the spine they were also excluded.

Objectives

The aim was to determine whether surgical stabilisation of the spine (by fusion or flexible stabilisation) was more or less effective at achieving worthwhile relief of symptoms over a two year period than an intensive rehabilitation programme based on principles of cognitive behaviour therapy.

Outcome measures

We assessed outcomes at baseline and 6, 12, and 24 months from randomisation by a trial research therapist in each centre. If the patient was unable to attend the follow-up appointments we mailed the questionnaire. We approached non-responders by phone, through their family doctor, and via national databases.

Primary outcome

The two primary measures at 24 months included a back pain specific questionnaire and a standardised walking test. The Oswestry low back pain disability index is scored from 0% (no disability) to 100% (totally disabled or bedridden) and designed to assess limitations of various activities of daily living.[12,13] The shuttle walking test is a standardised, progressive, maximal test of walking speed and endurance.[14–16]

Secondary outcomes

The short form 36 general health questionnaire (SF-36) includes 35 items summarised in two measures related to physical and mental health. Each scale ranges from 0 (worst health state) to 100 (best health state). The summary measures are transformed to give a population mean of 50 (SD 10). The SF-36 is recommended as an outcome assessment for spinal disorders because it provides strong psychometric support and extensive normative data.

Psychological assessment—We used the distress and risk assessment method (DRAM), which includes the modified Zung depression index and somatic perception questionnaire, to assess anxiety and depression.[17]

Complications—We recorded the intraoperative use of anaesthetic agents, implants, and radiological investigations; complications of surgery and any adverse effects of rehabilitation; postoperative complications, implant failure and repeat surgery; and personal items and devices purchased by the patient because of lower back pain. Work status was monitored. We recorded "obvious pseudoarthrosis" only where it was clear to the treating surgeon that fusion had failed and that this was a problem to the patient.

Sample size

We used the Oswestry disability index to determine the sample size. The trial was designed to be able to detect a difference in mean score between the intervention groups of as little as 4 points.[12,13] We estimated that 133 subjects would be required in each group to detect such a difference at the $\alpha = 0.05$ level with 80% power. We initially planned to recruit at least this number of patients in each of three separate clinical groups to allow reliable subgroup analysis, but most of the patients were recruited in one clinical category.

Interventions

Spinal stabilisation surgery—The particular technique used for spinal fusion was left to the discretion of the operating surgeon. This allowed choice of the most appropriate surgical approach, implant (if any), interbody cages, and bone graft material for that patient. A small number of surgeons used flexible stabilisation of the spine (the Graf or Global technique). This was recorded for each patient before randomisation.

Originally published in *BMJ* 2005; **330**. Reproduced with permission.

Intensive rehabilitation programme—Each centre was modelled on a daily outpatient programme of education and exercise running on five days per week for three weeks continuously. Further details of the programme are reported elsewhere.[15] Most centres offered 75 hours of intervention (range 60–110 hours), with one day of follow-up sessions at one, three, six, or 12 months after treatment. The rehabilitation programmes were led by physiotherapists but included clinical psychologists in all but one centre, as well as medical support. The daily exercises were individually tailored and paced to increase repetitions and duration, aiming to build on the participants' baseline ability. They included stretching of major muscle groups, spinal flexibility exercises, general muscle strengthening, spine stabilisation exercises, and cardiovascular endurance exercise using any mode of aerobic exercise (treadmill walking, step-ups, cycling, rowing). All but one centre included daily sessions of hydrotherapy. We used principles of cognitive behaviour therapy to identify and overcome fears and unhelpful beliefs that many patients develop when in pain.

Treatment allocation and recruitment
Surgeons approached patients who were candidates for spinal fusion. Each centre employed a trial research therapist to organise the trial locally, recruit patients, book treatment appointments, and carry out assessments. Patients were given verbal, written, and videotape (OMI, Oxford) explanations of the background and nature of the trial. The trial research therapists obtained written consent and carried out baseline assessments before randomisation.

Randomisation was generated centrally by computer program, with minimisation for various potential confounding factors: age, smoking, litigation, Oswestry score, clinical classification, and planned use of the Graf procedure.

Statistical methods
We carried out an intention to treat analysis. We used analysis of covariance (ANCOVA) to analyse quantitative outcomes at 24 months, with corresponding baseline values and treatment group as covariates.

We used multiple imputation to handle missing data. To impute the missing data we constructed multiple regression models including variables potentially related to the fact that the data were missing and also variables correlated with that outcome. We used Stata (StataCorp, College Station, Texas, USA)[18] and PROC MI in SAS (SAS Institute, Cary, NC, USA) to obtain similar answers, and only the former are presented.

Results
A total of 349 patients were randomised between June 1996 and February 2002 from 15 centres in the UK (176 allocated to surgery and 173 to rehabilitation). The figure shows the progression through the trial. Table 1 shows the baseline characteristics of patients who entered the trial.

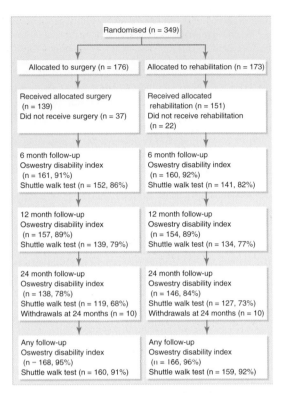

Flow of participants through each stage of the spine stabilisation trial, showing numbers completing the primary outcome measures (Oswestry score and shuttle walking test) at each follow-up stage

Compliance with treatment and follow-up
Table 2 shows data on participants' compliance with their treatment and follow-up. Forty eight (28%) patients randomised to rehabilitation had surgery by two years. Seven (4%) patients randomised to surgery had rehabilitation instead of surgery

Complications
Intraoperative complications occurred in 19 surgical cases (table 3). Eleven patients required further operations on their lumbar spine during the two year follow-up. We did not identify any specific complications of the rehabilitation programmes.

Clinical outcomes
Oswestry scores improved slightly more in favour of surgery (−4.1, 95% confidence interval −8.1 to −0.1, P = 0.045). After imputation for missing follow-up data the mean difference was −4.5 (−8.2 to −0.8, P = 0.02) (tables 4 and 5). No significant heterogeneity in the effect on the Oswestry score was observed between the predefined groups of patient (table 6). No other difference between groups in any of the other outcomes at 24 months reached significance, even when we used imputed values (tables 4 and 5).

Originally published in *BMJ* 2005; **330**. Reproduced with permission.

Table 1 Baseline characteristics of patients and clinical details at trial entry. Values are numbers of patients unless otherwise indicated

Characteristic	Surgery (n = 176)	Rehabilitation (n = 173)
Male	79 (44.9)	93 (53.8)
Female	97 (55.1)	80 (46.2)
Age:		
<30 years	24 (13.6)	20 (11.6)
30–39 years	63 (35.8)	67 (38.7)
40–49 years	56 (31.8)	66 (38.1)
≥50 years	33 (18.8)	20 (11.6)
Centre:*		
A	55 (31.3)	54 (31.2)
B	28 (15.9)	27 (15.6)
C	45 (25.6)	43 (24.9)
D	48 (27.3)	49 (28.3)
Mean duration of back pain years (range) in years	8 (1–35)	8 (1–35)
Current smokers	76 (43.2)	74 (42.8)
Litigation	25 (14.2)	21 (12.1)
Currently in paid employment	88 (50.0)	94 (54.3)
Back pain interfered patient's ability to work:	149 (84.7)	149 (86.1)
Had to give up job	65 (43.6)	67 (45.0)
Had to change job	19 (12.7)	10 (6.7)
Had to reduce hours	17 (11.4)	12 (8.0)
Had to take sick leave	59 (39.6)	69 (46.3)
Clinical details		
Clinical classification:		
Spondylolisthesis	20 (11.4)	18 (10.4)
Post-laminectomy	14 (8.0)	14 (8.1)
Chronic low back pain	142 (80.6)	141 (81.5)
Planned surgery type:		
Graf	27 (15.3)	28 (16.2)
Fusion	149 (84.7)	144 (83.2)
Missing	0	1 (0.6)
Planned fused level:		
Single level	100 (56.8)	109 (63.0)
>1 level	70 (39.8)	62 (35.8)
Missing	6 (3.4)	2 (1.2)
Mean score (SD)		
Oswestry disability index	46.5 (14.6)	44.8 (14.8)
Shuttle walking test in metres	254 (209)	247 (185)
SF-36 physical component score	19.4 (8.8)	20 (9.7)
SF-36 mental component score	43.2 (10.9)	44.2 (12.6)
Modified somatic perception questionnaire	9.0 (6.4)	7.7 (5.7)
Zung self rating depression scale	31.8 (10.4)	31.2 (11.8)
Distress and risk assessment method:		
Normal	14 (8.0)	14 (8.1)
At risk	65 (36.9)	85 (49.1)
Distressed depressive	87 (49.4)	69 (39.9)
Distressed somatic	9 (5.1)	2 (1.2)
Missing	1 (0.6)	3 (1.7)

*Refers to the three largest recruiting centres and a pool of the remaining centres.

Originally published in *BMJ* 2005; **330**. Reproduced with permission.

Table 2 Compliance with allocated intervention and further treatment

	Surgery (n = 176)	Rehabilitation (n = 173)
No. (%) patients who received allocated intervention	139 (79)	151 (87)
Time from randomisation to intervention received per No. of patients:		
<1 week	1	10
1–2 weeks	8	25
2 weeks–1 month	20	43
1–3 months	86	63
4–6 months	16	9
7–12 months	5	1
>12 months	3	0
Low attendance (1–49% available time)*	N/A	12
High attendance (50–100% available time)*	N/A	139
Median time from randomisation to intervention in months (range)	1.6 (0.2–15.4)	0.9 (0.1–10.2)
No (%) of patients who did not receive allocated treatment	**37 (21)**	**22 (13)**
Switched to the other treatment group	7	10
Physiotherapy	3	0
Medical treatment	11	2
No recorded treatment	16	10
No (%) of patients who required further treatment after allocated treatment	**97 (55.1%)**	**68 (39.3%)**
Further surgery or surgery *	11	38
Additional rehabilitation programme	7	0
Additional physiotherapy treatment	47	8
Additional medical treatment	32	22
No recorded additional treatment	42	83

*Rehabilitation only.

Table 3 Complication due to surgery (each subject could have more than one complication)

Complication	No of patients
At treatment site:	
Dural tear	5
Excessive bleeding	3
Implant problems	5
Bone fracture	1
Vascular injury	1
Loss of purchase or fixation	3
Broken drain	1
Associated with surgical approach:	
Vascular injury	1
Other (loss of swab 1, peritoneal tear 2)	3
Systemic:	
Haemorrhage	1
Further surgery (up to 2 years' follow-up)	11

A total of 19 patients had complications as a result of surgery.

Discussion

Patients with low back pain who are considered by surgeons to be candidates for spinal fusion may obtain similar benefits from an intensive rehabilitation programme as they do from surgery. Our large randomised controlled trial of spinal fusion surgery compared with intensive rehabilitation was limited by recruitment difficulties, some crossover between intervention groups, and incomplete follow-up at 24 months, but the results should help clinicians and service providers make decisions about the management of chronic low back pain. Both groups improved over time, but this effect may reflect a natural resolution of chronic low back pain or regression to the mean. The Oswestry scores improved significantly more in patients allocated to surgery than in those allocated to rehabilitation. Although this difference just exceeds the 4 points specified in the sample size calculation, clinically this difference is small considering the potential risks and additional costs of surgery. Analyses adjusting for baseline variations or per protocol analysis do not change this interpretation (data not shown). Overall, since the other primary outcome of the

Table 4 Mean (SD) outcome values at 24 months, and differences in changes from baseline to 24 months

	Surgery (n = 176)	Rehabilitation (n = 173)	Difference in change 0–24 months (95% CI)*	P value†
Oswestry disability index	**(n = 138)**	**(n = 146)**		
24 months	34.0 (21.1)	36.1 (20.6)	−4.1 (−8.1 to −0.1)	0.045
Shuttle walking test	**(n = 118)**	**(n = 126)**		
24 months	352 (244)	310 (202)	34 (−8 to 77)	0.12
SF-36 physical component score	**(n = 115)**	**(n = 131)**		
24 months	28.8 (14.9)	27.6 (14.6)	2.0 (−1.2 to 5.3)	0.21
SF-36 mental component score				
24 months	47.4 (12.2)	48.1 (12.6)	−0.2 (−2.9 to 2.6)	0.90
Domains of SF-36				
General health perception:				
Baseline	47.6 (20.5)	46.5 (22.0)		
24 months	57.7 (23.6)	53.8 (24.5)	3.2 (−1.9 to 8.2)	0.22
Physical functioning:				
Baseline	33.6 (19.0)	39.5 (22.1)		
24 months	50.0 (28.2)	49.8 (28.7)	4.8 (−1.2 to 10.8)	0.11
Role limitation (physical):				
Baseline	15.0 (27.1)	17.6 (30.5)		
24 months	39.6 (42.1)	38.6 (42.7)	2.4 (−7.5 to 12.3)	0.63
Role limitation (emotional):				
Baseline	43.2 (41.4)	51.2 (44.0)		
24 months	65.2 (42.7)	65.4 (43.4)	2.9 (−7.1 to 13.0)	0.57
Pain:				
Baseline	28.6 (17.3)	30.0 (16.0)		
24 months	48.1 (26.4)	44.9 (25.1)	4.1 (−1.67 to 10.0)	0.16
Social functioning:				
Baseline	41.1 (23.3)	42.8 (22.9)		
24 months	53.6 (26.2)	55.6 (26.2)	−0.9 (−6.5 to 4.7)	0.76
Mental health:				
Baseline	60.1 (19.9)	60.3 (21.6)		
24 months	66.5 (21.5)	68.4 (23.1)	−1.8 (−6.4 to 2.8)	0.45
Energy and vitality:				
Baseline	35.4 (20.0)	37.4 (21.7)		
24 months	46.7 (22.8)	46.4 (24.9)	1.5 (−3.8 to 6.7)	0.58

*Adjusted for baseline measures. Rehabilitation group is the reference group.
†Analysis of covariance adjusted for baseline measure.

Table 5 Summary of results from available cases and from multiple imputation analyses

	Available cases		Imputed analyses	
Outcome	Estimated difference (95% CI)	P value*	Estimated difference (% CI)	P value*
Oswestry disability index	−4.1 (−8.1 to −0.1)	0.04	−4.5 (−8.2 to −0.8)	0.02
Shuttle walking test	34 (−8 to 77)	0.12	25 (−16 to 66)	0.23
SF-36 (physical component score)	2.0 (−1.2 to 5.3)	0.21	2.5 (−0.4 to 5.5)	0.09
SF-36 (mental component score)	−0.2 (−2.9 to 2.6)	0.90	0.4 (−2.0 to 2.9)	0.73

*Analysis of covariance adjusted for baseline measure.

Originally published in *BMJ* 2005; **330**. Reproduced with permission.

Table 6 Mean Oswestry disability score (with standard deviations) at baseline and 24 months by different subgroups

Subgroup	Surgery	Rehabilitation
Centre		
A:		
Baseline	42.2 (14.9)	40.3 (12.1)
24 months	24.6 (20.7)	28.9 (17.3)
B:		
Baseline	46.7 (13.1)	46.9 (15.1)
24 months	31.4 (18.5)	43.7 (20.9)
C:		
Baseline	48.7 (14.0)	47.8 (15.8)
24 months	42.0 (18.8)	43.3 (19.7)
D:		
Baseline	49.3 (14.8)	45.8 (15.8)
24 months	39.7 (20.9)	33.6 (22.1)
Clinical classification		
Spondylolisthesis:		
Baseline	42.1 (15.1)	38.0 (13.8)
24 months	35.7 (25.4)	30.1 (19.9)
Post-laminectomy:		
Baseline	50.7 (14.2)	47.3 (10.2)
24 months	38.0 (18.4)	33.7 (14.8)
Chronic back pain:		
Baseline	46.7 (14.5)	45.4 (15.2)
24 months	33.3 (20.8)	37.2 (21.1)
Litigation		
No:		
Baseline	45.6 (14.9)	44.2 (15.1)
24 months	34.0 (21.7)	35.4 (20.9)
Yes:		
Baseline	52.0 (11.3)	49.1 (12.4)
24 months	34.1 (17.7)	41.5 (17.0)
Smoking		
No:		
Baseline	45.5 (14.6)	43.1 (14.9)
24 months	29.5 (19.1)	34.6 (19.3)
Yes:		
Baseline	47.8 (14.5)	46.9 (14.6)
24 months	40.6 (22.2)	38.4 (22.2)
Planned type of surgery		
Graf:		
Baseline	45.2 (12.6)	42.5 (17.2)
24 months	35.1 (18.9)	35.6 (24.3)
Fusion:		
Baseline	46.8 (14.9)	45.3 (14.4)
24 months	33.9 (21.5)	36.4 (19.8)

shuttle walking test and the other measures did not differ (even after imputation for missing values), the small difference observed in Oswestry scores should be interpreted cautiously. Furthermore, the confidence intervals can be used to rule out differences in Oswestry scores of more than 10 points

in favour of surgery and of more than 2 points in favour of rehabilitation. Consequently, they narrow substantially the range of plausible estimates for any benefit of surgery.

Comparison with related research

A Cochrane review in 1999 found a complete absence of randomised controlled evidence for spinal fusion.[5] Three randomised controlled trials have been reported subsequently. Möller and Hedlund reported a trial in isthmic spondylolisthesis, with 77 patients randomised to different forms of surgery and 34 patients randomised to an exercise programme.[19] The patients allocated to surgery reported greater benefits at two years in terms of Oswestry scores compared with those allocated to exercise, but instrumentation and bone grafting was not found to produce an advantage over bone grafting alone. A Swedish trial randomised 222 patients to three surgical groups of equal size and 72 patients to physiotherapy.[20] They reported decreased pain and disability in the surgical group compared with physiotherapy at two years but no difference in outcomes between the different surgical techniques. Little effect of physiotherapy was apparent at two years, although this may have been because of the type or intensity of treatment. Routine physiotherapy and intensive rehabilitation are not the same and should not be considered as such. Brox et al reported no differences between groups in a small trial of 64 patients comparing instrumented posterior fusion with rehabilitation followed to 12 months.[21] Improvements in outcomes were comparable with those in both arms of the present trial and in the surgical arm of the Swedish trial.

Evidence is moderate to strong that multidisciplinary rehabilitation including general exercise programmes of muscle strengthening, flexibility training, and cardiovascular endurance along with a cognitive behaviour approach improves function, reduces pain, and work loss in patients with chronic pain of the low back compared with usual care or non-multidisciplinary treatment.[8,22,23] This type of treatment was difficult to implement in the trial and, although recommended in recent European guidelines,[24] is not routinely available in the NHS.

Strengths and limitations of the study

The uncertainty principle had initially been expected to aid trial accrual by bringing the process of informed consent closer to standard medical practice. However, recruitment was slow and numbers enrolled smaller than planned. Eligibility was based on the uncertainty of outcome principle, but uncertainty does not come easily to surgeons when patients are demanding clear direction and advice. Factors influencing recruitment will be presented elsewhere. This pragmatic trial reflects current practice across the UK of experienced spine surgeons selecting patients for fusion. Surgeons may argue that we excluded the best candidates for surgery through "certainty" of outcome, but this certainty varied between surgeons. Evidence from the Swedish trial[25] shows that patients with low neuroticism, narrow discs, and a short time off work do best with surgery.

Originally published in *BMJ* 2005; **330**. Reproduced with permission.

Surgical issues

Surgeons were allowed their own choice of operation to improve the chance of clinical success. The Swedish trial showed no difference between three surgical techniques of fusion.[24] These results call into question what lumbar fusion is actually doing to patients with chronic back pain. Elucidation of this question was not the objective of this study. The results are highly relevant to spinal fusion surgery, as well as the new techniques of flexible stabilisation and disc replacement that are being applied to this group of patients.

Loss to follow-up

Loss to follow-up at 24 months (20%) limits the internal validity of the trial. We used multiple imputation as a sensitivity analysis to tackle potential bias resulting from the poor response rate. Overall estimates of the treatment effect were very similar with all methods of statistical analysis.

Blinding

The pre-randomisation outcomes were scored by the trial research therapists and later checked by computer. All subsequent outcomes were scored centrally. We were not able to blind the trial research therapists to patient allocation after the baseline assessment.

Limitation of outcomes

The available outcome measures are blunt instruments for assessing a complex condition. The minimum clinically important change in the Oswestry scores has been estimated by different observers as being somewhere between 4 and 17.[26] Debate continues among back pain experts over the question of what represents a clinically important change. Functional measures are difficult to apply in a multicentre setting, and although the use of muscle measurement techniques may be useful, it was not possible to use them in this trial because of financial limitations. Walking capacity was chosen as it is simple and cheap to measure and often a limitation for people with chronic low back pain.

Compliance with treatment protocol

The 48 (28%) patients who were randomised to rehabilitation and then had additional surgery by two years should be considered as an additional outcome of the trial and taken into account in the interpretation of the results. Although some patients and surgeons were clearly not satisfied with the results of rehabilitation, many more seem to have benefited and avoided surgical intervention.

Conclusion

Nearly three quarters of those patients allocated to rehabilitation avoided surgery by two years. Rehabilitation including a cognitive behaviour approach is not routinely or widely available to patients with chronic pain of the low back, and this trial implies that it should be. Rehabilitation programmes require finance, space, and training, but above all they need the strong support of all clinicians involved in the care of these patients.

What is already known on this topic

Limited evidence shows that patients with severe chronic low back pain treated with spinal stabilisation surgery have a better outcome in terms of pain and disability than with traditional conservative management

The results of spinal stabilisation surgery seem to be similar whatever surgical technique is used

Intensive multidisciplinary rehabilitation including a biopsychosocial approach improves pain and function in severe chronic low back pain compared with usual care or traditional conservative treatment

What this study adds

No clear evidence emerged that primary spinal fusion surgery was more beneficial than intensive rehabilitation using principles of cognitive behaviour therapy

Evidence exists to support intensive rehabilitation with cognitive behaviour principles as an alternative to spinal fusion surgery in the management of chronic low back pain

We thank the patients, who permitted a difficult decision to be made for them; referees, physiotherapist, and surgeons, inside and outside the trial (www.ndos.ox.ac.uk/SST), who helped develop the protocol; the Medical Research Council for supporting the study; NHS R&D (especially Richard Lilford) for supporting and promoting the study.

Contributors: JF was responsible for the overall study design, the organisation of the study, recruiting and operating on patients in the study, data analysis, and wrote the first draft of this report. HF was responsible for overall study design, the organisation of the study, the design and implementation of the rehabilitation programme, data analysis, and writing the first draft of the report. JWM was responsible for overall study design, the organisation of the study, recruiting and operating on patients in the study, data analysis, and editing the report. RC was responsible for overall study design, statistical advice and data analysis, and presented analyses to the data monitoring committee. LMY was responsible for statistical analysis. JF and HF are guarantors. KB was responsible for recruiting patients and data analysis. Of the contributors who are not listed as authors, Douglas Altman was responsible for statistical analysis and sat on the data monitoring committee. Alastair Gray was responsible for study design, the organisation of the study and economic analysis. Nicolas Maniadakis was responsible for economic data collection and analysis. Kate Johnston, Helen Campbell, and Oliver Rivero were responsible for economic analysis. Patricia Carver was responsible for data collection and analysis. L Morgan was responsible for data collection and database design. Kate Stevens, Victoria Erlanger, Rebecca Bale collected and entered data. Peter Smith developed and maintained the database.

Funding: The Medical Research Council supported the trial financially and was represented on the steering committee. The NHS (326) or private patient insurance (23) funded the treatment of patients. MRC grant number G94431172.

Competing interests: JF and JWM have received funding from Synthes for a spinal fellow.

Ethical approval: The trial was approved by a multicentre research ethics committee (twice; references 98/5/14 for original and 03/05/034 for long term follow-up) and 15 local research ethics committees.

References

1 Katz J. Lumbar spinal fusion: surgical rates, costs, and complications. *Spine* 1995;20:78S–83S.

2 Department of Health (England). Hospital episode statistics, 1998–2003. London: DoH, 1998–2003.

3 Cherkin D, Deyo R, Loeser J, Bush T, Waddell G. An international comparison of back surgery rates. *Spine* 1994;19:1201–6.

4 Deyo RA, Gray DT, Kreuter W, Mirza S, Martin, BI. United States trends in lumbar fusion surgery for degenerative conditions. *Spine* 2005 (in press).

5 Gibson J, Grant I, Waddell G. The Cochrane review of surgery for lumbar disc prolapse and degenerative lumbar spondylosis. *Spine* 1999;24:1820–32.

6 Mayer T, Gatchel R, Kishino N. Objective assessment of spine function following industrial injury. A prospective study with comparison group and one year follow up. *Spine* 1985; 10:482–93.

7 Lindstrom I, Ohlund C, Eek C. The effect of graded activity on patients with sub acute low back pain: A randomised prospective clinical study with an operant conditioning behavioural approach. *Phys Ther* 1992;72:279–93.

8 Guzman J, Esmail R, Karjalainen K, Malmivaara A, Irvin E, Bombardier C. Multidisciplinary rehabilitation for chronic low back pain: systematic review. *BMJ* 2001;322:1511–6.

9 NHS Standing Group. *Health technology (SGHT) report.* London: Department of Health, 1994.

10 Turner J, Ersek M, Herron L, Heselkorn J, Kent D, Ciol M, et al. Patient outcomes after lumbar spinal fusions. *JAMA* 1992;268:907–11.

11 Weijer C, Shapiro S, Cranley Glass K. For and against: clinical equipoise and not the uncertainty principle is the moral underpinning of the randomised controlled trial. *BMJ* 2000;321:756–8.

12 Fairbank J, Pynsent P. The Oswestry Disability Index. *Spine* 2000; 25:2940–53.

13 Roland M, Fairbank J. The Roland-Morris disability questionnaire and the Oswestry disability questionnaire. *Spine* 2000; 25:3115–24.

14 Taylor S, Frost H, Taylor A, Barker K. Reliability and responsiveness of the shuttle walking test in patients with chronic low back pain. *Physiother Res Int* 2001;6:170–8.

15 Frost H, Lamb S, Shackleton C. A functional restoration programme for chronic low back pain: a prospective outcome study. *Physiotherapy* 2000;86:285–93.

16 Pratt R, Fairbank J, Virr A. The reliability of the shuttle walking test, the Swiss spinal stenosis questionnaire, the Oxford spinal stenosis Score, and the Oswestry disability index in the assessment of patients with lumbar spinal stenosis. *Spine* 2002;27:84–91.

17 Main CJ, Wood PLR, Hollis S, Spanswick CC, Waddell G. The distress and risk assessment method: A simple patient classification to identify distress and evaluate the risk of poor outcome. *Spine* 1992;17:42–52.

18 Royston P. Multiple imputation of missing values. *Stata J* 2004; 4:227–41.

19 Möller H, Hedlund R. Surgery versus conservative treatment in adult isthmic spondylolisthesis. A prospective randomized study part 1. *Spine* 2000;25:1171–5.

20 Fritzell P, Hagg O, Wessburg P, Nordwall A, Group SLSS. Chronic back pain and fusion: a comparison of three surgical techniques: a prospective multicentre randomized study from the Swedish Lumbar Spine Study Group. *Spine* 2002;27:1131–41.

21 Brox J, Sørensen R, Friis A, Nygaard Ø, Indahl A, Keller A, et al. Randomized clinical trial of lumbar instrumented fusion and cognitive intervention and exercises in patients with chronic low back pain and disc degeneration. *Spine* 2003;28:1913–21.

22 Schonstein E, Kenny D, Keating J, Koes B, Herbert R. Physical conditioning programs for workers with back and neck pain: a Cochrane systematic review. *Spine* 2003;28(19):E391–5.

23 Liddle S, Baxter G, Gracey J. Exercise and chronic low back pain: what works? *Pain* 2004;107:176–90.

24 European Commission Rersearch Directorate General. COST B13 Management Committee. *European guidelines for the management of low back pain.* www.backpaineurope.org, 2005 (accessed 17 May 2005).

25 Hägg O, Fritzell P, Elkselius L, Nordwall A. Predictors of outcome in fusion surgery for chronic low back pain. A report from the Swedish lumbar spine study. *Eur Spine J* 2003;12:22–33.

26 Taylor S, Taylor A, Foy M, Fogg A. Responsiveness of common outcome measures for patients with low back pain. *Spine* 1999;24:1805–12.

Originally published in *BMJ* 2005; **330**. Reproduced with permission.

Survival analyses

Aims

To understand the different ways in which survival analyses can be used, and to decide whether appropriate figures have been used to report survival rates.

Learning objectives
On completion of this unit, participants will be able to:
- interpret results reported as per cent survival, Kaplan–Meier statistics or hazard ratios;
- decide whether the assumptions for survival analyses have been met;
- compute a hazard ratio;
- judge whether graphical representations of survival rates are appropriate.

Glossary

Term	Definition
Event	Outcome of interest which is typically death but can be a non-fatal or favourable outcome, e.g. discharge from hospital.
Censored observations	Used to describe participants who withdraw from the study or who do not experience the outcome of interest.
Kaplan–Meier statistic	Statistic used to compare the event rate over time between two or more study groups. Also called a log-rank test.
Hazard ratio	The risk of the event in a study group divided by the risk of the event in a reference group.

Background

Rates of survival can be measured in longitudinal studies which include both cohort studies and randomised controlled trials in which participants are followed for a length of time. In a cohort study, the influence of an exposure on survival rates can be compared between study groups, whereas in randomised controlled trials the efficacy or effectiveness of a new treatment compared with a standard treatment in increasing survival rates can be measured.

In this Unit, we will use the term 'event' to describe the outcome of interest. In survival analyses, the event is classically a non-favourable outcome such as death, disease onset or treatment failure. However, survival analyses can also be applied to other types of events, such as discharge from hospital, disease remission or a lifestyle choice – for example cessation of breast-feeding or uptake of contraception. In some studies, several outcomes may be combined to define an event. For example, an event that summarises whether death, acute myocardial infarction or cardiac arrest has occurred is often used in clinical trials.[1]

In this Unit, we discuss three ways in which data relating to survival events can be summarised, that is, as frequency rates, Kaplan–Meier statistics or hazard ratios.

Per cent survival
Given that survival is a binary outcome, the number of events at a certain point in time can be summarised using percentages, as discussed in Unit 2. Survival rates are very similar to incidence rates except that for survival, the event usually signals the cessation of a condition, whereas for incidence, the outcome signals the onset of a condition. Frequency statistics are often used to summarise survival rates, for example, as one-, two- and five-year survival rates in patients who undergo a surgical procedure. Survival rates expressed as percentages in this way can be compared between exposure groups or treatment groups using a chi-square test to obtain a P value (see Unit 3) or by estimation using confidence intervals (see Unit 1).

Kaplan–Meier statistics
Although survival rates at a single point in time provide useful summary statistics, they do not take advantage of the complex nature of data collected longitudinally. If the event is regarded as being positive or negative regardless of the amount of time that participants have been in the study, important information is lost. To utilise data collected about both the occurrence and the timing of events, Kaplan–Meier statistics are used.

Rather than simply comparing events at arbitrary time points, Kaplan–Meier statistics are used to compare the event rate over time between the study groups.[2] Kaplan–Meier statistics are based on non-parametric methods and have the advantage that they do not require the survival time to be normally distributed or the event rate to be constant over time. A feature of Kaplan–Meier statistics is that they allow for some participants to be followed for longer periods of time than others, and for the event to have not yet occurred in all participants.[3] Obviously, a participant who has been in the study for only 6 months does not have the same chance for the event to occur as a participant who has been in the study for 12 months. In Kaplan–Meier analyses, the occurrence of the event, the time to the event and the different length of follow-up for each participant is taken into account, and therefore allowance is made for participants who leave the study early or who have had less opportunity for the event to occur.

Participants who leave the study or do not experience the event during the follow-up period are called 'censored' observations.[2] The term 'censored' is also used to describe participants who are lost to follow-up, for example because they withdraw from the study, die without the investigators' knowledge or die from causes other than the condition being studied. Classifying participants who leave the study before experiencing the event as being 'censored' allows them to be included in the analysis. The participants who complete the time frame of the study without experiencing the event are also regarded as being censored.

Survival analyses are often shown plotted as Kaplan–Meier curves as in Figure 9.1. In this figure, the curve for 30 people in a new treatment group is compared with the curve for 26 people in a control group who receive standard care.[4] Each time an event occurs, the per cent that are event free is reduced and the curve steps down. Each time a person is censored, that is, leaves the study, the time to being censored is marked as a cross-hatch on the line and the curve does not step down. However, censoring reduces the number of people contributing to the curve, so each event after the censor represents a higher percentage of the remaining people. Because censoring results in a decrease in the number of people at risk, the curve becomes less reliable over the study period, especially if there are many people who are censored at the beginning of the curve.

The curve can be used to calculate the probability of survival at any time interval and also over a time period. In Figure 9.1, for the new treatment group in the interval from 0 to 9 days, 3 people are censored as indicated by the cross-hatches, therefore 27 (30 – 3) people are at risk of experiencing the event on day 9. On day 9, one person experienced the event as indicated by the step down. At the end of day 9, the probability of surviving is the number of people who have not experienced the event divided by the number of people at risk, that is, 26/27 or 0.963. At the start of the next time interval before the next event, that is days 9 to 12, 26 people are at risk, 1 person is censored on day 9 and 1 person experiences the event on day 12. At the end of this interval, 25 (26 –1 person censored) people are at risk and 1 person experienced the event. Therefore, the proportion surviving this interval is 24 (25 – 1 person who experienced the event) divided by 25, the number of people at risk, or 0.960. The estimated survival to any time point is equal to the probability of surviving the preceding intervals. Therefore, the estimated survival rate at day 12 is 0.963 multiplied by 0.960, to give 0.924. This procedure continues until the last event or the completion of the study.

The most commonly reported statistic to test whether the survival rates are different between study groups is the log-rank statistic. This statistic is similar in some ways to a chi-square test in that the number of observed events is compared to the number of expected events. The method to calculate the number of expected events is shown later in this Unit. For the data in Figure 9.1, the log-rank statistic has a P value of 0.07, indicating no significant difference between survival rates in the new treatment and control groups. When marginal P values such as this occur, it is important to assess whether the finding can be regarded as a type II error, as described in Unit 1.

It is recommended that survival plots are not extended into times when the number of participants remaining is unduly small, and that the plots are curtailed when less than 10–20% of the participants are still in follow-up.[1] The decision of when to restrict the x-axis time period is difficult, but the right-hand side of the plot should not represent only a few participants in which there is greater uncertainty. When the number in either group is small, a single event can have a large difference on the per cent of patients who

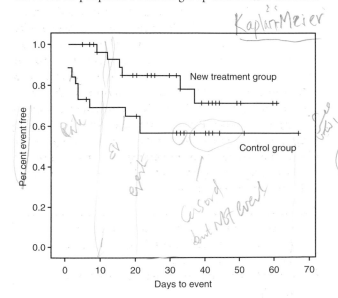

Figure 9.1 Time to an event in the new treatment group and the control group.

remain event free. Thus, a large step down in the curve can occur which may visually increase the between-group difference considerably, but which may only have a small effect on the *P* value.

In the trial shown in Figure 9.1, there was a fixed follow-up time of 72 days. There were 6 events and 24 censored cases in the new treatment group at 59 days, and 11 events and 15 censored cases in the control group at 65 days. The *x*-axis could be restricted to 42 days when 20% of the sample or 11 participants remained enrolled, but this would make little difference to the figure because no events occurred after 36 days. No matter how the *x*-axis is restricted when displaying the data in a figure, all participants must be included in the calculation of the log-rank statistic regardless of the number remaining at any point in time.

> ## TAKE HOME LIST
>
> The three different ways to analyse data from studies in which information is collected about whether a specified event occurs over time are:
>
> - to compare the rate of the event between the study groups at set time points, e.g. the rate of deaths at 1, 3 and 5 years following surgery;
>
> - to use Kaplan–Meier statistics to compare event rates over time between study groups;
>
> - to calculate the hazard ratio at set time points.

Hazard ratios

Although Kaplan–Meier statistics are widely used to compare event rates, they do not provide any direct information about the size of the difference between the groups.[5] Although some estimate of an effect size can be obtained by comparing survival frequencies, as described above, it is also possible to calculate a relative risk which compares the event rates in the two groups at a single point in time. This statistic has the same interpretation as relative risk, as described in Unit 4, but in survival analyses the risk statistic is called the hazard ratio. The hazard ratio will be less than 1 if the treatment is beneficial.[6]

Although some statistics programs do not report the hazard ratio directly, it can be obtained using Cox regression or easily calculated. The formula for the hazard ratio at any time point is:

$$\text{Hazard ratio} = \frac{(O_T/E_T)}{(O_C/E_C)}$$

where *O* is the observed number, *E* is the expected number, the subscript T refers to the treatment group and the subscript C refers to the control group. The expected number of events is the number that would occur if there was an equal risk in both groups.[7] If both groups have an equal risk, the expected number of events is the observed number of events in each group. The expected number of events in a study group is calculated as follows:

Expected = Total number of events
     × (Group size/Total sample size)

For example, if there are 100 participants in each group and the observed number of events is 30 in the new treatment group and 50 in the control group, then the expected number of events in each group will be 80 × (100/200) or 40. The hazard ratio can then be calculated as (30/40)/(50/40), or 0.6, indicating a decreased risk of the event in the new treatment group.

This hazard ratio of 0.6 should not be interpreted to mean that the new treatment group are 0.6 times less likely to die, although it does mean that they are 'protected' from the event occurring when compared to the control group. A hazard ratio of 0.6 is more correctly interpreted to mean that the participants in the new treatment group, who are still alive at a certain time point, have 0.6 times the chance of experiencing the event at the next time point, compared to participants in the control group.[8]

Assumptions

There are three assumptions for Kaplan–Meier analyses and calculating the hazard ratio. As with other independent samples statistics, the first assumption is that the groups are independent, that is, each participant is included only once and in only one group. The other two assumptions described below relate to possible reasons for differences between the groups, and are not so important in clinical trials in which randomisation is expected to balance the important prognostic factors, but can be important in observational studies.

The second assumption is that participants' survival prospects remain constant, that is participants who are enrolled early in the study have the same survival prospects as those who are enrolled towards the end of the study. Thus, factors that influence participants' survival prospects, such as new treatments, should not be introduced over the study period. Time-related differences in survival rates can also occur if participants enrolled early on have a different underlying prognosis from participants enrolled towards the end of the study. If the sample size is large enough, this assumption can be tested by comparing event rates in participants enrolled at different times during the study.

> The assumptions for survival analyses are that:
> - the observations are independent, that is, each person can be included once only;
> - survival prospects remain constant over the study period;
> - censored participants have the same survival prospects as the non-censored participants.

The third assumption is that participants who are censored have the same survival prospects as participants who continue in the study, that is the risk of the event must not be related to the reason for censoring or loss to follow-up.[3] For example, participants who experience more debilitating symptoms in a new treatment group should not be preferentially lost to follow-up compared with participants who experience fewer symptoms in the control treatment group. This assumption is not easy to test and the judgment may have to rely on background knowledge and clinical insight.[7]

Minimising bias

The measurements of both the event and the time to the event must be accurate to avoid bias in the estimates from a survival analysis. It is important that the event is clearly defined and that it is measured precisely. When an event occurs that is not due to the condition being investigated, it is important to give careful consideration to whether it is treated in the analyses as an event or as a withdrawal (censored observation).

It is also important that the measurement of the time to the event is precise. This can be achieved through regular observations during the study rather than surmising that the event occurred between two points in time.[3] For accurate estimates of survival statistics, it is not adequate to make routine clinical examinations, for example at 6-month intervals, and assume that the event occurred at the 6-month follow-up when it actually occurred at an earlier time.

As with all analyses, if the total number of participants in any group is small, say less than 30, the standard errors around the summary statistics will be large, and therefore the survival estimates will be imprecise and type II errors may occur.

Reading and questions

Reprint

Pocock SJ, Clayton TC, Altman DG. Survival plots of time-to-event outcomes in clinical trials: good practice and pitfalls. Lancet 2002;359:1686–1689. (See p. 136.)

The reprint by Pocock *et al.* (2002) discusses the ways in which the display of survival plots is potentially open to visual misinterpretation that may mask the correct clinical message. In the reprint, some common pitfalls in the ways in which survival plots can be presented are discussed and some guidelines about preferred statistical practice are suggested. After reading the reprint answer the following questions.

Questions

1 When is it preferable for survival curves to be plotted going upwards to display the cumulative proportion who have experienced the event over time?

2 When is plotting the data going downwards the most useful way to display the results?

3 How can a break in the *y*-axis scale make the curve potentially open to misinterpretation?

4 How far should the *x*-axis that displays time be extended?

5 What problems can occur when there are only a small number of participants remaining at the end of the trial?

Worked example

Set article

Gibbs JL, Monro JL, Cunningham D, Rickards A. Survival after surgery or therapeutic catheterisation for congenital health disease in children in the United Kingdom: analysis of the central cardiac audit database for 2000–1. BMJ 2004;328;611. (See p. 141.)

In the set article, Gibbs *et al.* (2004) report 30-day and 1-year survival rates in children who have undergone treatment for congenital heart disease. The data were collected in a cardiac audit database in which data from all 13 tertiary centres at which cardiac surgery is performed on children in the United Kingdom is centralised. Children who underwent surgery are classified into three groups: neonates (less than 1 month of age), infants (1 month to 1 year of age) and children (1 to 16 years of age).

The authors show a survival plot in Figure 1 that describes survival rates following bypass in each of the three age groups. No *P* value is given, so we have to rely on the confidence intervals presented in the table to estimate whether there is a difference in survival rates between age groups. The authors report 30-day and 1-year survival rates with 99% confidence intervals. Although the 99% confidence intervals are wider than 95% confidence intervals, the same principles of comparing overlap, as discussed in Unit 2, apply; but in this case no overlap infers a *P* value of at least < 0.01 rather than < 0.05. The 1-year survival rates for bypass surgery that are reported in the table are shown graphically in Figure 9.2. The reported

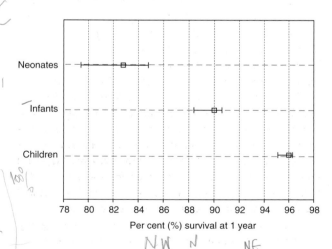

Figure 9.2 Per cent survival after bypass surgery at 1 year with 99% confidence intervals.

Table 9.1 Survival at 30 days for neonates, infants and children undergoing bypass surgery

Group	No. of procedures	% survival at 30 days	95% CI	No. of events	Hazard ratio
Neonate	383	87.1	83.7, 90.5	34	5.2
Infant	909	94.4			
Child	1353	97.5			—
Neonate	30	87.1			
Infant	75	94.4			
Child	110	97.5			—

Table 9.2 Survival at 1 year for neonates, infants and children undergoing bypass surgery

Group	No. of procedures	% survival at 1 year	95% CI	No. of events	Hazard ratio
Neonate	383	82.8	79.0, 86.6	54	4.3
Infant	909	90.0			
Child	1353	96.0			—
Neonate	30	82.8			
Infant	75	90.0			
Child	110	96.0			—

confidence intervals were based on a binomial distribution and are asymmetric around the survival rate, unlike confidence intervals based on a normal distribution which would have been symmetric. Comparison of the confidence intervals shows that they do not overlap, indicating a significant difference in 1-year survival rates between each of the age groups with $P < 0.01$.

Because the x-axis range in this figure is from 78% to 98% survival, rather than from 0 to 100%, it tends to make the differences between the three ages groups look more dramatic than they actually are. In fact, the gaps between the confidence intervals are only 4 to 6%.

The survival rates for bypass surgery at 30 days and 1 year are summarised in Tables 9.1 and 9.2. Calculate the 95% confidence intervals around the percentages based on a normal distribution using the formula given in Unit 2. These confidence intervals will be symmetrical around the survival rate. Also calculate the 95% confidence intervals for the bottom three rows of Tables 9.1 and 9.2, which have the sample size that would be expected from a single centre. Next, plot the 1-year estimates for both the total sample and the single centre on the graph shown in Figure 9.2.

Finally, calculate the number of events in each group and the hazard ratio for death to occur in the neonates and infants, each compared to the 'child' group as the reference group. Note that the hazard ratio does not change with sample size, but in this exercise the hazard ratios will be slightly different because of rounding errors.

By comparing the 95% confidence intervals and using the plotted estimates and the hazard ratios, answer the following questions.

- How do your 95% confidence intervals compare with the 99% confidence intervals reported?
- What happens when the sample size is smaller?
- Would you revise the conclusion about a between age group difference if the data from only one centre had been reported?
- Could the interpretation of age group differences from the 13 centres or from only one centre be regarded as a type I or type II error?
- The authors report that: "For infants, mortality after treatment for heart disease at 1 year was double that at 30 days". From the data presented in the article, how do they reach this conclusion?
- How would you interpret the hazard ratios?

Critical appraisal

Work through the critical appraisal checklist to review the paper by Gibbs *et al.* (2004) and decide whether the results and the conclusions are valid and justified.

Critical appraisal checklist for an article that reports survival data	
A. Study design	
1. Is the event clearly defined?	
2. Could the event be subject to recall bias?	
3. Has time been measured accurately?	
4. Could any factors have preferentially changed the participant's survival prospects over the course of the study?	
B. Statistical methods	
5. Is the sample size sufficient in each group?	
6. Are there sufficient people in each group to make conclusions towards the end of the study?	
7. Do the authors provide evidence that the assumptions for survival analysis have been met?	
C. Results	
8. Is the figure reported appropriately?	
9. Has the y-axis been truncated to visually inflate the differences between the groups?	
D. Interpretation	
10. Do the authors show survival rates for different subgroups? If yes, how do they interpret these rates?	
11. Have the survival rates been interpreted correctly?	

Quick quiz

Tick the correct answer for each of the following questions.

1 Kaplan–Meier statistics are most appropriate when:
(a) the time of follow-up is normally distributed;
(b) many people drop out of the study;
(c) most people have been followed for a long period of time;
(d) people have been followed for different periods of time.

2 If Kaplan–Meier statistics are used, information of the event should be collected from participants:
(a) at regular 6-month intervals;
(b) as often as possible;
(c) at planned medical check-ups;
(d) at planned home visits.

3 A censored observation in the data occurs:
(a) before the follow-up data are collected;
(b) when the data are not entered into the database;
(c) if a participant misses a study visit;
(d) when a person has withdrawn from the study.

4 If the y-axis of a Kaplan–Meier curve is shortened this will:
(a) visually magnify differences between study groups;
(b) visually minimise differences between study groups;
(c) visually make no difference;
(d) visually make the figure easier to read.

References

1. Pocock SJ, Clayton TC, Altman DG. Survival plots of time-to-event outcomes in clinical trials: good practice and pitfalls. Lancet 2002;359:1686–1689.
2. Altman DG, Bland JM. Statistics notes: Time to event (survival) data. BMJ 1998;317:468–469.
3. Bland JM, Altman DG. Statistics notes: Survival probabilities (the Kaplan–Meier method). BMJ 1998;317:1572.
4. Peat JK, Barton B. Survival analyses. In: Medical Statistics. A guide to data analysis and critical appraisal. Harayana, India: BMJ Books Blackwell Publishing, 2005; pp 296–305.

5. Altman DG. Analysis of survival times. In: Practical statistics for medical research. London: Chapman & Hall, 1996; pp 365–387.

6. Altman DG, Andersen, PK. Calculating the number needed to treat where the outcome is time to an event. BMJ 1999;319:1492–1495.

7. Bull K, Spiegelhalter DJ. Survival analysis in observational studies. Stat Med 1997;16:1041–1074.

8. Spruance SL, Reid JE, Grace M, Samore M. Hazard ratio in clinical trials. AAC 2004; 48:2787–2792.

DEPARTMENT OF MEDICAL STATISTICS

Survival plots of time-to-event outcomes in clinical trials: good practice and pitfalls

Stuart J Pocock, Tim C Clayton, Douglas G Altman

Survival plots of time-to-event data are a key component for reporting results of many clinical trials (and cohort studies). However, mistakes and distortions often arise in the display and interpretation of survival plots. This article aims to highlight such pitfalls and provide recommendations for future practice. Findings are illustrated by topical examples and also based on a survey of recent clinical trial publications in four major journals. Specific issues are: should plots go up or down (we recommend up), how far in time to extend the plot, showing the extent of follow-up, displaying statistical uncertainty by including SEs or CIS, and exercising caution when interpreting the shape of plots and the time-pattern of treatment difference.

In many clinical trials, the primary outcome for comparison of treatments is the time to occurrence of a disease-related event. The most widely adopted method of displaying such results is by means of Kaplan-Meier survival plots, which show the proportion of patients who experience (or do not experience) the event by time since randomisation. The event itself could be death (hence the term "survival plot" is used loosely), but is often time to a non-fatal event (eg, disease recurrence in cancer) and can sometimes be a favourable outcome such as discharge from hospital. Combined endpoints are used increasingly in clinical trials (eg, death, acute myocardial infarction, or cardiac arrest), and in such cases, the survival plot shows the time to the first event.

The statistical methods for producing survival plots and for calculating p values, estimates of treatment effects, and associated CIs are all well documented.[1–3] However, the display and interpretation of survival plots are prey to several potential distortions and deceptions that can make the right message difficult to work out, as reported in a previous survey of survival analyses in cancer trials.[4] In this article, we concentrate on treatment comparisons in clinical trials, although many of the same problems apply to survival plots in general. Our aim is to reveal some of the more common pitfalls and to give some guidelines to authors, journal editors, and readers on what constitutes desirable statistical practice.

As a practical basis for our concerns and conclusions, we identified all 35 clinical trials with survival plots that were published in four general medical journals during July to October, 1999 (19 in *The Lancet*, ten in the *New England Journal of Medicine*, four in the *British Medical Journal*, and two in the *Journal of the American Medical Association*). These trials constituted 41% of the 86 individually randomised parallel-group trials published in the four journals.

Should plots go up or down?

A survival plot going down displays the proportion of patients free of the event (which of course declines over time), whereas a plot going up shows the cumulative proportion experiencing the event by time. In principle, both contain the same information, but the visual perceptions with regard to comparison of treatment groups can be quite different.

For instance, figure 1 shows three ways of displaying the same data on time to non-fatal myocardial infarction or death in the RITA-2 trial.[5] The first plot, going up, indicates clearly the excess of events in the group randomised to percutaneous transluminal coronary angioplasty (PTCA) compared with the group continuing on medical treatment. This plot has the same style as in the trial's publication,[5] which also gave the numbers and percentages of patients with myocardial infarction or death: 32 of 504 (6.3%) and 17 of 514 (3.3%) for the PTCA and medical treatment groups, respectively (p = 0.02). The second plot, going down and using the whole vertical axis from 0 to 100%, makes the difference look much less pronounced (the corresponding proportions event-free being 93.7% and 96.7%, respectively) and mainly emphasises that most patients did not experience the event. The third plot, going down but with a break in the vertical axis seems to fill the space more informatively, but relies on the reader recognising the break in scale: if they do not, the impression is left that PTCA is harmful to a large proportion of patients. Hence having such a break in the scale is not a good style to adopt.

In practice, only one of these options can be displayed in a trial report. We recommend the first option—the plot going

Lancet 2002; **359:** 1686–89

Medical Statistics Unit, London School of Hygiene and Tropical Medicine, London WC1E 7HT, UK (Prof S J Pocock PhD, T Clayton MSc); **Centre for Statistics in Medicine, Oxford, UK** (Prof D G Altman DSc)

Correspondence to: Prof Stuart J Pocock
(e-mail: stuart.pocock@lshtm.ac.uk)

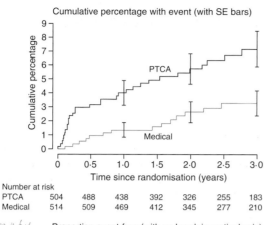

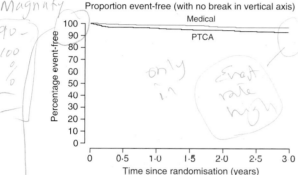

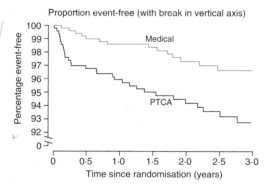

Figure 1 Time to non-fatal myocardial infarction or death in RITA-2 trial: three ways to display same data.

up—as the most reliably informative, especially if the event rate is lower than, say, 30%. To maximise the clarity of information, the highest value on the vertical axis should be a round number slightly greater than the highest value represented by the steepest curve—ie, 9% in figure 1. Some might argue that the full scale (0–100%) should always be included, but this inhibits the ability to discriminate between treatments. For instance, the ELITE 2 trial[6] included such a plot, which helped to hide the apparent survival inferiority of losartan compared with captopril. Admittedly, the treatment difference was not statistically significant, but any claim of potential equivalence was perhaps falsely magnified by the choice of survival plot going down over the full 100% scale.[7] The important survival superiority of pravastatin over placebo in the LIPID trial[8] was hard to discern because of this same injudicious choice of survival plot going down over the full 100% scale, since death rates in all groups were, in fact, less than 10% after 5 years. Incidentally, the investigators claim that this choice was introduced by the journal, not the authors themselves. Such plots going down are useful only for trials in which the event rate is high, such as those in cancers with poor prognosis. For instance, for a neuroblastoma trial,[9] the same style of survival plot was perfectly clear, since the median survival was less than 2 years in a study with follow-up over 5 years for those still alive.

The applicability of trial findings should not rely on relative treatment differences alone (eg, proportional reduction in mortality), but must also include absolute treatment differences (eg, number needed to treat per life saved[10,11]). Provision of both survival plots would perhaps be ideal, one going up to reveal the detail and the relative treatment difference, and one going down to clarify the small absolute risk and hence small absolute difference in treatments. In trial reports for which space is at less of a premium and in regulatory submissions, such an approach is to be encouraged for the key outcomes, but it is unrealistic for journal publications.

In the 35 trials we surveyed, 12 had plots going up, 15 had plots going down all the way to zero, and eight had plots going down but with a break in scale. This disparity in approach is undesirable.

How far in time to extend the plot?

Follow-up times in any one trial can vary substantially because patients are usually recruited over a long period, and some patients can be lost to follow-up. Length of follow-up is taken into account in the Kaplan-Meier life-table method[1–3] for estimating the proportion of patients who experience an event by time since randomisation. Technically, any survival plot can be extended right through to the longest follow-up time, and five trials we surveyed did just that. However, this extension is not good statistical practice, since for any such plot the eye is drawn to the right (ie, where the plot finishes), which is where there is least information and greatest uncertainty. In small trials, much of the right-hand part of the plot can depict just a few patients.

For instance, figure 2 is a reproduction of the plot of time to end-stage renal failure in a trial comparing ramipril with conventional treatment.[12] The visual impression is that treatments are similar up to 48 months, but thereafter the conventional group develops a striking excess of end-stage renal failures, reaching an estimated 50% failure, by 60 months. However, the median follow-up was 31 months and only 25% of patients assigned conventional treatment reached 48 months' follow-up. The number reaching 60 months is not stated but must be very few. Thus, for both treatment groups,

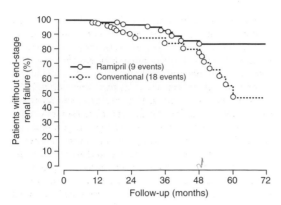

Figure 2 Kaplan-Meier estimation of renal survival among patients on ramipril or conventional treatment. Relative risk 2·72 (95% CI 1·22–6·08), p = 0·01.

there are inadequate data to estimate reliably the failure rates beyond 48 months' follow-up.

In general, we recommend that survival plots be halted once the proportion of patients free of an event, but still in follow-up, becomes unduly small. In our experience, this view is not universally held, but we hope that our recommendation is a good basis for debate.

What constitutes "unduly small" is open to debate and depends on the context. It will often be reasonable to curtail the plot when only around 10–20% are still in follow-up. For example, suppose in a trial of 500 patients, 100 had the event of interest by 2 years of follow-up, but of the remaining 400 patients, only 80 (20%) were still in follow-up beyond 2 years. In this case, restriction of the plot to 2 years' follow-up might be sensible. Such a restriction is just for the plot; all events should be retained in analysis (eg, nine *vs* 18 events in the ramipril trial should remain the basis for the statistical inference given in the legend of figure 2). In this example, the authors' dilemma is clear, since all the "action" happens beyond 48 months. However, were the later follow-up to be included in the plot, it should include a note highlighting the small number of patients on which the data were based. These problems do not arise for trials with an intended fixed length of follow-up (usually quite short), as was the case for 21 of the trials we surveyed.

Showing the extent of follow-up

So, readers need to be informed about the extent of follow-up, and stating the median follow-up time is often useful. Another helpful device is to display the numbers of patients event-free and still in follow-up in each treatment group at relevant time points, as shown in figures 1 and 3. These numbers at risk of the event convey to the reader the increasing unreliability of estimates as time gets further from randomisation; most trials we surveyed included this information. The numbers on the time axis of the published 4S trial plot[13] reproduced in figure 3 show a case for not extending the

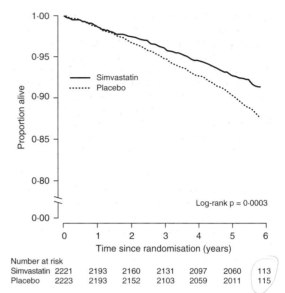

Number at risk							
Simvastatin	2221	2193	2160	2131	2097	2060	113
Placebo	2223	2193	2152	2103	2059	2011	115

Figure 3 Kaplan-Meier curves for all-cause mortality in 4S trial.

graph to 6 years. Since only a small minority of patients reached 6 years' follow-up, the apparent extra boost in treatment difference in that last year is less reliably estimated. Incidentally, plots going downwards with an axis break like figure 3 make focusing on the main finding harder. We needed a ruler and calculator to work out that mortality rates after 5 years were 7.4% on simvastatin and 9.7% on placebo.

Displaying statistical uncertainty

Most outcome results of clinical trials include measures of statistical uncertainty—eg, either SEs or CIs—for each treatment group, or a CI for the comparison of groups. However, survival plots often fail to include such measures. Hence the visual impression of any treatment differences, and how they vary over time, can look much more convincing than is really the case, especially if the clinical trial has few outcome events.

For any time since randomisation, the SE (or 95% CI) for the estimated proportion of patients with (or without) the event can be calculated.[2,3] In principle, such error bands could be displayed at all time points for each treatment group, but displaying the SE or 95% CI at a few regularly spaced time points on the plot for each treatment group is clearer. For instance, figure 1 (top panel) shows the SE bars for the estimated event rate for each treatment at 1, 2, and 3 years' follow-up. As is common in such plots, the smaller numbers of patients in follow-up at later time points is reflected in the increasing SE over time.

Although these SEs display each plot's uncertainty, they do not directly display the uncertainty of the treatment difference, which is usually of primary interest. In fact, the SE of the treatment difference in event rates is equal to the square root of the sum of the two squared SEs, but there is no conventionally accepted style (nor any easy way) of displaying this on a survival plot. One simple rule of thumb is that if the treatment difference at a particular time is less than the sum of the two plotted SEs (ie, if the plotted SEs overlap), the difference is well within the bounds of random chance. If the difference is more than twice the sum of the SEs (ie, the 95% CIs do not overlap) it is highly significant. Whether SEs or 95% CIs should be plotted is open to debate, but authors should always make clear which is being used.

One problem here is the focus on the difference between treatments at particular arbitrary time points. The overall evidence of a treatment difference is usually given by the estimated hazard ratio (sometimes called relative risk) and its 95% CI,[14] and by a log-rank test of significance,[2,3] as shown in the legend of figure 2. Thus, an alternative to plotting SEs is to present overall treatment comparisons and their uncertainty on the survival plot or its legend. Most authors do neither, leaving any comment on statistical uncertainty to the text only. In fact, only one of the 35 trial reports we surveyed included CIs at regular time points on the survival plot, five plots included the hazard ratio and its CI, and 16 plots incorporated the log-rank p value. 18 plots included none of the above. We recommend that future authors include in each survival plot some indication of statistical uncertainty (panel).

Interpreting the shape of survival plots

The easiest patterns to interpret are those that show no apparent difference between treatments or when there is a steady divergence between treatments over time. However, in many instances, more complex patterns seem to exist: the treatment difference might look greater early on (figure 1), the divergence between treatments might start later on (figures 2 and 3), or the survival curves might cross. Such putative treatment–time interactions need cautious interpretation since there are rarely sufficient data to consolidate their true existence.

For instance, in the ramipril trial (figure 2), most of ramipril's benefit seems to have occurred late: nine ramipril failures versus 11 conventional treatment failures before 48 months, compared with zero failures versus seven failures, respectively, after 48 months. However, the strength of evidence for this effect is limited, since the number of failures is small, the statistical test for treatment–time interaction is of borderline significance, and such a post-hoc (data-driven) analysis is disputable. So, the overall conclusion needs to rest on events during the total follow-up rather than after any specific time point.

Even for the much larger 4S trial (figure 3), caution is required in interpreting the visual impression that the treatment effect does not occur until after 18 months' follow-up. There seem to have been 55 deaths in each group in the first 18 months, and a striking treatment difference thereafter, with 201 versus 127 deaths favouring simvastatin.[13] A test for treatment–time interaction (ie, of whether the hazard ratio is different before and after 18 months) is significant (p = 0.03), but its validity can be questioned because the 18-month time-split for the data has been selected post hoc after seeing the survival plot. Thus, even in such a large trial, to expect reliable estimation of when a treatment effect first begins is unrealistic.[15] Indeed, recent evidence from the Heart Protection Study indicates that there is an observable treatment difference in survival even in early follow-up, which becomes more rapidly divergent beyond 2 years (www.hpsinfo.org).

Summary of recommendations

- Survival plots are best presented going upwards, to maximise detail without needing a break in the scale
- Plots should only be extended through the period of follow-up achieved by a reasonable proportion of participants
- The extent of follow-up should be explained—eg, by listing at regular intervals under the time axis the number still at risk in each treatment group
- Plots should include some measure of statistical uncertainty, otherwise any visual signs of treatment differences might look more convincing than they really are. Either SEs or CIs should be displayed at regular time points, or an overall estimate of treatment difference (eg, relative risk) with its 95% CI should be given
- Authors and readers should be cautious in interpreting the shape of survival plots. The lack of follow-up and poorer estimation to the right-hand end, the lack of any prespecified hypothesis, and the lack of statistical power to explore subtleties of treatment difference other than the overall comparison should be recognised

References

1 Kaplan EL, Meier P. Nonparametric estimation from incomplete observations. *J Am Stat Assoc* 1958; **53:** 457–81.

2 Collett D. Modelling survival data in medical research, section 2.1. London: Chapman and Hall, 1994.

3 Altman DG. Practical statistics for medical research, chapter 13. London: Chapman and Hall, 1991.

4 Altman DG, De Stavola BL, Love SB, Stepniewska KA. Review of survival analyses published in cancer journals. *Br J Cancer* 1995; **72:** 511–18.

5 RITA-2 Trial Participants. Coronary angioplasty versus medical therapy for angina: the second Randomised Intervention Treatment of Angina (RITA-2) trial. *Lancet* 1997; **350:** 461–68.

6 Pitt B, Poole-Wilson A, Segal R, et al. Effect of losartan compared with captopril on mortality in patients with symptomatic heart failure: randomised trial—the Losartan Heart Failure Survival Study ELITE II. *Lancet* 2000; **355:** 1582–87.

7 Hall A. Comparison of losartan and captopril in ELITE II. *Lancet* 2000; **356:** 851.

8 Tonkin AM, Colquhoun D, Emberson J, et al. Effects of pravastatin in 3260 patients with unstable angina: results from the LIPID study. *Lancet* 2000; **356:** 1871–75.

9 Matthay KM, Villablanca JG, Seeger RC, et al. Treatment of high-risk neuroblastoma with intensive chemotherapy, radiotherapy, autologous bone marrow transplantation, and 13-*cis*-retinoic acid. *N Engl J Med* 1999; **341:** 1165–73.

10 Altman DG, Anderson PK. Calculating the number needed to treat for trials where the outcome is time to an event. *BMJ* 1999; **319:** 1492–95.

11 Lubsen J, Hoes A, Grobbee D. Implications of trial results: the potentially misleading notions of number needed to treat and average duration of life gained. *Lancet* 2000; **356:** 1757–59.

12 Ruggenenti P, Perna A, Gherardi G, et al. Renoprotective properties of ACE-inhibition in non-diabetic nephropathies with non-nephrotic proteinuria. *Lancet* 2000; **354:** 359–64.

13 Scandinavian Simvastatin Survival Study Group. Randomised trial of cholesterol lowering in 4444 patients with coronary heart disease: the Scandinavian Simvastatin Survival Study (4S). *Lancet* 1994; **344:** 1383–89.

14 Altman DG, Machin D, Bryant TN, Gardner MJ, eds. Statistics with confidence, chapter 9. London: BMJ Publishing, 2000.

15 Boutitie F, Gueyffier F, Pocock SJ, Boissel J-P. Assessing treatment-time interaction in clinical trials with time to event data: a meta-analysis of hypertension trials. *Stat Med* 1998; **17:** 2883–903.

Survival after surgery or therapeutic catheterisation for congenital heart disease in children in the United Kingdom: analysis of the central cardiac audit database for 2000–1

John L Gibbs, James L Monro, David Cunningham, Anthony Rickards

Abstract

Objectives   To analyse simple national statistics and survival data collected in the central cardiac audit database after treatment for congenital heart disease and to provide long term comparative statistics for each contributing centre.

Design   Prospective, longitudinal, observational, national cohort survival study.

Setting   UK central cardiac audit database.

Main outcome measures   Survival at 30 days and one year after treatment in the year April 2000–March 2001, assessed by using both volunteered life status and independently validated life status through the Office for National Statistics, using the patient's unique NHS number, or the general register offices of Scotland and Northern Ireland. Institutional results following a group of six benchmark operations and three benchmark catheterisation procedures.

Results   Since April 2000 data have been received from all 13 UK tertiary centres performing cardiac surgery or therapeutic cardiac catheterisation in children with congenital heart disease. Altogether 3666 surgical procedures and 1828 therapeutic catheterisations were performed. Central tracking of mortality identified 469 deaths, 194 occurring within 30 days and 275 later. Forty two of the 194 deaths within 30 days were detected by central tracking but not by volunteered data. For surgery overall, survival at 30 days was 94.9%, falling to 91.2% at one year; this effect was most marked for infants. For therapeutic catheterisation survival at 30 days was 99.1%, falling to 98.1% at one year. Survival of individual centres or individual operators did not differ from the national average after benchmark procedures.

Conclusions   Independent data validation is essential for accurate survival analysis. One year survival gives a more realistic view of outcome than traditional perioperative mortality. Currently no detectable difference exists in survival between any of the 13 UK tertiary congenital heart disease centres, but confidence intervals for small centres are wide, limiting our power to detect underperformance from analysis of a single year's data. Appropriately resourced, focused national audit is capable of accurate data collection on which nationwide, long term quality control can be based.

Introduction

Monitoring of survival rates after cardiac surgery was introduced in the United Kingdom in 1977 with voluntary submission of data to the Society of Cardiothoracic Surgeons of Great Britain and Ireland. The central cardiac audit database was established by the British Cardiac Society, the Society of Cardiothoracic Surgeons, and the British Paediatric Cardiac Association to provide national analysis of outcomes of cardiac surgery and therapeutic cardiac catheterisation. It differs in three major aspects from previous national audit projects: data are collected electronically in a secure format; mortality and reintervention are tracked centrally by using

doi 10.1136/bmj.38027.613403.F6

Central Cardiac Audit Database, Department of Paediatric Cardiology, Leeds General Infirmary, Calverley, Leeds LSI 3EX
jgibbs@boltblue.com

John L Gibbs *lead clinician for congenital heart disease*

Society of Cardiothoracic Surgeons of England and Ireland, Southampton General Hospital, Southampton SO16 6YD

James L Monro *past president*

Central Cardiac Audit Database, Royal Brompton Hospital, London SW3 6NP

David Cunningham *technical director*
Anthony Rickards *director*

Correspondence to: J Gibbs
(email: jgibbs@boltblue.com)

(Accepted 2 December 2003)

Originally published in *BMJ* 2004; **328**. Reproduced with permission.

a unique patient identifier (the NHS number); and independent data validation is used. In 2000 the Department of Health funded the central cardiac audit database to collate data from all centres for congenital heart disease in the United Kingdom. This report contains the first year's data (1 April 2000 to 31 March 2001), with centrally tracked one year survival. The results are presented on behalf of the Society of Cardiothoracic Surgeons, the British Paediatric Cardiac Association, and all contributing centres, each of which gave consent to publication of identifiable, centre specific data.

Methods
Data collection
We designed a minimum dataset of 20 fields with the simple aims of the project in mind. All 13 congenital heart disease centres in England, Scotland, and Northern Ireland participated. To ensure patient confidentiality the central cardiac audit database employs advanced data encryption technology to control access to data through a secure key system. We used lists with fixed choices consisting of all but the rarest and most complex combinations of diagnoses and procedures to minimise the potential complexities of diagnostic and procedural coding for congenital heart disease.

Data validation
The minimum dataset included date of death, but we linked with the Office for National Statistics by using NHS numbers to assess mortality wherever possible. We compared volunteered mortality data with centrally tracked data. In Northern Ireland and Scotland we used the general register offices to track mortality centrally.

The central cardiac audit database includes other forms of independent data validation carried out by visiting centres, when two weeks' submitted data, chosen at random, are compared with hospitals' written medical records, with operating theatres' records, and with laboratory records on cardiac catheterisation.

We checked entries in the logbooks for operating theatres and catheter laboratories for the entire year in each centre, to ensure complete ascertainment of caseload. We also compared submitted data with nationally held hospital episode statistics whenever these were accessible.

Data analysis
We used the online Lotus Domino version of the central cardiac audit database to collect data and transferred these

Survival for neonates, infants, all children under 1 year, and children between 1 year and 16 years undergoing surgery or therapeutic catheterisation

Age	No. of procedures	% survival at 30 days (99% CI)	% survival at 1 year (99% CI)
All surgery (bypass and non-bypass)			
All ages	3666	94.9 (94.5 to 95.1)	91.2 (90.6 to 91.5)
Neonate and infant:	2073	93.1 (92.4 to 93.4)	87.7 (85.2 to 89.8)
Neonate	780	90.9 (89.4 to 91.5)	86.1 (84.1 to 87.2)
Infant	1293	94.5 (93.6 to 94.7)	88.7 (87.4 to 89.4)
Child	1561	97.7 (97.0 to 97.7)	96.1 (95.4 to 96.2)
Bypass surgery			
All ages	2664	94.7 (94.2 to 94.9)	91.8 (91.1 to 92.1)
Neonate and infant:	1292	92.1 (91.1 to 92.5)	87.8 (84.6 to 90.3)
Neonate	383	87.1 (84.3 to 88.4)	82.8 (79.4 to 84.8)
Infant	909	94.4 (93.3 to 94.7)	90.0 (88.4 to 90.6)
Child	1353	97.5 (96.8 to 97.5)	96.0 (95.1 to 96.1)
Non-bypass surgery			
All ages	1002	95.5 (94.6 to 95.7)	89.7 (88.3 to 90.4)
Neonate and infant:	781	94.6 (93.4 to 94.9)	87.6 (83.4 to 90.8)
Neonate	397	94.7 (92.5 to 95.0)	89.3 (86.5 to 90.3)
Infant	384	94.6 (92.5 to 94.9)	85.9 (82.7 to 87.3)
Child	208	98.8 (95.0 to 98.8)	97.4 (93.2 to 97.5)
Catheter intervention			
All ages	1828	99.1 (98.7 to 99.1)	98.1 (97.6 to 98.1)
Neonate and infant:	472	98.3 (96.7 to 98.3)	96.1 (92.5 to 97.9)
Neonate	178	98.8 (94.9 to 98.8)	97.3 (93.0 to 97.4)
Infant	294	98.0 (95.4 to 98.0)	95.3 (92.4 to 95.6)
Child	1320	99.4 (98.8 to 99.4)	98.8 (98.1 to 98.7)

Survival is calculated based only on cases where follow up reaches 30 days or one year and no further intervention has taken place. The Wilson score method was used to calculate 99% confidence intervals for survival.

Originally published in *BMJ* 2004; **328**. Reproduced with permission.

for analysis to SPSS 10.0 for Microsoft Windows. We used Wilson's score method to calculate confidence intervals for survival.[1,2] We used 99% confidence intervals (table) to make allowances for the high number of multiple comparisons, to minimise false positive results. We did not consider an individual survival value to be significantly different from the mean if the confidence intervals overlapped the mean.

We used analysis of survival after "benchmark" operations to compare results from different centres, to eliminate the effect of different case mix. We chose six benchmark procedures for surgery (repairs of atrial septal defect, ventricular septal defect, atrioventricular septal defect, tetralogy of Fallot, simple transposition of the great arteries, and coarctation) and three for therapeutic catheterisation (atrial septal defect closure, arterial duct closure, and pulmonary balloon valvoplasty). We did not undertake detailed risk stratification as no validated method exists.

We calculated 30 day postoperative survival to facilitate comparison with results from previous UK registry data and to comply with practice in the United States.[3] Central tracking of mortality has, however, also allowed us to plot one year survival curves, in contrast to previous registry analyses. We included foreign nationals but censored them from survival analysis after the perioperative period unless specific follow up data were available (central tracking was not possible for this group). We analysed individual operators' results anonymously, but each centre agreed to be identified. We have not calculated freedom from reintervention statistics for this report as follow up is currently too short to allow meaningful interpretation of results.

Results

Data collection and quality
Overall completeness of the dataset was 96.8%, with completeness for individual data fields ranging from 75% (for NHS number) to 100%. Data were received for a total of 5494 procedures, of which 3666 were surgical and 1828 were therapeutic catheterisations.

We have reported all cause mortality, choosing not to attempt detailed investigation of cause of death and its relation to treatment. We found substantial differences in volunteered and centrally tracked mortality, with seven of 11 centres in England under-reporting death within 30 days. Central tracking of mortality identified 469 deaths, 194 occurring within 30 days and 275 later. Forty two of the 194 deaths within 30 days were detected by central tracking but were not in the volunteered data. Nineteen of these patients were discharged alive but subsequently died within 30 days of the operation. The remainder had been incorrectly coded as alive at discharge; using reported discharge status would have underestimated 30 day mortality by 22%. Data on hospital episode statistics were available for 2716 patients and under-reported death within 30 days by 9%, classifying 1% of surviving patients as deceased. Hospital episode statistics data also under-reported the total number of procedures by 10%. During validation visits we found a total of 143 procedures to be missing from the data submissions to the central cardiac

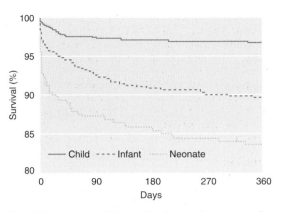

Figure 1 One year survival after cardiopulmonary bypass surgery for age groups <1 month, 1 month–1 year, and 1–16 years for the United Kingdom.

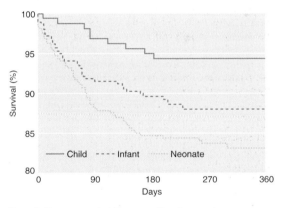

Figure 2 One year survival for non cardiopulmonary bypass surgery for age groups <1 month, 1 month–1 year, and 1–16 years for the United Kingdom.

audit database, predominantly related to systematic errors in data collection. The visits resulted in submission of missing or revised data from all of the 13 centres.

Survival
Figures 1–3 show national survival curves after cardiopulmonary bypass surgery, non-cardiopulmonary bypass surgery or therapeutic catheterisation. The table shows survival at 30 days and one year after all procedures. We assessed benchmark procedure survival anonymously for individual operators (41 surgeons and 63 cardiologists) as well as for different centres. No significant difference from the national mean survival was detectable for any individual. Figures 4 and 5 and figures A-I (see bmj.com), respectively, show individual centre's survival data for pooled and individual benchmark procedures.

Originally published in *BMJ* 2004; **328**. Reproduced with permission.

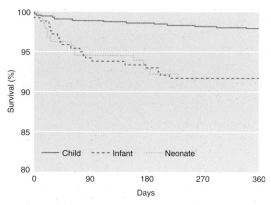

Figur 3 One year survival for therapeutic catheterisation for age groups <1 month, 1 month–1 year, and 1–16 years for the United Kingdom.

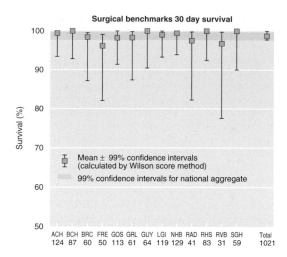

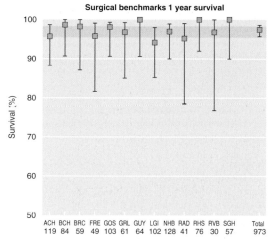

Figure 4 Survival at 30 days and at one year reported by individual centre, with 99% confidence intervals for all benchmark surgical procedures. The shaded areas represent the national means with 99% confidence intervals. If a centre's confidence intervals overlap the shaded area their survival does not differ statistically from the national mean. For a list of the abbreviations see bmj.com.

Discussion
Data quality
We found a striking difference in deaths identified by centres' own records and by central tracking. This was most marked when death occurred after the perioperative period, but deaths were missing from submitted data even when death occurred within 30 days. It seems inevitable that previous registry reports (including the register of the Society of Cardiothoracic Surgeons, used in the Bristol inquiry) that have relied on voluntary reporting of death have also under-reported mortality, casting doubt on their validity. The introduction of the NHS number as a unique and permanent patient identifier and the ability to establish electronic linkage with the Office for National Statistics is a major advance in tracking patients' outcomes.

Risk stratification
The use of benchmark procedures minimises the effect of varying case mix for the purposes of comparison of outcomes in different centres. Attempts have been made to establish a consensus view of risk assessment in the United States[4] and case complexity in the United Kingdom.[5] These protocols, applied to the data in the central cardiac audit database that have been accumulated over several years, should facilitate development and validation of risk stratification for the future.

Patient confidentiality
We did not include patients' consent for data submission to the central cardiac audit database in our protocol. Our current understanding of the Data Protection Act 1998 is that patients' consent is not required if anonymised data are used for the purpose of research or audit. The exception to anonymising data is the NHS number, which we have protected by encryption with a key held only by the data managers and used only for record linkage. In the United Kingdom we have

an almost unique opportunity to carry out effective and believable national audit because we have a single health care system with an Office for National Statistics where the life status of an individual patient, based on their NHS number, is known.

With appropriate precautions central tracking is possible while maintaining patient confidentiality.

Diagnostic and procedure coding
Several groups have devised coding systems for congenital heart disease.[3,6,7] The central cardiac audit database plans to adopt the coding system of the Association for European

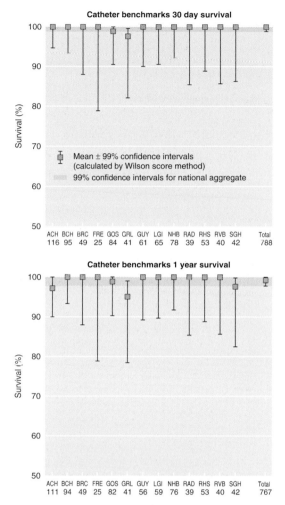

Catheter benchmarks 30 day survival

Survival (%)

Mean ± 99% confidence intervals
(calculated by Wilson score method)

99% confidence intervals for national aggregate

ACH	BCH	BRC	FRE	GOS	GRL	GUY	LGI	NHB	RAD	RHS	RVB	SGH	Total
116	95	49	25	84	41	61	65	78	39	53	40	42	788

Catheter benchmarks 1 year survival

Survival (%)

ACH	BCH	BRC	FRE	GOS	GRL	GUY	LGI	NHB	RAD	RHS	RVB	SGH	Total
111	94	49	25	82	41	56	59	76	39	53	40	42	767

Figure 5 Survival at 30 days and at one year reported by individual centre, with 99% confidence intervals for all benchmark catheter procedures. The shaded areas represent the national means with 99% confidence intervals. If a centre's confidence intervals overlap the shaded area their survival does not differ statistically from the national mean. For a list of the abbreviations see bmj.com.

Paediatric Cardiology[7] from 2004, to facilitate future international compatibility of data.

Outcomes after treatment

Centre specific data analysis shows that quality of treatment is high throughout the United Kingdom; no centre and no individual operator has detectably different survival from the national mean after benchmark procedures. We have been unable to assess accurately how our results compare with those of other nations, although our data seem to compare favourably with unvalidated registry reports from North America and Europe.

What is already known on this topic

The validity of previous voluntary registers of survival after surgery has long been held to be potentially inaccurate

The Bristol inquiry report highlighted the inadequacy of current national audit, particularly for the treatment of congenital heart disease

What this study adds

Volunteered survival data are of little value, sometimes overestimating survival by as much as 20%

Data validation is essential for national or local audit of survival and has been made far easier by the introduction of the NHS number and the ability to use it to create electronic links to the Office for National Statistics

Traditionally reported perioperative (30 day) mortality can give a misleadingly optimistic view of prognosis to both professionals and the public; for infants mortality after treatment for heart disease at one year was double that at 30 days

The central cardiac audit database places validated, centre specific survival results for treatment of children with congenital heart disease in the public domain

We believe that this study is the first to present validated, centre specific survival data for nationwide treatment of congenital heart disease. Population based, 45 year, actuarial survival has been reported for the whole of Finland,[8] but individual centres' performance was not included. Most previous reports have concentrated on multicentre, mean perioperative mortalities (defined as death within 30 days of operation),[9] and a similar approach was used for the register of the Society of Cardiothoracic Surgeons.[10] Although this simplistic approach may be convenient, our data show how misleading 30 day results may be as a descriptor of overall outcome.

We calculated 99% confidence intervals for the purpose of assessing survival in different centres. Even at this level, having performed a total of 178 comparisons, we think that it is likely that we will generate spuriously significant results: we calculate that the chance of at least one spuriously significant difference in survival is 83% (this would have been 99.99% had we used 95% confidence intervals).

This early data analysis has concentrated on survival, which is a crude indicator of overall performance. For smaller centres, as well as for individual operators, analysis of a single year's data has limited power to detect underperformance by institutions or individual operators and year on year analysis will be necessary to provide more robust reassurance. Freedom from reintervention is likely to be a powerful indicator of overall performance, but several years' data will be required before our capability to track reintervention can be put to use.

Conclusions

Independent validation of data is essential for accurate survival analysis. One year survival statistics give a more realistic view of outcome than traditional perioperative mortality. At present survival is no different between any of the 13 UK tertiary centres for congenital heart disease, but confidence intervals are wide, limiting our power to detect underperformance from analysis of a single year's data. Appropriately resourced, focused, national audit is capable of accurate data collection on which nationwide, long term, quality control can be based.

The paper was written on behalf of the Society of Cardiothoracic Surgeons of Great Britain and Northern Ireland, the British Paediatric Cardiac Association, and the congenital heart disease units of Alder Hey Hospital, Liverpool; Birmingham Children's Hospital; Bristol Royal Hospital for Sick Children; Freeman Hospital, Newcastle; Glenfield Hospital, Leicester; Great Ormond Street Hospital, London; Guy's Hospital, London; John Radcliffe Hospital, Oxford; Leeds General Infirmary; Royal Brompton and Harefield NHS Trust, London; Royal Hospital for Sick Children, Glasgow; Royal Victoria Hospitals, Belfast; and Southampton General Hospital.

Contributors: JLG, DC, and AR initiated the study. DC analysed the data. JLG, JLM, and AR drafted the report. All four authors are guarantors on behalf of the 13 centres that contributed data.

Funding: The National Health Service Information Authority (NHSIA) funded the central data collection, data validation, and data analysis.

Competing interests: None declared.

References

1 Wilson EB. Probable inference, the law of succession, and statistical inference. *J Am Stat Assoc* 1927;22:209–12.

2 Newcombe R. Two sided confidence intervals for the single proportion: a comparative evaluation of seven methods. *Stat Med* 1998;17:857–72.

3 Mavroudis C, Jacobs JP. Congenital heart surgery nomenclature and database project: Overview and minimum dataset. *Ann Thorac Surg* 2000;69:S2–17.

4 Jenkins KJ, Gauvreau K, Newburger JW, Spray TL, Moller JH, Iezzoni LI. Consensus-based method for risk adjustment for surgery for congenital heart disease. *J Thorac Cardiovasc Surg* 2002;123:110–18.

5 Gallivan S, Davis KB, Stark JF. Early identification of divergent performance in congenital cardiac surgery. *Eur J Cardiothorac Surg* 2001;20:1214–9.

6 Lacour-Gayet F, Maruszewski B, Mavroudis C, Jacobs JP, Elliott MJ. Presentation of the international nomenclature for congenital heart surgery. The long way from nomenclature to collection of validated data at the EACTS. *Eur J Cardiothorac Surg* 2000;18:128–35.

7 Franklin RC, Anderson RH, Daniels O, Elliott M, Gewillig MH, Ghisla R, et al. Report of the coding committee of the Association for European Paediatric Cardiology. *Cardiol Young* 2000;10 (suppl 1):1–26.

8 Nieminen HP, Jokinen EV, Sairanen HI. Late results of pediatric cardiac surgery in Finland: a population-based study with 96% follow-up. *Circulation* 2001;104:570–5.

9 Stark J, Gallivan S, Lovegrove J, Hamilton JR, Monro JL, Pollock JC, et al. Mortality rates after surgery for congenital heart defects in children and surgeons' performance *Lancet* 2000;355:1004–7.

10 Aylin P, Alves B, Best N, Cook A, Elliott P, Evans SWJ, et al. Comparison of UK paediatric cardiac surgical performance by analysis of routinely collected data 1984–1996: was Bristol an outlier? *Lancet* 2001;358:181–7.

UNIT 10

Diagnostic and screening statistics

Aims

To understand how to calculate and interpret the results of statistics that describe the utility of diagnostic tests used in clinical practice and screening tests used in populations.

Learning objectives

On completion of this unit, participants will be able to understand:

- the differences between the application of diagnostic and screening tests;
- why positive and negative predictive values have limited applicability;
- why sensitivity, specificity and likelihood ratios are robust statistics for describing the utility of diagnostic and screening tests;
- the ways in which sample size affects the precision of diagnostic and screening statistics.

Background

In clinical medicine, it is often important to know the efficiency of a screening or diagnostic test in predicting a medical condition. In general, a screening test is used to identify non-symptomatic people in a population who may have a disease. On the other hand, a diagnostic test is used to identify a disease in patients who have presented to a clinical practice because they have symptoms that are consistent with a disease or because they have a positive result from a screening test. Diagnosis is the second step in the pathway to confirm or reject the indication of abnormality.[1]

The objectives of diagnostic and screening tests may include the detection or exclusion of disease and the assessment of prognosis.[2] For example, a psychological test could be used as a diagnostic test to help a clinician decide whether a patient has evidence of clinical depression. An X-ray may be used to identify the presence of pneumonia or a bone fracture. In community settings, screening tests such as mammograms are used for the early detection of disease in the general population.

For diagnostic or screening tests to be efficient, it is important to have accurate information about their utility. Most diagnostic and screening tests are inherently imperfect, so knowledge of the degree of accuracy in predicting disease is important for helping health care practitioners to interpret the value of a positive or a negative test result and to decide whether to recommend further diagnostic tests or treatments.

Glossary

Term	Definition
Screening test	Test used for early identification of disease in a population without symptoms.
Diagnostic test	Test used to confirm disease in people who present with signs or symptoms.
Gold standard	Test regarded as the most accurate method available for classifying people as disease positive or negative.

For estimating the utility of diagnostic or screening tests, we use statistics that describe how closely the test result and the presence or absence of the disease are related. These statistics come from a special class of methods that are used to describe the within-subject agreement between two measurements. In evaluating diagnostic and screening tests, it is essential that a 'gold standard' is used to classify the presence or absence of the disease. If a gold standard test is not available, a proxy gold standard can be used, but the result from the test being evaluated must not be included in the proxy definition.[3] It is also essential that the people who record the results of the diagnostic or screening test result are blinded to the 'gold standard' test result, that is, the disease status of the patient. Blinding avoids bias that may result from expectation if people who are responsible for interpreting the test result have prior knowledge of whether the disease is present or absent.

147

Table 10.1 Diagnostic statistics

	Disease present	Disease absent	Total
Test positive	a	b	a + b
Test negative	c	d	c + d
Total	a + c	b + d	N

Diagnostic and screening statistics

In computing diagnostic and screening statistics, the variable indicating disease status is best coded as 0 (or 1) for disease present as measured by the gold standard or test positive, and 1 (or 2) for disease absent or test negative. When using this coding schedule, the most commonly used statistical packages will provide a table as shown in Table 10.1 where the group with disease present is represented in the left-hand data column of the table and the group who do not have the disease is represented in the right-hand data column. Similarly, the group who are test positive are represented on the top data row of the table and the group who are test negative are represented on the bottom data row of the table. The layout of disease positive and negative groups in Table 10.1 is commonly used in clinical epidemiology, and is essentially the same format that we have used to calculate statistics, such as a chi-square value and odds ratio as discussed in Units 3 and 4.

Positive and negative predictive values

In estimating the utility of a test, both positive predictive value (PPV) and negative predictive value (NPV) can be calculated. From Table 10.1, these values are calculated as follows:

Positive predictive value (PPV) = $a/(a + b)$
Negative predictive value (NPV) = $d/(c + d)$

PPV is the proportion of test-positive patients in whom the disease is present and NPV is the proportion of test-negative patients in whom the disease is absent. As such, these two tests 'look forwards' in that PPV is the probability that a patient will have a disease if they have a positive test result and NPV is the probability that a patient will not have a disease if they have a negative test result.

The statistics PPV and NPV indicate the probability that the test will make a correct diagnosis,[4] and therefore it seems intuitive that these values would be useful statistics. However, PPV and NPV have serious limitations because their interpretation is based on the proportion of the sample with and without disease, and they are therefore influenced by the prevalence of the disease in the sample. The PPV becomes larger when the per cent of patients in the sample who have the disease is high and lower when the per cent of patients in the sample who have the disease is small. As such, PPV

and NPV are heavily influenced by the sampling criteria and the inherent characteristics of the population in addition to the utility of the test.

For this reason, these statistics should only be calculated if the study sample is a random population sample. These statistics should not be calculated from a case-control study in which groups of patients and healthy people are recruited independently. This design is commonly used in studies designed to assess diagnostic tests. If PPV and NPV are calculated from a study in which a selected sample is enrolled, and therefore the per cent with disease is different from the prevalence of disease in the population, the results can rarely be generalised to other settings with different patient profiles or compared against the diagnostic utility of other diagnostic tests.

TAKE HOME LIST

- PPV and NPV can only be generalised to other settings when they are calculated from a random population sample.

- PPV and NPV will change if the prevalence of the disease changes. When the per cent of patients in the sample who have the disease increases, PPV will increase and NPV will decrease.

- PPV is inflated when the frequency of people with disease in the sample is higher than in the general population.

Sensitivity and specificity

Because PPV and NPV have serious limitations in their interpretation, the statistics most often used to describe the utility of diagnostic and screening tests are sensitivity and specificity.[5] These diagnostic statistics can be computed from Table 10.1 as follows:

Sensitivity = $a/(a + c)$
Specificity = $d/(b + d)$

Sensitivity indicates how likely a patient is to have a positive test if they have the disease and specificity indicates how likely the patient is to have a negative test if they do not have the disease. Thus, these two statistics 'look backwards' in that they describe the proportion of patients in each disease category who are test-positive or test-negative. Sensitivity is computed from only the people in whom the disease is present and specificity is computed from only the people in whom the disease is absent and therefore neither statistic is influenced by the prevalence of the disease in the sample.

The notation shown in Table 10.1 can be extended to show the terminology often used with sensitivity and specificity as shown in Table 10.2. Because the interpretation of sensitivity

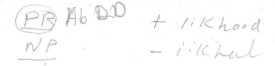

Table 10.2 Terms used in diagnostic statistics

	Disease present	Disease absent	Total
Test-positive	a	b	
	TP	FP	
	(true +ve)	(false +ve)	
	Sensitivity	1 – Specificity	
Test-negative	c	d	
	FN	TN	
	(false –ve)	(true –ve)	
	1 – Sensitivity	Specificity	
Total	a + c	b + d	N

Glossary

Term	Definition
Positive predictive value	Proportion of test-positive people who have the disease.
Negative predictive value	Proportion of test-negative people who do not have the disease.
Sensitivity	Proportion of disease-positive people who are test-positive.
Specificity	Proportion of disease-negative people who are test-negative.
Likelihood ratio	Probability of a positive test in a person with the disease compared to the probability of a positive test in a person without disease.

and specificity is not necessarily intuitive, it is often helpful if the classification of true-positives (TP), false-positives (FP), true-negatives (TN) and false-negatives (FN) are calculated for each quadrant of table.[6] The false-negative group is the proportion of patients who have the disease and who have a negative test result. The false-positive group is the proportion of patients who do not have the disease and who have a positive test result.

From Table 10.2, it can be seen that the rate of false-negatives (FN) is the complement of the rate of true-positives (TP) for patients who have the disease. Similarly, the rate of false-positives (FP) is the complement of the rate of true-negatives (TN) for patients who do not have the disease. It is important to note that there is a trade-off between the rate of true-positives and the rate of true-negatives, that is, between sensitivity and specificity. As sensitivity increases, specificity will decrease and vice versa.

Unravelling the meanings of the terms used for diagnostic and screening tests can be confusing and informative diagrams can help in understanding the concepts.[7] The terminology used for sensitivity and specificity is not logical in that the 'opposites' rule applies in remembering the meaning of

the terms. Sensitivity describes the rate of true test-positives in the group with the disease. However, sensitivity has a 'n' in it and applies to the true-positive group, which begins with 'p'. Similarly, specificity describes the rate of true-test negatives in the group without the disease but has a 'p' in it and applies to the true-negative group, which begins with 'n'.

In the field of clinical epidemiology, SnNout and SpPin are terms that have been coined to aid in the interpretation of sensitivity and specificity.[8] The term SnNout stands for Sensitivity-Negative-out. The interpretation is that if the test has a high sensitivity (true-positive rate) and therefore a low false-negative rate, a negative test result will rule out the disease or diagnosis. A test that is used to screen a population in which many people will not have the disease needs to have high sensitivity so that it will identify most people with the disease. It is counter-intuitive that although sensitivity needs to be high in a test to rule out a disease, this statistic is calculated solely from the column of patients with the disease.

The term SpPin stands for Specificity-Positive-in. The interpretation is that if the test has a high specificity (true-negative rate) and therefore a low false-positive rate, a positive result will rule in the disease. A test that is used to diagnose a disease in patients with symptoms needs to have a low false-positive rate so that it will identify most people who do not have the disease. Although specificity needs to be high for a diagnostic test to rule in a disease, this statistic is calculated solely from the column of patients without the disease.

The interpretation of sensitivity and specificity may not seem directly useful, but these statistics have the advantage that they can be compared between different clinical settings and between studies with different inclusion criteria and in which the prevalence of the disease may be different. Sensitivity and specificity can also be used to compare the diagnostic and screening utility of different tests. Although sensitivity and specificity are not directly affected by prevalence and are therefore less influenced by sampling bias than PPV and NPV, they may still change if the same test is applied in different clinical settings with different types of patients, for example primary, secondary or tertiary health care settings.[9]

TAKE HOME LIST

- Sensitivity and specificity are not influenced by the prevalence of disease in the sample and can be compared between different settings and different tests.

- A high sensitivity will help to rule out a disease.

- Sensitivity is computed from the group of people with the disease.

- A high specificity will help to rule in a disease.

- Specificity is computed from the group of people without the disease.

Interpretation of sensitivity and specificity in screening tests

Although mammography is widely used as a screening test for the early identification of breast cancers, the sensitivity of this test ranges from 75% to 90% depending on the age and family history of the person being screened.[10] However, mammography also has a high specificity of 90–95%.[11] The interpretation of these statistics is that the rate of false-negative results (missed tumours) in a screened population will be 10–25% and the rate of false-positive results (falsely detected tumours) will be 5–10%. On average, it is thought that about 7% of women who are screened will be called back to undergo a diagnostic test, such as a needle biopsy, for a false-positive result and that 10–20% of cancers will be missed with mammography. The incidence of breast cancer, as well the specificity and sensitivity of mammograms, is lower in women under 50. Thus, the cost effectiveness of screening women under 50 years of age who have false-positive results and who are found later to be cancer free has been questioned.[12] In addition, false-positive results may cause anxiety and stress, as well as the need for unnecessary tests such as surgical biopsies, which induce additional costs to the health care system.[12] Although magnetic resonance imaging (MRI) is a more sensitive test in that it has a higher rate of true-positive results than mammograms, the cost of MRI screening makes it prohibitive for use as a screening tool.[13] MRI screening for breast cancer also has a slightly lower specificity than mammograms and therefore produces more false-positive results, hence the need for further diagnostic tests such as biopsies. In health care practice, the balance between the costs and invasiveness of screening and diagnostic tests and the potential effects of false-positive and false-negative results on people who are tested need to be carefully considered.

Likelihood ratio

When applying diagnostic and screening statistics in clinical practice, sensitivity and specificity have limited clinical use for an individual patient, since these statistics are based on the tests when used in the population.[14] In addition, a problem with sensitivity and specificity is that each is calculated from separate parts of the data and therefore the use of one statistic in isolation from the other ignores all of the information available. To combine the information from both statistics, the values can be converted into a likelihood ratio in which data from the total sample is used to estimate the relative predictive value of the test. The likelihood ratio always refers to the likelihood of a patient having a disease.[14] When a patient has a positive test, the positive likelihood ratio (LR+) can be calculated as follows:

$$\text{Likelihood ratio (LR+)} = \text{Probability of a positive result in people with disease/Probability of a positive result in people without disease}$$
$$= \text{True-positives/False-positives}$$
$$= \text{Sensitivity/(1 − Specificity)}$$

Thus, the positive likelihood ratio is simply the ratio of the true-positive rate to the false-positive rate. This statistic provides clinical information about an individual person because it indicates how likely a positive result will be found in a person with the disease compared to a person without the disease. A positive likelihood ratio greater than 1 indicates that a positive test result is associated with the presence of the disease, whereas a positive likelihood ratio of less than 1 indicates that a positive test result is associated with the absence of a disease. For example, a positive likelihood ratio equal to 10 indicates that the person with the disease is about 10 times more likely to have a positive test result than a person without the disease.

Similarly, when a patient has a negative test result, the negative likelihood ratio (LR−) can be calculated as follows:

$$\text{Likelihood ratio (LR−)} = \text{Probability of a negative result in people with disease/Probability of a negative result in people without disease}$$
$$= \text{False-negatives/True-negatives}$$
$$= \text{(1 − Sensitivity)/Specificity}$$

A negative likelihood ratio of less than 1 indicates that a negative result is less likely to occur in a person with the disease compared to a person without the disease. A negative likelihood ratio greater than 10 rules in the disease, while a negative likelihood ratio of less than 0.1 generally rules out the disease.[15] Because a likelihood ratio is derived from sensitivity and specificity, it also has the advantage that valid comparisons of diagnostic and screening statistics between different study samples and between different diagnostic tests can be made.

In practice, a nomogram can be used to convert the pre-test probability of disease in a patient into a post-test probability using the likelihood ratio.[16] The pre-test probability will usually be the prevalence of the disease in the clinical setting that the patient attends. A nomogram is a graphical tool that uses the result of a diagnostic test to calculate a person's probability of having the disease. In a nonogram, the pre-test probability that the person has the disease is entered on the left axis and is then joined by a line to the likelihood ratio on the middle axis. The line is then extended to show the post-test probability of disease on the right axis.

Sample size considerations

The study sample size from which any statistic is calculated has important implications for quantifying the uncertainty around the estimate. Because PPV, NPV, sensitivity and specificity are essentially proportions, uncertainty can be estimated by calculating 95% confidence intervals as discussed in Unit 2. The confidence interval for each statistic is calculated using the sample size as the denominator.

The sample size for sensitivity is the number who are disease-positive and for specificity is the number who are disease-negative.

The 95% confidence intervals can be surprisingly wide when the number in a disease-positive or disease-negative group is small. For this reason, the number of participants in studies designed to measure diagnostic and screening statistics must be large enough to report all of the estimates with precision. Although the sample size in each of the disease-present and disease-absent groups influences the width of the 95% confidence intervals for sensitivity and specificity, few investigators appear to consider sample size requirements when designing studies to calculate diagnostic and screening statistics.[17] Thus, there have been calls for better methods to be used in the assessment of the utility of diagnostic and screening tests including the use of systematic reviews to increase precision.[2] In addition, a comprehensive checklist for the accurate reporting of diagnostic and screening utility has been developed by a steering group called the Standards for Reporting of Diagnostic Accuracy (STARD).[18]

Reading and questions
Reprint
Grimes DA, Schultz KF. Uses and abuses of screening tests. Lancet 2002;359:881–884. (See p. 154.)

The reprint by Grimes and Schultz (2002) discusses the advantages and the disadvantages to screening tests and the terms – PPV, NPV, sensitivity and specificity which describe the utility of a test. After reading the reprint by Grimes and Schultz (2002), answer the following questions.

1 What are the limitations in classifying people as either disease-present or disease-absent?
2 How does a low prevalence rate of disease in a population affect the PPV?
3 What would a PPV of 0.50 indicate?
4 What are the advantages and disadvantages of screening tests in the population?
5 What problems may arise from early diagnosis as a result of a positive screening test?

Worked example
Set article
Nassar N, Roberts C, Cameron CA, Olive EC. Diagnostic accuracy of clinical examination for detection of non-cephalic presentation in late pregnancy: Cross sectional analytic study. BMJ 2006;333:578–580. (See p. 159.)

The set article by Nassar et al. (2006) reports the diagnostic accuracy of a clinical examination in detecting non-cephalic (breech, transverse or oblique lie) presentations in late pregnancy. This is a nicely designed study in which

Table 10.3 Sensitivity and specificity for detecting fetal presentation

	Non-cephalic	Cephalic	Total
Examination positive	91 (true +ve = 91/130 = 0.70)	74 (false +ve = 74/1503 = 0.05)	165
Examination negative	39 (false –ve = 39/130 = 0.30)	1429 (true –ve = 1429/1503 = 0.95)	1468
Total	130	1503	1633

a total of 1633 women underwent clinical examination to assess fetal presentation. Ultrasonography was then used as the gold standard to confirm the fetal position. To reduce bias, the ultrasonographers were blinded to results of the clinical examination.

Using Table 10.2 as a template, the numbers from which overall sensitivity and specificity are calculated were taken from the table in the paper and are shown in Table 10.3. Thus,

PPV = 91/165 = 0.55
NPV = 1429/1468 = 0.97
Sensitivity = 91/130 = 0.70
Specificity = 1429/1503 = 0.95
Positive likelihood ratio = 0.70/0.05 = 14.0

Exercise

Using the section of the table in the reprint that stratifies sensitivity and specificity by maternal body mass index, create tables similar to Table 10.3 to complete Table 10.4 on page 152.

After completing Table 10.4, answer the following questions:
- Are the statistics PPV and NPV appropriate to describe diagnostic utility in the sample studied?
- What populations would these statistics generalise to?
- Does calculation of the likelihood ratio influence how you would interpret the results of the study?
- Do you agree with the authors' conclusion that an ultrasound is only required to determine fetal position in late pregnancy in overweight and obese women?

Critical appraisal

The checklist describes some of the questions that can be asked when critically appraising a report of diagnostic statistics. Work through the checklist to review the paper by Nassar et al. (2006) and decide whether the results warrant a change in clinical practice.

Table 10.4 PPV, NPV and likelihood ratio for detecting fetal presentation

	Sensitivity	Specificity	PPV	NPV	Likelihood ratio
Overall	0.70	0.95	0.55	0.97	14.0
Body mass index					
Thin	0.69	0.95			
Normal weight	0.73	0.96			
Overweight	0.68	0.97			
Obese	0.38	0.89			

Critical appraisal checklist for an article that reports diagnostic statistics	
A. Study design	
1. Was a 'gold standard' used to classify the diagnosis?	
2. Were the test results withheld from the people who decided the diagnosis?	
3. Were standard protocols used for collecting information of both the test and the diagnosis?	
4. Was the interval between the test and the diagnosis short enough so that the diagnosis would not have changed?	
5. Are the inclusion and exclusion criteria clearly described?	
6. Were the participants recruited randomly, by consecutive sampling or by another method?	
B. Statistical methods	
7. Is full information of the positive and negative predictive values and of sensitivity and specificity presented?	
8. Are confidence intervals around these estimates shown?	
C. Results	
9. Is a cross-tabulation provided to aid in the interpretation of the statistics?	
10. Are there sufficient numbers of participants to describe the diagnostic statistics with precision?	
D. Interpretation	
11. Is the clinical applicability of the diagnostic statistics interpreted correctly?	

Quick quiz

Tick the correct answer for each of the following questions.

1 A high sensitivity for a diagnostic test means that:
   (a) your doctor is tuned into your needs;
   (b) if your test is positive, you have a disease;
   (c) the 'true-positive' rate for the test is high;
   (d) you probably do not have the disease.

2 A high specificity for a diagnostic test means that:
   (a) the test is specific for the diagnosis of the disease;
   (b) most people who are test-negative do not have the disease;
   (c) most people who do not have the disease are test-negative;
   (d) a positive result indicates that you probably do have the disease.

3 If the positive predictive value (PPV) is high, a positive test result means that:

(a) the disease is almost certainly present;

(b) the disease is more likely to be present if the PPV was calculated from a random population sample;

(c) you cannot be certain that the disease is absent;

(d) another test is needed to decide the presence of the disease.

4 If the negative predictive value (NPV) is low, a negative test result means that:

(a) another test is needed to rule out the disease;

(b) you almost certainly do not have the disease;

(c) you cannot be certain that the disease is present;

(d) there is a low probability that the disease is absent.

References

1. Kerr C. Assessment of screening tests. In Kerr CB, Taylor R, Heard GS, eds, Handbook of public health methods, McGraw-Hill, Sydney, Australia, 1998; pp 623–626.

2. Knottnerus JA, van Weel C, Muris JWM. Evidence base of clinical diagnosis: Evaluation of diagnostic procedures. BMJ 2002;324: 477–480.

3. Greenhalgh T. How to read a paper. Papers that report diagnostic or screening tests. BMJ 1997;315:540–543.

4. Altman DG, Bland JM. Diagnostic tests 2: predictive values. BMJ 1994;309:102.

5. Altman DG, Bland JM. Diagnostic tests 1: sensitivity and specificity. BMJ 1994;308:1552.

6. Jaeschke R, Guyatt GH, Sackett DL. Users' guides to the medical literature. III. How to use an article about a diagnostic test. B. What are the results and will they help me in caring for my patients? The Evidence-Based Medicine Working Group. JAMA 1994;271: 703–707.

7. Loong T-W. Understanding sensitivity and specificity with the right side of the brain. BMJ 2003;327:716–719.

8. Sackett DL. On some clinically useful measures of the effects of treatment. Evidence-Based Med 1996;1:37–38.

9. Sackett DL, Haynes RB. Evidence base of clinical diagnosis: The architecture of diagnostic research. BMJ 2002;324:539–541.

10. http://en.wikipedia.org/wiki/mammography.

11. http://www.acpm.org/breast.htm.

12. Lidbrink E, Elfving J, Frisell J, Jonsson E. Neglected aspects of false positive findings of mammograph in breast screening: analysis of false positive cases from the Stockholm trial. BMJ 1996;312: 273–276.

13. Kriege M, Brekelmans CT, Boetes C, et al. Efficacy of MRI and mammography for breast-cancer screening in women with a familial or genetic predisposition. N Engl J Med 2004;351:427–437.

14. Attia J. Moving beyond sensitivity and specificity: using likelihood ratios to help interpret diagnostic tests. Aust Prescr 2003;26:111–113.

15. Jaescheke R, Guyatt G, Lijmer J. Diagnostic tests. In Guyatt G, Rennie D, editors. Users' guide to the medical literature: A manual for evidence based clinical practice. AMA Press, Chicago, 2002; pp 121–140.

16. Deeks JJ, Altman DG. Diagnostic tests 4: likelihood ratios. BMJ 2004;329:168–169.

17. Bachmann LM, Puhan MA, ter Riet G, Bossuyt PM. Sample sizes of studies on diagnostic accuracy: Literature survey. BMJ 2006;332:1127–1129.

18. Bossuyt PM, Reitsma JB, Bruns DE, Gatsonis CA, Glasziou PP, Irwig LM, et al. Towards complete and accurate reporting of studies of diagnostic accuracy: The STARD initiative. BMJ 2003;326:41–44.

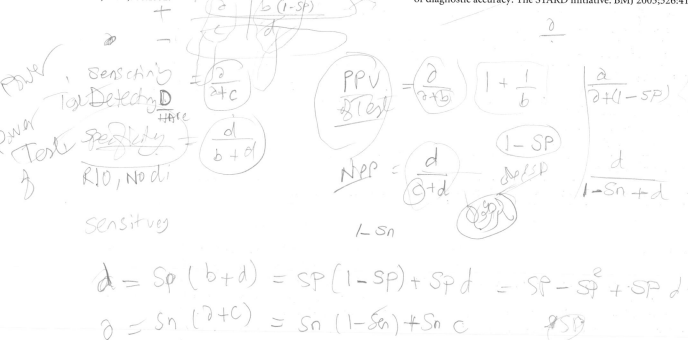

Uses and abuses of screening tests

David A Grimes, Kenneth F Schulz

Screening tests are ubiquitous in contemporary practice, yet the principles of screening are widely misunderstood. Screening is the testing of apparently well people to find those at increased risk of having a disease or disorder. Although an earlier diagnosis generally has intuitive appeal, earlier might not always be better, or worth the cost. Four terms describe the validity of a screening test: sensitivity, specificity, and predictive value of positive and negative results. For tests with continuous variables—eg, blood glucose—sensitivity and specificity are inversely related; where the cutoff for abnormal is placed should indicate the clinical effect of wrong results. The prevalence of disease in a population affects screening test performance: in low-prevalence settings, even very good tests have poor predictive value positives. Hence, knowledge of the approximate prevalence of disease is a prerequisite to interpreting screening test results. Tests are often done in sequence, as is true for syphilis and HIV-1 infection. Lead-time and length biases distort the apparent value of screening programmes; randomised controlled trials are the only way to avoid these biases. Screening can improve health; strong indirect evidence links cervical cytology programmes to declines in cervical cancer mortality. However, inappropriate application or interpretation of screening tests can rob people of their perceived health, initiate harmful diagnostic testing, and squander health-care resources.

Screening is a double-edged sword, sometimes wielded clumsily by the well-intended. Although ubiquitous in contemporary medical practice, screening remains widely misunderstood and misused. Screening is defined as tests done among apparently well people to identify those at an increased risk of a disease or disorder. Those identified are sometimes then offered a subsequent diagnostic test or procedure, or, in some instances, a treatment or preventive medication.[1] Looking for additional illnesses in those with medical problems is termed case finding;[2,3] screening is limited to those apparently well.

Screening can improve health. For example, strong indirect evidence lends support to cytology screening for cervical cancer. Insufficient use of this screening method accounts for a large proportion of invasive cervical cancers in industrialised nations.[4] Other beneficial examples include screening for hypertension in adults; screening for hepatitis B virus antigen, HIV-1, and syphilis in pregnant women; routine urine culture in pregnant women at 12–16 weeks' gestation; and measurement of phenylalanine in newborns.[5] However, inappropriate screening harms healthy individuals and squanders precious resources. The nearly universal antenatal screening

for gestational diabetes (a diagnosis in search of a disease)[6] in the USA[7] exemplifies the widespread confusion about the nature and aim of screening. Here, we review the purposes of screening, the selection of tests, measurement of validity, the effect of prevalence on test outcome, and several biases that can distort interpretation of tests.

Ethical implications

What are the potential harms of screening?

Screening differs from the traditional clinical use of tests in several important ways. Ordinarily, patients consult with clinicians about complaints or problems; this prompts testing to confirm or exclude a diagnosis.[8] Because the patient is in pain and requests our help, the risk and expense of tests are usually deemed acceptable by the patient. By contrast, screening engages apparently healthy individuals who are not seeking medical help (and who might prefer to be left alone). Alternatively, consumer-generated demand for screening, such as for osteoporosis and ovarian cancer, might lead to expensive programmes of no clear value.[5,9] Hence, the cost, injury, and stigmatisation related to screening are especially important (though often ignored in our zeal for earlier diagnosis); the medical and ethical standards of screening should be, correspondingly, higher than with diagnostic tests.[10] Bluntly put: every adverse outcome of screening is iatrogenic and entirely preventable.

Screening has a darker side that is often overlooked.[2] It can be inconvenient (the O'Sullivan screen for gestational diabetes), unpleasant (sigmoidoscopy or colonoscopy), and

Lancet 2002; **359**: 881–84

Family Health International, PO Box 13950, Research Triangle Park, NC 27709, USA (D A Grimes MD, K F Schulz PhD)

Correspondence to: Dr David A Grimes
(e-mail: dgrimes@fhi.org)

expensive (mammography). For example, a recent Markov model revealed that new screening tests for cervical cancer that are more sensitive than the Papanicolaou test (and thus touted as being better) will drive up the average cost of detecting an individual with cancer.[11] Paradoxically, these higher costs could make screening unattainable by poor women who are at highest risk.[4] The net effect might be more instances of cancer.

A second wave of injury can arise after the initial screening insult: false-positive results and true-positive results leading to dangerous interventions.[2] Although the stigma associated with correct labeling of people as ill might be acceptable, those incorrectly labeled as sick suffer as well. For example, labeling productive steelworkers as being hypertensive led to increased absenteeism and adoption of a sick role, independent of treatment.[12,13] More recently, women labeled as having gestational diabetes reported deterioration in their health and that of their infants over the 5 years after diagnosis.[14] By what right do clinicians rob people of their perceived health, and for what gain?[2]

Screening can also lead to harmful treatment. Treatment of hyperlipidaemia with clofibrate several decades ago provides a sobering example. Treatment of the cholesterol count (a risk factor, rather than an illness itself) inadvertently led to a 17% increase in mortality among middle-aged men given the drug.[2] This screening misadventure cost the lives of more than 5000 men in the USA alone.[2] Because of these mishaps, reviews of screening practices have recommended that clinicians be more selective.[5,15]

Criteria for screening
If a test is available, should it be used?
The availability of a screening test does not imply that it should be used. Indeed, before screening is done, the strategy must meet several stringent criteria. One checklist separates criteria in three parts: the disease, the policy, and the test.[1] The disease should be medically important and clearly defined, and its prevalence reasonably well known. The natural history should be known, and an effective intervention must exist. Concerning policy, the screening programme must be cost effective, facilities for diagnosis and treatment must be readily available, and the course of action after a positive result must be generally agreed on and acceptable to those screened. Finally, the test must do its job. It should be safe, have a reasonable cut-off level defined, and be both valid and reliable. The latter two terms, often used interchangeably, are distinct. Validity is the ability of a test to measure what it sets out to measure, usually differentiating between those with and without the disease. By contrast, reliability indicates repeatability. For example, a bathroom scale that consistently measures 2 kg heavier than a hospital scale (the gold standard) provides an invalid but highly reliable result.

Although an early diagnosis generally has intuitive appeal, earlier might not always be better. For example, what benefit would accrue (and at what cost) from early diagnosis of Alzheimer's disease, which to date has no effective treatment?

Sackett and colleagues[2] have proposed a pragmatic checklist to help decide when (or if) seeking a diagnosis earlier than usual is worth the expense and bother. Does early diagnosis really benefit those screened; for example, in survival or quality of life? Can the clinician manage the additional time required to confirm the diagnosis and deal with those diagnosed before symptoms developed? Will those diagnosed earlier comply with the proposed treatment? Has the effectiveness of the screening strategy been established objectively?[5,15] Finally, are the cost, accuracy, and acceptability of the test clinically acceptable?

Assessment of test effectiveness
Is the test valid?
For over half a century,[16] four indices of test validity have been widely used: sensitivity, specificity, and predictive values of positive and negative. Although clinically useful (and far improved over clinical hunches), these terms are predicated on an assumption that is often clinically unrealistic—ie, that all people can be dichotomised as ill or well. (Indeed, one definition of an epidemiologist is a person who sees the entire world in a 2 × 2 table.) Often, those tested simply do not fit neatly into these designations: they might be possibly ill, early ill, probably well, or some other variant. Likelihood ratios, which incorporate varying (not just dichotomous) degrees of test results, can be used to refine clinicians' judgments about the probability of disease in a particular person.

For simplicity, however, assume a population has been tested and assigned to the four mutually exclusive cells in figure 1. Sensitivity, sometimes termed the detection rate,[10] is

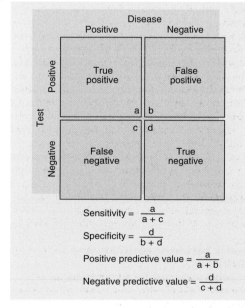

Figure 1 Template for calculation of test validity.

the ability of a test to find those with the disease. All those with disease are in the left column. Hence, the sensitivity is simply those correctly identified by the test (a) divided by all those sick (a+c). Specificity denotes the ability of a test to identify those without the condition. Calculation of this proportion is trickier, however. By analogy to sensitivity, many assume (incorrectly) that the formula here is b/(b+d). However, the numerator for specificity is cell d (the true negatives), which is divided by all those healthy (b+d).

Although sensitivity and specificity are of interest to public-health policymakers, they are of little use to the clinician. Stated alternatively, sensitivity and specificity (population measures) look backward (at results gathered over time).[8] Clinicians have to interpret test results to those tested. Thus, what clinicians need to know are the predictive values of the test (individual measures, which look forward). To consider predictive values, one needs to shift the orientation in figure 1 by 90 degrees: predictive values work horizontally (rows), not vertically (columns). In the top row are all those with a positive test, but only those in cell a are sick. Thus, the predictive value positive is a/(a+b). The "odds of being affected given a positive result (OAPR)" is the ratio of true positives to false positives, or a to b.[10] For example, in figure 1, the OAPR is 75/5, or 17/1. This corresponds to a positive predictive value of 89%. Advocates of use of the OAPR note that these odds better describe test effectiveness than do probabilities (predictive values). In the bottom row of figure 1 are those with negative tests, but only those in cell d are free of disease. Hence, the predictive value negative is d/(c+d).

Learning (and promptly forgetting) these formulas was an annual ritual for many of us in our clinical training. If readers understand the definitions above and can recall the 2 × 2 table shell, then they can quickly figure out these formulas when needed. As a mnemonic, disease goes at the top of the table shell, since it is our top priority. By default, test goes on the left border.

Through the years, researchers have tried to simplify these four indices of test validity by condensing them into a single term.[8] However, none adequately depicts the important trade-offs between sensitivity and specificity that generally arise. An example is diagnostic accuracy, which is the proportion of correct results.[3] It is the sum of the correctly identified ill and well divided by all those tested, or (a+d)/(a+b+c+d). Cells b and c are noise in the system. Another early attempt, Youden's J, is simply the predictive value positive plus the predictive value negative minus one.[17] The range of values extends from zero (for a coin toss with no predictive value) to 1.0, where predictive values of both positive and negative tests are perfect.

Trade-offs between sensitivity and specificity
Where should the cut-off for abnormal be?
The ideal test would perfectly discriminate between those with and without the disorder. The distributions of test results for the two groups would not overlap. More commonly

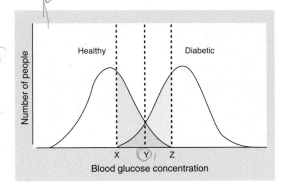

Figure 2 Hypothetical distribution of blood glucose concentrations in people with and without diabetes. Setting cut-off for abnormal at X yields perfect sensitivity at the expense of specificity. Setting cut-off at Z results in perfect specificity at the cost of lower sensitivity. Cut-off Y is a compromise.

in human biology, test values for those with and without a disease overlap, sometimes widely.[18] Where one puts the cut-off defining normal versus abnormal determines the sensitivity and specificity. For any continuous outcome measurement—for example, blood pressure, intraocular pressure, or blood glucose—the sensitivity and specificity of a test will be inversely related. Figure 2 shows that placing the cut-off for abnormal blood glucose at point X produces perfect sensitivity; this low cut-off identifies all those with diabetes. However, the trade-off is poor specificity: those in the part of the healthy distribution in pink and purple are incorrectly identified as having abnormal values. Placing the cut-off higher at point Z yields the opposite result: all those healthy are correctly identified (perfect specificity), but the cost here is missing a proportion of ill individuals (portion of the diabetic distribution in purple and blue). Placing the cutoff at point Y is a compromise, mislabeling some healthy people and some people with diabetes.

Where the cut-off should be depends on the implications of the test, and receiver-operator characteristic curves are useful in making this decision.[19] For example, screening for phenylketonuria in newborns places a premium on sensitivity rather than on specificity; the cost of missing a case is high, and effective treatment exists. The downside is a large number of false-positive tests, which cause anguish and further testing. By contrast, screening for breast cancer should favour specificity over sensitivity, since further assessment of those tested positive entails costly and invasive biopsies.[20]

Prevalence and predictive values
Can test results be trusted?
A badly understood feature of screening is the potent effect of disease prevalence on predictive values. Clinicians must know the approximate prevalence of the condition of interest in the population being tested; if not, reasonable interpretation is impossible. Consider a new PCR test for

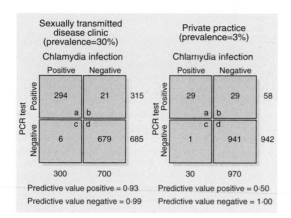

Figure 3 Predictive values of a PCR test for *Chlamydia trachomatis* in high-prevalence and low-prevalence settings.

chlamydia, with a sensitivity of 0.98 and specificity of 0.97 (a superb test). As shown in the left panel of figure 3, a doctor uses the test in a municipal sexually transmitted disease clinic, where the prevalence of *Chlamydia trachomatis* is 30%. In this high-prevalence setting, the predictive value of a positive test is high, 93%—ie, 93% of those with a positive test actually have the infection.

Impressed with the new test, the doctor now takes it to her private practice in the suburbs, which has a clientele that is mostly older than age 35 years (figure 3, right panel). Here, the prevalence of chlamydial infection is only 3%. Now the same excellent test has a predictive positive value of only 0.50. When the results of the test are positive, what should the doctor tell the patient, and what, in turn, should the patient tell her husband? Here, flipping a coin has the same predictive positive value (and is considerably cheaper and simpler than searching for bits of DNA). This message is important, yet not widely understood: when used in low-prevalence settings, even excellent tests have poor predictive positive value. The reverse is true for negative predictive values, which are nearly perfect in figure 3. Although failing to diagnose sexually transmitted diseases can have important health implications, incorrectly labeling people as infected can wreck marriages and damage lives.

Tests in combination
Should a follow-up test be done?
Clinicians rarely use tests in isolation. Few tests have high sensitivity and specificity, so a common approach is to do tests in sequence. In the instance of syphilis, a sensitive (but not specific) reagin test is the initial screen. Those who test positive then get a second, more specific test, a diagnostic treponemal test. Only those who test positive on both receive the diagnosis. This strategy generally increases the specificity

compared with a single test and limits the use of the more expensive treponemal test.[20] Testing for HIV-1 is an analogous two-step procedure.

Alternatively, tests can be done in tandem (parallel or simultaneous testing).[3,21] For example, two different tests might both have poor sensitivity, but one might be better at picking up early disease, whereas the other is better at identifying late disease. A positive result from either test would then lead to diagnostic assessment. This approach results in higher sensitivity than would arise with either test used alone.

Benefit or bias?
Does a screening programme really improve health?
Even worthless screening tests seem to have benefit.[2] This cruel irony underlies many inappropriate screening programmes used today. Two common pitfalls lead to the conclusion that screening improves health; one is an artifact and the other a reflection of biology.

Lead-time bias
Lead-time bias refers to a spurious increase in longevity associated with screening. For example, assume that mammography screening leads to cancer detection 2 years earlier than would have ordinarily occurred, yet the screening does not prolong life. On average, women with breast cancer detected through screening live 2 years longer than those with cancers diagnosed through traditional means. This gain in longevity is apparent and not real: this hypothetical screening allows women to live 2 years longer with the knowledge that they have cancer, but does not prolong survival, an example of zero-time shift.[2]

Length bias
Length bias is more subtle than lead-time bias: the longevity association is real, but indirect. Assume that community-based mammography screening is done at 10-year intervals. Women whose breast cancers were detected through screening live 5 years longer on average from cancer initiation to death than those whose cancers were detected through usual means. That screening is associated with longer survival implies clear benefit. However, in this hypothetical example, this benefit indicates the inherent variability in cancer growth rates and not a benefit of screening. Women with indolent, slow-growing cancers are more likely to live long enough to be identified in decennial screening. Conversely, those with rapidly progressing tumours are less likely to survive until screening.

The only way to avoid these pervasive biases is to do randomised controlled trials and then to assess age-specific mortality rates for those screened versus those not screened.[10] Moreover, the trials must be done well. The quality of published trials of mammography screening has raised serious questions about the utility of this massive and hugely expensive enterprise.[22–24]

Conclusion
Screening can promote or impair health, depending on its application. Unlike a diagnostic test, a screening test is done

Originally published in *The Lancet* 2002; **259**: 881–4. Reproduced with permission.

in apparently healthy people, which raises unique ethical concerns. Sensitivity and specificity tend to be inversely related, and choice of the cut-off point for abnormal should indicate the implications of incorrect results. Even very good tests have poor predictive value positive when applied to low-prevalence populations.

Lead-time and length bias exaggerate the apparent benefit of screening programmes, underscoring the need for rigorous assessment in randomised controlled trials before use of screening programmes.

Acknowledgments

We thank Willard Cates and David L Sackett for their helpful comments on an earlier version of this report. Much of this material stems from our 15 years of teaching the Berlex Foundation Faculty Development Course.

References

1 Cuckle HS, Wald NJ. Principles of screening. In: Antenatal and neonatal screening. Oxford: Oxford University Press, **1984**: 1–22.

2 Sackett DL, Haynes RB, Guyatt GH, Tugwell P. Clinical epidemiology: a basic science for clinical medicine, 2nd edn. Boston: Little, Brown and Company, 1991.

3 Lang TA, Secic M. How to report statistics in medicine. Philadelphia: American College of Physicians, 1997.

4 Sawaya GF, Grimes DA. New technologies in cervical cytology screening: a word of caution. *Obstet Gynecol* 1999; **94**: 307–10.

5 US Preventive Services Task Force. Guide to clinical preventive services, 2nd edn. Baltimore: Williams and Wilkins, 1996.

6 Enkin M, Keirse MJNC, Neilson J, et al (eds). A guide to effective care in pregnancy and childbirth, 3rd edn. Oxford: Oxford University Press, 2000.

7 Gabbe S, Hill L, Schmidt L, Schulkin J. Management of diabetes by obstetrician–gynecologists. *Obstet Gynecol* 1998; **91**: 643–47.

8 Feinstein AR. Clinical biostatistics XXXI: on the sensitivity, specificity, and discrimination of diagnostic tests. *Clin Pharmacol Ther* 1975; **17**: 104–16.

9 NIH Consensus Development Panel on Ovarian Cancer. Ovarian cancer: screening, treatment, and follow-up. *JAMA* 1995; **273**: 491–97.

10 Wald N, Cuckle H. Reporting the assessment of screening and diagnostic tests. *Br J Obstet Gynaecol* 1989; **96**: 389–96.

11 Myers ER, McCrory DC, Subramanian S, et al. Setting the target for a better cervical screening test: characteristics of a cost-effective test for cervical neoplasia screening. *Obstet Gynecol* 2000; **96**: 645–52.

12 Haynes RB, Sackett DL, Taylor DW, Gibson ES, Johnson AL. Increased absenteeism from work after detection and labeling of hypertensive patients. *N Engl J Med* 1978; **299**: 741–44.

13 Taylor DW, Haynes RB, Sackett DL, Gibson ES. Longterm follow-up of absenteeism among working men following the detection and treatment of their hypertension. *Clin Invest Med* 1981; **4**: 173–77.

14 Feig DS, Chen E, Naylor CD. Self-perceived health status of women three to five years after the diagnosis of gestational diabetes: a survey of cases and matched controls. *Am J Obstet Gynecol* 1998; **178**: 386–93.

15 Canadian Task Force on the Periodic Health Examination. The Canadian guide to clinical preventive care. Ottowa: Minister of Supply and Services Canada, 1994.

16 Yerushalmy J. Statistical problems in assessing methods of medical diagnosis, with special reference to X-ray techniques. *Pub Health Rep* 1947; **62**: 1432–49.

17 Youden WJ. Index for rating diagnostic tests. *Cancer* 1950; **3**: 32–35.

18 Griffith CS, Grimes DA. The validity of the postcoital test. *Am J Obstet Gynecol* 1990; **162**: 615–20.

19 Begg CB. Biases in the assessment of diagnostic tests. *Stat Med* 1987; **6**: 411–23.

20 Hennekens CH, Buring JE. Epidemiology in medicine. Boston: Little, Brown and Company, 1987.

21 Riegelman RK, Hirsch RP. Studying a study and testing a test, 2nd edn. Boston: Little, Brown and Company, 1989.

22 Gotzsche PC, Olsen O. Is screening for breast cancer with mammography justifiable? *Lancet* 2000; **355**: 129–34.

23 Olsen O, Gotzsche PC. Cochrane review on screening for breast cancer with mammography. *Lancet* 2001; **358**: 1340–42.

24 Horton R. Screening mammography: an overview revisited. *Lancet* 2001; **358**: 1284–85.

Diagnostic accuracy of clinical examination for detection of non-cephalic presentation in late pregnancy: cross sectional analytic study

Natasha Nassar, Christine L Roberts, Carolyn A Cameron, Emily C Olive

Abstract

Objective   To examine the diagnostic accuracy of clinical examination to determine fetal presentation in late pregnancy.

Design   Cross sectional analytic study with index test of clinical examination and reference standard of ultrasonography.

Setting   Antenatal clinic in tertiary obstetric hospital in Sydney, Australia.

Participants   1633 women with a singleton pregnancy between 35 and 37 weeks' gestation attending antenatal clinics.

Intervention   Fetal presentation assessed by clinical examination during routine antenatal care, followed by ultrasonography to confirm the diagnosis.

Main outcome measures   Sensitivity, specificity, and positive and negative predictive values of clinical examination compared with ultrasonography. Diagnostic rates by maternal characteristics.

Results   Ultrasonography identified non-cephalic presentation in 130 (8%) women, comprising 103 (6.3%) with breech and 27 (1.7%) with transverse or oblique lie. Sensitivity of clinical examination for detecting non-cephalic presentation was 70% (95% confidence interval 62% to 78%) and specificity was 95% (94% to 96%). The positive predictive value and negative predictive value were 55% and 97%, respectively.

Conclusions   Clinical examination is not sensitive enough for detection and timely management of non-cephalic presentation.

Introduction

Antenatal detection of non-cephalic presentation—comprising breech presentation and transverse or oblique lie—in late pregnancy is important for timely management and clinical decision making. For breech presentation, women and their clinicians must decide whether to try external cephalic version to increase the likelihood of vaginal birth or plan a caesarean section, with optimal gestation being 37 and 39 weeks, respectively.[1] Diagnosis of non-cephalic presentation after the onset of labour is associated with increased maternal and infant morbidity and mortality.[2]

Fetal presentation is generally assessed by palpating the abdomen (clinical examination), though we do not know the accuracy of this in late pregnancy.[3–6] We conducted a cross sectional analytic study to compare clinical examination with the reference standard of ultrasonography.

Methods

Patients, setting, and data collection

We carried out the study at an antenatal clinic in a tertiary obstetric hospital between September 2003 and December 2004. Women with a singleton pregnancy at 35–37 weeks' gestation were eligible. A midwife, resident, registrar, or obstetrician, all of whom were aware of the study, provided routine antenatal care. All eligible women underwent clinical examination to assess fetal presentation. Subsequently, those who consented to participate underwent ultrasonography to confirm the diagnosis. The ultrasound examination was conducted with a portable hand held machine following a standard protocol. The operators were blinded to the result of the clinical examination until after the ultrasonography.

We collected data from the antenatal record and recorded it von a standard data abstraction form. We assessed the accuracy of clinical examination in diagnosing fetal presentation by calculating sensitivity specificity, and positive and negative predictive values.

Editorial by Nicholson

Centre for Perinatal Health Services Research, School of Public Health, University of Sydney NSW 2006, Australia

Natasha Nassar *research associate*
Christine L Roberts *research director*
Carolyn A Cameron *research associate*
Emily C Olive *research fellow in obstetrics*

Correspondence to: N Nassar
(email: natashan@ichr.uwa.edu.au)

This article was posted on bmj.com on 4 August 2006:
http://bmj.com/cgi/doi/10.1136/bmj.38919.681563.4F

Originally published in *BMJ* 2006; **333**: 578–80. Reproduced with permission.

Sensitivity and specificity (as %) of clinical examination for detecting fetal presentation

Characteristic	Non-cephalic, correctly diagnosed		Cephalic, correctly diagnosed	
	No. of cases	Sensitivity (95% CI)	No. of cases	Specificity (95% CI)
Overall	91/130	70 (62 to 78)	1429/1503	95 (94 to 96)
Maternal age (years):				
<35	55/84	65 (64 to 66)	1100/1158	95 (94 to 96)
≥35	34/44	77 (75 to 79)	319/336	95 (94 to 96)
Gestational age (weeks):				
34–35	32/41	78 (76 to 80)	316/343	92 (91 to 93)
36	29/44	66 (64 to 68)	492/512	96 (95 to 97)
37–38	28/43	65 (63 to 67)	615/641	96 (95 to 97)
Parity:				
Nulliparous	49/73	67 (65 to 68)	779/820	95 (94 to 96)
Multiparous	42/57	74 (72 to 75)	643/677	95 (94 to 96)
Body mass index:				
Thin	9/13	69 (62 to 76)	109/115	95 (94 to 96)
Normal weight	49/67	73 (72 to 74)	862/898	96 (95 to 97)
Overweight	19/28	68 (65 to 71)	234/241	97 (96 to 98)
Obese	3/8	38 (26 to 49)	139/156	89 (88 to 90)
Country of birth:				
Australia/New Zealand/Europe	52/72	72 (71 to 73)	855/900	95 (94 to 96)
Asia	18/39	46 (67 to 72)	407/424	96 (95 to 97)
Other	8/11	69 (37 to 54)	144/152	95 (94 to 96)

Numbers may not add up to totals because of missing data.

Sample size and analysis

To determine a sensitivity of 75% (with a 95% confidence interval plus or minus 10%) we required 100 women with a breech presentation. As 6–8% of singleton pregnancies are breech at 35–37 weeks' gestation,[7] we needed between 1250 and 1700 women to gain a sample of 100 with a breech presentation. We investigated predictive factors associated with correct diagnosis of fetal presentation using contingency tests and used sensitivity analyses to examine specific accuracy rates by maternal characteristics. $P<0.05$ was considered significant and analyses were conducted with SAS version 8.2 (SAS Institute, Cary, NC).

Results

Of the 1707 eligible women approached, 65 women refused to take part because of lack of time or concern about having had too many ultrasound examinations during their pregnancy, and nine women were excluded owing to missing data. The average age of the 1633 participating women was 31 years (SD 5.4); 55% were nulliparous; 31% were overweight or obese; and 61% were white. Over 60 care providers participated, with 55% of examinations performed by residents or registrars, 28% by midwives, and 17% by obstetricians.

Ultrasonography identified non-cephalic presentation in 130 (8%) women, comprising 103 (6.3%) with breech and 27 (1.7%) with transverse or oblique lie. The sensitivity of clinical examination for identifying non-cephalic presentation was 70% and specificity was 95% (table). A similar rate of sensitivity was found for breech presentation (70%, 61% to 78%). The positive and negative predictive values were 55% and 97%, respectively

The sensitivity of clinical examination for determining non-cephalic presentation was not associated with any particular maternal characteristics, but there was a trend of increasing sensitivity for women with a previous pregnancy (multiparous) and lower body mass index (table). The proportion of women in whom cephalic presentation was correctly diagnosed (specificity) was significantly greater with increasing gestational age and decreasing body mass index ($P < 0.05$) (table).

Discussion

In this large study in a general maternity population we found that clinical examination was, generally, not sensitive enough to accurately diagnose fetal presentation in late pregnancy. Although clinical examination increased the probability of diagnosis from 8% (prior probability or prevalence) to 55% (posterior probability or positive predictive value),[8] only 70% of non-cephalic presentations were detected. If we apply our findings to a general maternity population of 1000 women, clinical examination would identify 101 women as having a non-cephalic presentation but in only 56 would this be correct; and 24 women with non-cephalic presentation would be missed altogether.

Originally published in *BMJ* 200w6; **333**: 578–80. Reproduced with permission.

Strengths and limitations of the study

We included a large unselected sample and used appropriate timing of the clinical examination relevant for management of non-cephalic presentation in late pregnancy. Previous reports of the sensitivity of clinical examination for detecting non-cephalic presentation have ranged from 28–88%. These studies were small, underpowered, and included selected high risk pregnancies and low gestational ages (range 20–42 weeks).[3–6] Our observed prevalence of non-cephalic presentation was consistent with rates found in longitudinal studies of fetal presentation,[9] suggesting that our findings may be applied in other obstetric settings.

We did not collect information on individual clinicians and were unable to ascertain whether particular individuals may have biased results. As all examiners were aware of the study and assessments were recorded and verified, we assumed that assessors would be vigilant. Nevertheless, it is possible that some clinicians may not have been as attentive because diagnoses were going to be checked with ultrasonography.

Room for improvement

Introduction of routine ultrasonography to assess fetal presentation in late pregnancy would improve diagnostic accuracy. However, costs, resource availability, and feasibility need to be considered, as well as the potential deskilling of care providers in performing clinical examination. A cost effectiveness analysis would be necessary before implementation and change in clinical obstetric practice. However, lower rates of accuracy found among overweight or obese women suggest that formal ultrasonography in late pregnancy for these women is required.

Clinical examination to assess fetal presentation is a relatively simple procedure and, with ongoing diligence and regular audit and feedback, accuracy may be increased. Variability in accuracy rates by examiner and level of experience also suggest there is room for improvement by all pregnancy care providers.[3,5,10]

What is already known on this topic

There is limited information about the accuracy of clinical examination for detection of fetal presentation in late pregnancy.

What this study adds

Compared with ultrasonography, the sensitivity of clinical examination is inadequate for detection and timely management of non-cephalic presentation.

We thank the staff and the women at Royal Prince Alfred Women and Babies Hospital who participated in the study for their time and cooperation. We particularly thank Hala Phipps, Sarah Charlton, and Julie Bedford for recruiting women and performing the ultrasound examinations.

Contributors: See bmj.com.

Funding: Australian National Health and Medical Research Council (NHMRC) project grant (211051). NN was funded by an Australian NHMRC Public Health Postgraduate Research Scholarship. CLR was funded by an Australian NHMRC Public Health Practitioner Fellowship.

Competing interests: None declared.

Ethical approval: Approved by the Central Sydney Area Health Service Research Ethics Committee (Protocol number: X03-0185).

References

1 Hofmeyr GJ, Kulier R. External cephalic version for breech presentation at term. *Cochrane Database Syst Rev* 2000; 2: CD000083.

2 Waterstone M, Bewley S, Wolfe C. Incidence and predictors of severe obstetric morbidity: case-control study. *BMJ* 2001; 322:1089–93.

3 Watson WJ, Welter S, Day D. Antepartum identification of breech presentation. *J Reprod Med* 2004;49:294–6.

4 Thorp JM Jr, Jenkins T, Watson W. Utility of Leopold maneuvers in screening for malpresentation. *Obstet Gynecol* 1991; 78:394–6.

5 McFarlin BL, Engstrom JL, Sampson MB, Cattledge F. Concurrent validity of Leopold's maneuvers in determining fetal presentation and position. *J Nurse Midwifery* 1985;30:280–4.

6 Lydon-Rochelle M, Albers L, Gorwoda J, Craig E, Qualls C. Accuracy of Leopold maneuvers in screening for malpresentation: a prospective study. *Birth* 1993;20:132–5.

7 Roberts CL, Nassar N, Raynes-Greenow CH, Peat B. Update on the management of term breech deliveries in NSW, Australia. *Aust N Z J Obstet Gynaecol* 2003;43:173.

8 Altman DG, Bland JM. Diagnostic tests 2: predictive values. *BMJ* 1994;309:102.

9 Scheer K, Nubar J. Variation of fetal presentation with gestational age. *Am J Obstet Gynecol* 1976;125:269–70.

10 Nassar N. Breech presentation: facilitating informed decision-making [dissertation]. Sydney, NSW: University of Sydney, 2005.

Originally published in *BMJ* 2006; 333: 578–80. Reproduced with permission.

Answers

Answers to guide quizzes

Unit 1: C, B, D, A
Unit 2: B, A, C, D
Unit 3: B, C, D, D
Unit 4: D, C, A, D
Unit 5: B, D, C, B
Unit 6: B, A, C, B
Unit 7: C, B, D, D
Unit 8: A, C, B, D
Unit 9: D, B, D, A
Unit 10: C, B, B, D

Answers to exercises

Unit 1

Table 1.1 Mean and 95% CI cognitive scores at baseline in 1394 women with type 2 diabetes

	N	Mean	SD	SE	Lower 95% CI	Upper 95% CI
TICS (8–41 points)	1394	33.2	2.9	0.08	33.1	33.4
TICS 10 word list	1394	2.0	1.9	0.05	1.9	2.1
East Boston memory test – immediate recall	1394	9.3	1.8	0.05	9.2	9.4
East Boston memory test – delayed recall	1394	8.9	2.1	0.06	8.8	9.0

- What factors influence the 95% confidence intervals and in what way?

Confidence intervals are influenced by the precision with which the summary statistic has been measured as estimated by the standard error, and the size of the standard error is directly influenced by sample size. Thus, as the sample size increases, the confidence intervals become smaller for the same mean value and standard deviation. Similarly, the confidence intervals become larger as the sample size decreases.

• Why are the confidence intervals so narrow?

In Table 1.1 the confidence intervals are narrow because the sample size at 1394 participants is large.

Table 1.2 Mean and 95% CI cognitive scores at baseline in 50 women with type 2 diabetes

	N	Mean	SD	SE	Lower 95% CI	Upper 95% CI
TICS (8–41 points)	50	33.2	2.9	0.41	32.4	34.0
TICS 10 word list	50	2.0	1.9	0.27	1.5	2.5
East Boston memory test – immediate recall	50	9.3	1.8	0.25	8.8	9.8
East Boston memory test – delayed recall	50	8.9	2.1	0.30	8.3	9.5

• What happens to the 95% confidence intervals when the sample size is smaller?

The means and standard deviations in this table are the same as those in Table 1.1, however, because the sample size is smaller (only a subset of 50 participants are included in this analysis), the standard errors around the estimates and the 95% confidence intervals are consequently larger.

• Why does this happen?

The precision of an estimate based on a small sample is less than the precision of an estimate based on a large sample. Consequently, the range or width of the confidence interval increases as the sample size decreases because we are less certain of the approximation of the sample mean to the true population mean.

Unit 2

Table 2.4 Prevalence rates and 95% CI

	Number positive	Total number	P	Prevalence (95% CI)
Prevalence rate 1	187	428	0.44	43.7 (38.9 to 48.5)
Prevalence rate 2	90	428	0.21	21.0 (17.2 to 24.9)
Prevalence rate 3	150	428	0.35	35.0 (30.5 to 39.6)
Prevalence rate 4	165	428	0.39	38.6 (33.9 to 43.2)

• If the four prevalence rates had been collected at yearly intervals over a 4 year period, what inferences could be made about significant differences between them by comparing the confidence intervals?

The decrease in prevalence rate from year 1 (rate 1) to year 2 (rate 2) is significantly different because there is no overlap between the range of the two 95% confidence intervals. The increase from year 2 (rate 2) to year 3 (rate 3) would represent a significant increase over the 12 month period since the 95% confidence intervals for the rates do not overlap with each other. The change in prevalence between year 3 (rate 3) and year 4 (rate 4) would not be statistically significant because there is substantial overlap of the 95% confidence intervals.

Unit 3

Grade of tetanus on day 6 by treatment group

	Grade III or IV tetanus	Grade I or II tetanus	Total
Treatment (study) group	7 (15%)	39 (85%)	46
Control group	29 (56%)	23 (44%)	52
Total	36	62	98

Contingency table for tetanus grade I–II and tetanus grade III–IV on day 6

Observed (O)	Row total	Column total	Total sample size	Expected (E)	O–E	$(O–E)^2/E$
7	46	36	98	16.90	−9.90	5.80
39	46	62	98	29.10	9.90	3.37
29	52	36	98	19.10	9.90	5.13
23	52	62	98	32.90	−9.90	2.98
					SUM	17.27

- Is the Pearson's chi-square value statistically significant and consistent with the difference in severity rates between treatment groups?

Yes – a Pearson's chi square value of over 3.84 is statistically significant for a 2×2 table and the value of 17.27 shows a highly significant difference between groups of $P<0.0001$. This occurs because the rate of grade III or IV tetanus is 15% in the treatment group compared to 56% in the control group – a large between-group difference of 41%.

Grade of tetanus on day 6 by treatment group with 25 patients enrolled in each group

	Grade III or IV tetanus	Grade I or II tetanus	Total
Treatment (study) group	4 (15%)	21 (85%)	25
Control group	14 (56%)	11 (44%)	25
Total	25	25	50

Observed (O)	Row total	Column total	Total sample size	Expected (E)	O–E	$(O–E)^2/E$
4	25	18	50	9.00	−5.00	2.78
21	25	32	50	16.00	5.00	1.56
14	25	18	50	9.00	5.00	2.78
11	25	32	50	16.00	−5.00	1.56
					SUM	8.68

- If the number of patients enrolled was 25 in each group with approximately the same percentages and rates as day 6, would the difference in severity rates between groups on day 6 still be statistically significant? Would this result lead you to change the conclusion drawn by the authors?

If 25 patients had been enrolled in each group and the between-group difference remained at 41%, the Pearson's chi square value would be lower at 8.68 with a P value of 0.003. This still indicates a statistically significant difference in severity rates between the groups, but the difference is not as highly significant as when the number of participants was 98. It would be concluded that patients in the study group who were treated with anti-tetanus immunoglobulin by intrathecal and intramuscular routes had a significantly lower rate of grade III or IV tetanus than patients in the control group who were treated by the intramuscular route. This conclusion is consistent with the authors' conclusion, that is, that patients treated with anti-tetanus immunoglobulin by the intrathecal route show better clinical progression than patients treated by the intramuscular route.

Unit 4

Association between redness at 1 day and size of needle

	Redness present	Redness absent	Total
Long thin (23G, 25 mm) needle	15	38	53
Short, wide (25G, 16 mm) needle	36	21	57
Total	51	59	110

Association between redness at 2 days and size of needle

	Redness present	Redness absent	Total
Long thin (23G, 25 mm) needle	5	48	53
Short, wide (25G, 16 mm) needle	22	35	57
Total	51	59	110

Association between redness at 3 days and size of needle

	Redness present	Redness absent	Total
Long thin (23G, 25 mm) needle	2	51	53
Short, wide (25G, 16 mm) needle	16	41	57
Total	18	92	110

Table 4.3 Relative risk and odds ratios for redness over three days

	Protection		Risk	
	Relative risk	Odds ratio	Relative risk	Odds ratio
6 hours	0.66	0.44	1.51	2.25
1 day	0.45	0.23	2.23	4.34
2 days	0.24	0.17	4.09	6.03
3 days	0.13	0.10	7.44	9.95

1 For risk, what can you infer from the estimates of relative risk and odds ratios over time?

The estimates of relative risk and odds ratios follow approximately the same pattern, in that the values of protection and risk increase over time. The estimates suggest that long thin needles not only decrease the short-term risk of redness at 6 hours but have an increasingly protective effect on longer term risk of redness of up to 3 days in infants undergoing routine vaccination. The relative risk of 7.44 suggests that infants are 7 times more likely to have redness at 3 days if a short, wide needle is used.

2 Does the difference between the estimates of relative risk and odds ratios vary with the frequency of the outcome?

The frequency of redness (outcome) in the long thin needle and short wide needle groups respectively is as follows: day 1, 28% vs 63%; day 2, 9% vs 39% and day 3, 4% vs 28%. Odds ratios are unreliable in studies such as this when events are common (say >20%) or when an event rate is high in one group. Thus, at day 1 when the outcome is common in both groups and the control group has an event rate of 63%, the odds ratio for risk is almost double the relative risk. However, at days 2 and 3 when the event rates become lower, the difference between the relative risk and odds ratio becomes smaller in relative terms. It is clear from the columns for risk that the odds ratio always over-estimates the relative risk.

3 Why do you think this happens?

The calculations of the odds ratio and relative risk are different. The odds ratio is the odds of an outcome occurring in one group, divided by the odds of the outcome occurring in another group. The relative risk is the ratio of the probability of an outcome in one group divided by the probability of the outcome in another group. Therefore, the difference between odds ratios and relative risk values depends upon the odds or probability of the outcome in both groups. Only when the outcome occurs infrequently (<10%) will the odds ratio approximate the relative risk.

Unit 5

	Complications	No complications	Total
Study group	33	25	58
Control group	46	16	62
Total	79	41	120

	Respiratory infection	No respiratory infection	Total
Study group	29	29	58
Control group	42	20	62
Total	71	49	120

	Respiratory failure or mechanical failure	No respiratory failure or mechanical failure	Total
Study group	22	36	58
Control group	34	28	62
Total	56	64	120

	Died	Did not die	Total
Study group	4	54	58
Control group	10	52	62
Total	14	106	120

Table 5.3 ARR and NNT for complications and mortality for tetanus by intrathecal and intramuscular route or the intramuscular route

Outcome	CER	EER	ARR	NNT
Complications	0.74	0.57	0.17	5.8
Respiratory infection	0.68	0.50	0.18	5.6
Respiratory failure or mechanical ventilation	0.55	0.38	0.17	5.9
Death	0.16	0.07	0.09	10.8

- How do the NNT values compare and which NNT value would be the most important for deciding which treatment to use?

The NNT values are similar at approximately 6 for complications and respiratory conditions, with a higher NNT value of approximately 11 for death. The most important NNT value to use to decide which treatment is superior would be death, as the patient's life is the primary concern, although more patients would need to receive the treatment to prevent one death than to prevent one complication or respiratory condition. Comparison of the CER and EER rates for death indicates that the occurrence of death is 9% lower in patients treated for tetanus by intrathecal and intramuscular route and this is reflected in the ARR of 0.09.

- In the study, there were 10 deaths in the control group and 4 deaths in the new treatment group. If the reverse had happened, that is, there was 10 deaths in the new treatment group compared to 4 in the control group, what would the NNT be?

	Died	Did not die	Total
Study group	10	48	58
Control group	4	58	62
Total	14	106	120

With 10 deaths in the new treatment group and 4 deaths in the control group the NNT would be −9.27, which is rounded to a whole number, −9. A negative NNT value is equivalent to the number needed to harm (NNH), that is, the number of people who need to be exposed to the risk factor to cause harm to one additional person. A negative NNT indicates that the new study treatment is harmful in that it is less effective than the control group treatment, in this case, anti-tetanus immunoglobulin by the intramuscular route. This value indicates that by treating 9 patients by the intrathecal and intramuscular route, 1 additional patient will die.

- What type of analyses does the paper report (intention-to-treat, available-case analysis or treatment-received)? How does this influence how you would interpret the results?

The authors state that participants who did not complete the therapeutic procedure were analysed according to the group to which they were allocated. For two patients who were assigned to treatment via the intrathecal route, it was not possible for them to be punctured. Therefore, they received treatment by the intramuscular route only but were included in the analysis for the intrathecal group. There is no mention of how any missing outcomes were dealt with. However, since patients were analysed according to the group to which they were allocated regardless of whether they completed the treatment or received only part of the treatment assigned, this suggests that an intention-to-treat analysis was conducted. This type of analysis provides a conservative, unbiased estimate of the treatment effect.

Unit 6

Table 6.2 Other back pain-related NHS contacts for surgery and rehabilitation

	Surgery (N = 176)		Rehabilitation (N = 173)		
	Mean cost (SD)	95% range	Mean cost (SD)	95% range	P value
Surgery outpatient clinics	190 (159)	−128, 508	82 (119)	−156, 320	≤0.001
Physiotherapy outpatient clinics	286 (523)	−760, 1332	301 (584)	−867, 1469	NS
Unplanned hospital admissions	451 (1881)	−3311, 4213	2128 (3522)	−4916, 9172	≤0.001
Other back pain-related hospital admissions	130 (910)	−1690, 1950	73 (555)	−1037, 1183	NS
Total other back pain-related NHS contact costs	1707 (2451)	−3195, 6609	3009 (4001)	−4993, 11011	≤0.001

- Do you think that the SD describes the distribution of the data accurately?

The authors say that cost data is modestly skewed but do not indicate the degree of skewedness. The standard deviations are large indicating a large amount of variation. In fact, the standard deviation is larger than the mean value for all variables (except for surgery outpatient clinics costs for patients who had surgery) and when the 95% ranges are computed they show that the ranges of the data include some large negative (implausible) values. This suggests that the data are quite skewed and, clearly, the standard deviation does not describe the spread of the data accurately. Thus, the standard deviation will not be an accurate measure of variability to use when computing summary statistics or comparing differences between the groups.

- The authors say that skew in the cost data was modest and therefore that parametric confidence intervals were used. However, they do not say how the *P* values in Table 3 were derived. Do you think that the distributions of cost in each group were approximately normal so that a *t*-test could be used to generate valid *P* values?

T-tests are robust to a mild degree of skewness, especially when group sizes are equal. However, computing the 95% range estimates in Table 6.2 suggest that the data are quite skewed and that the standard deviations do not describe the characteristics of the data accurately. In this case, it would be appropriate to use medians and inter-quartile ranges to describe the centre of the data and the range of data values and non-parametric statistics to avoid any bias in *P* values when comparing the groups.

- Are the *P* values reported consistent with the 95% confidence intervals around the mean cost differences in Table 3 in the set article?

A statistically significant mean difference will have a confidence interval that does not contain zero. As can be seen from Table 3 the 95% confidence intervals of the significant mean differences do not contain the value zero and so are consistent with the reported *P* values. Similarly, the 95% confidence intervals of the non-significant mean values do overlap the zero value.

Refer to Figure 1. By comparing the confidence intervals what would you conclude about:

- the between-group differences;

At each time interval, there is considerable overlap of the confidence intervals of the surgical group and rehabilitation group; therefore, there would not be a statistically significant difference between the groups.

- the change in mean utility levels over the period of the study.

Overall, the mean utility levels increase over time, with a minimal change in mean utility between 6 months and 12 months. Comparison of the overlap of the 95% confidence intervals indicates that mean utility levels for the surgery group at 6, 12 and 24 months are significantly higher than at baseline, with no significant difference between mean values at 6, 12 and 24 months. For the rehabilitation group, the mean utility value at baseline only slightly overlaps with the confidence intervals at 6 and 12 months. Therefore, the mean difference from baseline to 6 months and 12 months may be marginally significant but the lack of overlap of 95% confidence intervals between baseline and 24 months shows that the mean utility level at 24 months is significantly higher than at baseline.

Unit 7
Worked Example

Table 7.1 Predicted FVC and per cent predicted FVC

Height (m)	Age (years)	Gender	Measured FVC (L)	Predicted FVC (L)	Per cent predicted FVC (%)
1.50	20	Female	3.8	3.19	119.0
1.74	20	Female	3.8	4.37	87.0
1.50	60	Female	3.8	1.99	190.7
1.74	60	Female	3.8	3.17	120.0
1.58	20	Male	3.8	4.14	91.9
1.82	20	Male	3.8	5.43	70.0
1.58	60	Male	3.8	2.94	129.5
1.82	60	Male	3.8	4.23	89.9

- How would you interpret the coefficient for the binary variable 'gender'?

The positive sign for the coefficient for gender indicates that FVC increases as the coding for gender increases. The coding for gender is female = 0 and male = 1 so the coefficient of 0.59 indicates that on average males have a FVC that is 0.59 L higher than females.

- Are your calculations of predicted FVC in accordance with the signs and sizes of the regression coefficients?

The regression equation indicates that that FVC will be larger for people who are taller, younger or male. The calculation of predicted values for people with given characteristics is shown in Table 7.1. As expected, the highest predicted FVC value is for a tall, young male. In contrast, the lowest predicted FVC value is for a short, older female. The coefficient for height is 0.62 and positive, indicating that FVC increases by 0.62 L for each metre increase in height cubed. For the first two people shown in Table 7.1, they are both female and are the same age, with one female 0.24 m taller. Using the regression equation, the difference for predicted FVC for these two females is 1.18. The contribution of height to FVC for the female who is 1.50 m is 2.10 L (i.e. 0.62×1.50^3) and 3.27 L for the female who is 1.74 m tall, a difference of 1.18 L. Height cubed of these two females is 3.8 m and 5.27 m respectively – a difference of 1.89 m. This difference multiplied by the coefficient of height, 0.62, equals 1.17 L which approximately equals the predicted FVC difference of 1.18 L. Similarly, as the age of the individual increases by one year, the predicted FVC values decrease by 0.03 L and males have a FVC that is 0.59 L higher than females. Therefore, the predicted FVC values are in accordance with the signs and sizes of the regression coefficients.

- What do the estimates of per cent predicted FVC indicate?

Per cent predicted values tell us how close a person is to their predicted value, that is, the mean value in the population of people with the same characteristics. Per cent predicted values close to 100% indicate the person's measured or actual value is very close to his/her predicted value. Per cent predicted values above 100% indicate that a person's actual value is higher than his/her predicted value. Conversely, per cent predicted values lower than 100% indicate that a person's measured value is lower than his/her predicted value. When measuring lung function, low per cent predicted values, for example values less than 80%, are often used in clinical settings to indicate that a person has compromised lung function, for example as a result of a respiratory condition or a history of smoking.

- What clinical importance would you attach to these estimates of per cent predicted FVC?

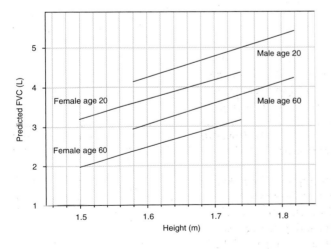

Figure 7.6 Regression lines for predicted FVC values for males and females.

If a model is accurate in that it is based on a large random sample of the population, it can be used in a clinical setting to predict FVC values and develop normal reference values. From the per cent predicted values calculated in Table 7.1, we can conclude that the one person with a predicted FVC of less than 80% has a much lower lung function than other people in the population with the same characteristics and that this may be an indicator of lung disease. However, the other people have a FVC which is close to or higher than their predicted value.

Exercise

• What populations can these results be generalised to?

The results can be generalised only to an infant sample with similar characteristics to the current sample, that is, preterm infants born between 25 and 35 weeks gestation.

• Can the *r* values be compared across the four figures to assess which measure of nutrient intake is the 'best' predictor of faecal E1?

The range of values on either axis influences the size of the correlation coefficient. The correlation coefficient becomes larger and therefore more significant as the range of a variable increases. In the four figures, the range of values is the same on each *x*-axis but each figure has a different range for the *y*-axis. Therefore, the *r* values cannot be compared across the four figures to determine the best predictor of faecal E1.

• Are the measurements displayed correctly on the *x*- and *y*-axis, that is, are the outcome and explanatory variables correctly classified?

The outcome variable is generally plotted on the *y*-axis and the explanatory variable on the *x*-axis. In the graphs of Figure 2, the outcome variable is the amount of faecal pancreatic enzyme elastase 1 which is plotted on the *x*-axis and the explanatory variables are plotted along the *y*–axis, which is counter-intuitive. Regression lines are used in prediction and it seems unlikely that clinicians would want to predict information such as total energy intake from faecal EI.

• Are the lines of best fit that are shown on the figures valid assessments of the relationships given the presentation of the explanatory and outcome variable on the *x*-axis and *y*-axis?

The equation for the lines of best fit would be exactly the same as shown in the figures if the outcome variable was plotted on the *y*-axis and the explanatory variable was plotted on the *x*-axis. However, the regression equations for the figures as shown would provide an estimate of error around the predictor, for example total energy intake, rather than around the outcome, that is faecal EI.

• Do you think that each line meets the assumptions for using regression?

Simple linear regressions are shown and most of the assumptions appear to have been met although it is hard to decide if the relationships are linear, if the residuals are normally distributed or if the variance is constant over the models. The authors would have needed to have ascertained that these assumptions were met during data analyses and to have reported this in the paper. However there is one outlier that appears to be influential and it seems that the lines of best fit would be different if the outlier was removed or recoded to have less influence.

Unit 8

Table 8.5 Mean outcome values at follow-up, effect size and mean difference

Outcome	Surgery group Mean (SD) (n = 176)	Rehabilitation group Mean (SD) (n = 173)	Effect size (SDs)	Mean difference (95% CI)	t- value	P value
Disability index	(n = 138) 34.0 (21.1)	(n =146) 36.1 (20.6)	−0.10	−2.1 (−7.0, 2.8)	0.85	0.40
Shuttle walk	(n = 118) 352 (244)	(n =126) 310 (202)	0.19	42 (−14.1, 98.1)	1.47	0.14
SF-36 physical	(n = 115) 28.8 (14.9)	(n =131) 27.6 (14.6)	0.08	1.2 (−2.5, 4.9)	0.64	0.52
SF-36 mental	47.4 (12.2)	48.1 (12.6)	−0.06	−0.7 (−3.8, 2.4)	0.44	0.66

- What does a negative effect size mean?

A negative effect size means that the treatment resulted in a lower mean outcome in the treatment group compared to the control group. If the outcome is scored so that a higher value means better health, a negative mean difference would indicate an effect that was opposite to the predicted direction. In Table 8.5, the negative effect size of −0.10 SDs for the disability index indicates that the rehabilitation treatment programme had a smaller effect on lower back pain (as measured by the disability index) when compared to surgery.

- Do the P values reflect the effect size between the groups?

An effect size of 0.2 is considered to be a small treatment effect. Therefore, because all of the effect sizes in Table 8.5 are below 0.2 this suggests that there is little difference between the means of the two treatment groups. This is reflected by the P values which are all greater than 0.05 and indicate a non-significant difference between groups.

- Do any of the P values suggest that a type II error has occurred?

The effect sizes are small. If the effect sizes were large and the P values were non-significant, we may judge that a type II error had occurred. In this study, the sample sizes are quite large and the differences have not reached statistical significance because they are small. Therefore, we could conclude that a type II error is unlikely to have occurred.

- How do the P values that you have computed compare with the P values in Table 4 of Fairbank *et al.* (2005)? Can you explain why they are higher or lower?

The P values in Table 8.5 are different – two values are higher and two are lower than the P values reported in Table 4 of the article. The P values computed in the article were derived from an ANCOVA, which adjusted for baseline differences. The P values in Table 8.5 were derived from an independent t-test that does not account for differences at baseline. Whenever different analyses are conducted on the same data, a discrepancy between P values can be expected because the questions being asked are slightly different.

- Do you agree with the authors' interpretation of their data?

The calculated results support the author's conclusion that there is no difference between the treatment groups at the 24-month follow-up.

Unit 9

Table 9.1 Survival at 30 days for neonates, infants and children undergoing bypass surgery

Group	No. of procedures	% survival at 30 days	95% CI	No. of events	Hazard ratio
Neonate	383	87.1	83.7, 90.5	49	5.2
Infant	909	94.4	92.9, 95.9	46	2.0
Child	1353	97.5	96.7, 98.3	34	—
Neonate	30	87.1	75.1, 99.1	4	5.2
Infant	75	94.4	89.2, 99.6	4	2.0
Child	110	97.5	94.6, 100.4	3	—

Table 9.2 Survival at 1 year for neonates, infants and children undergoing bypass surgery

Group	No. of procedures	% survival at 1 year	95% CI	No. of events	Hazard ratio
Neonate	383	82.8	79.0, 86.6	66	4.3
Infant	909	90.0	88.0, 92.0	91	2.5
Child	1353	96.0	95.0, 97.0	54	—
Neonate	30	82.8	69.3, 96.3	5	4.3
Infant	75	90.0	83.2, 96.8	8	2.5
Child	110	96.0	92.3, 99.7	4	—

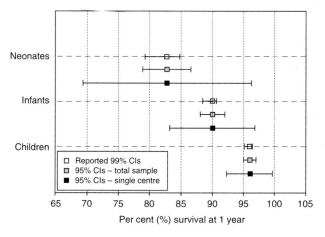

Figure 9.2 Per cent bypass surgery at 1 year with 99% and 95% confidence intervals.

- How do your calculated 95% confidence intervals compare with the 99% confidence intervals reported?

The 99% confidence intervals reported in the article cover a slightly smaller range than the 95% confidence intervals calculated. For example, the 95% confidence interval around the survival rate of 87.1% for neonates at 30 days is 83.7 to 90.5, while the reported 99% confidence interval is 84.3 to 88.4. This is not intuitive because the 99% CIs should indicate a wider range than the 95% CIs because it is a range in which we are less certain that the true population value lies. However, the 99% confidence intervals reported in the article are calculated using the Wilson score method and are asymmetric while the 95% confidence interval calculated in Tables 9.1 and 9.2 are symmetric. It is difficult to make valid comparisons of statistics when they are computed using different methods.

- What happens when the sample size is smaller?

As the sample size gets smaller the confidence intervals become wider for the same summary statistics. This occurs because we have less confidence in the accuracy of the result from a small sample compared to a large sample.

- Would you revise the conclusion about a between-age-group difference if the data from only one centre had been reported?

If data was only collected from one centre the conclusion would be that there is no significant difference between the groups for survival rates. Comparison of the 95% confidence intervals from a single centre indicates that the intervals of three groups overlap, indicating that there are substantial similarities between the groups in terms of survival.

- Could the interpretation of age group differences from the 13 centres or from only 1 centre be regarded as type I or type II error?

The likelihood of a type II error is usually related to the sample size. With data from only one centre, which indicates that there is no significant difference between groups, it is very likely that a type II error might have occurred as a result of insufficient power because of small sample size to show that between-group differences are statistically significant. By combining the data from all 13 centres, the sample size is much larger and the chance of a type II error occurring is reduced. However, as noted by the authors, a total of 178 between-group comparisons were conducted in this report and it is likely that a spuriously significant result was generated simply by chance, that is, a type I error may have occurred.

- The authors report that "For infants, mortality after treatment for heart disease at 1 year was double that at 30 days". From the data presented in the article, how do they reach this conclusion?

At 30 days the mortality rate in infants is 100−94.4 or 5.6% and the mortality rate at 1 year is 100−90 or 10%. Thus, the mortality rate at 1 year is approximately double the mortality rate at 30 days.

- How would you interpret the hazard ratios?

In Table 9.1, the hazard ratio of 5.2 indicates that neonates who had surgery at 30 days had approximately five times the chance of surviving at the next time point compared to older children who had similar surgery. Similarly, the hazard ratio of 2.0 indicates that infants who had surgery at 30 days had approximately twice the chance of surviving at the next time point compared to older children who had similar surgery.

Unit 10

Diagnostic table for detecting fetal presentation for thin participants classified

	Non-cephalic	Cephalic	Total
Examination positive	9	6	15
Examination negative	4	109	113
Total	13	115	128

Diagnostic table for detecting fetal presentation for normal weight participants

	Non-cephalic	Cephalic	Total
Examination positive	49	26	85
Examination negative	18	862	880
Total	67	898	965

Diagnostic table for detecting fetal presentation for overweight participants

	Non-cephalic	Cephalic	Total
Examination positive	19	7	26
Examination negative	9	234	243
Total	28	241	269

Diagnostic table for detecting fetal presentation for obese participants

	Non-cephalic	Cephalic	Total
Examination positive	3	17	20
Examination negative	5	139	144
Total	8	156	164

Table 10.4 PPV, NPV and likelihood ratio for detecting fetal presentation

	Sensitivity	Specificity	PPV	NPV	Likelihood ratio
Overall	0.70	0.95	0.55	0.97	14.0
Body mass index					
Thin	0.69	0.95	60.0	96.5	13.3
Normal weight	0.73	0.96	57.6	98.0	18.2
Overweight	0.68	0.97	73.1	96.3	23.4
Obese	0.38	0.89	15.0	96.5	3.4

- Are the statistics PPV and NPV appropriate to describe diagnostic utility in the sample studied?

The proportion of the sample with and without the disease influences the statistics PPV and NPV. In this sample, there is a large discrepancy between the number of cases presenting with the disease ($n = 1503$) compared to the number who do not have the disease ($n = 130$). Thus, PPV is more likely to be higher in the cephalic group than the non-cephalic group. Therefore, PPV and NPV may not be the appropriate statistics to describe diagnostic utility in this sample.

- What populations would these statistics generalise to?

The statistics PPV and NPV can only be generalised to population samples when they are based on a random population sample. The sample in this paper is recruited from one hospital setting and therefore is likely to be biased in terms of demographic factors such as socioeconomic status etc. The results should only be generalised to other women who attend similar settings.

- Does calculation of the likelihood ratio influence how you would interpret the results of the study?

The likelihood ratios show that the test is most predictive in the group of overweight women. This is the group in whom specificity is also higher than in the other groups.

- Do you agree with the authors' conclusion that an ultrasound is only required to determine fetal position in late pregnancy in overweight and obese women?

The results seem to suggest that the use of ultrasound would be warranted in overweight women in whom there is a high specificity, high PPV and high likelihood ratio. The value of using the test in obese women compared to thin or normal weight women is not so clear.

Glossary

95% confidence interval
Range in which we can be approximately 95% certain that the true population value lies.

Absolute risk reduction (ARR)
The reduction in risk (probability of the outcome) that is conferred by the new treatment.

Available case analysis
Only participants with final study outcomes are included in the data analysis but participants are maintained in the group to which they were allocated. The results may be influenced by bias and confounders.

Censored observations
Used to describe participants who withdraw from the study or who do not experience the outcome of interest.

Chi-square test
A statistic used to test whether the rate of an outcome is significantly different between two or more exposure groups. The test provides a probability that the outcome and the exposure are independent.

Chi-square test for trend
A statistic used to test whether there is a linear trend for an outcome to increase or decrease over the range of an ordered categorical exposure variable.

Control event rate (CER)
The frequency of the outcome in the control (current best practice treatment or placebo) group.

Cross-over trial
A study in which participants receive two or more treatments given consecutively, usually in a random order. The response to the first treatment can be contrasted with the response to the second treatment in the same participants.

Diagnostic test
Test used to confirm disease in people who present with signs or symptoms.

Effect size
The distance between two mean values, described in units of their standard deviations, that describes the relative magnitude of the difference between two groups.

Event
Outcome of interest, which is typically death but can be a non-fatal or favourable outcome, e.g. discharge from hospital.

Experimental event rate (EER)
The frequency of the outcome in the experimental (new treatment) group.

Experimental study
A study which is conducted to test the effect of a treatment or intervention.

Explanatory variable
A characteristic that is hypothesised to influence the outcome variable. In clinical studies the explanatory variable is often the group to which patients have been randomised. In cross-sectional and cohort studies, explanatory variables are often exposure variables.

Gold standard
Test regarded as the most accurate method available for classifying people as disease-positive or -negative.

Hazard ratio
The risk of the event in a study group divided by the risk of the event in a reference group.

Incidence
The number of new cases of a condition that develop in a population during a defined time period.

Independent samples *t*-test
Test to measure whether a continuous outcome variable with a normal distribution is significantly different between two groups, e.g. between male and female or between an intervention and a control group.

Intention-to-treat analysis

All participants are analysed in the group to which they were allocated regardless of subsequent events such as non-compliance or withdrawal from the study. This provides a conservative estimate of treatment effect that is not influenced by confounders.

Kaplan–Meier statistic

Statistic used to compare the event rate over time between two or more study groups. Also called a log-rank test.

Likelihood ratio

Probability of a positive test in a person with the disease compared to the probability of a positive test in a person without disease.

Line of best fit

Regression line through a set of data points calculated to minimise the sums of the squared residuals.

Negative predictive value

Proportion of test-negative people who do not have the disease.

Normal values

Range of values in which the majority of people in a population are expected to lie.

Null hypothesis

A hypothesis stating that there is no difference between the study groups.

Number-needed-to-treat (NNT)

The number of people who need to receive a new treatment to prevent one adverse event occurring.

Observational study

A study which is conducted to measure rates of disease in a population or to measure associations between exposures (risk factors) and disease.

Odds

The probability of an event (p) occurring divided by the probability of that event not occurring ($1-p$).

Odds ratio

Ratio of the odds of the outcome occurring in one group divided by the odds of the outcome occurring in another group.

Outcome variable

The outcome measurement in a study, that is, the variable of interest such as the primary illness or disease status indicator.

Outlier

Data points at the extremities of the range or separated from the normal range of the data values. Data points more than three standard deviations from the mean are usually considered to be outliers.

P value

Probability that a difference between study groups would have occurred if the null hypothesis was true.

Paired t-test

A parametric test that measures whether the means of two related continuous measurements are different from one another, typically measurements taken from the same participants on two occasions.

Parametric statistics

Statistics used when the outcome measurement has a distribution that is approximately normal.

Phase I trial

Initial trial of a new treatment to assess safety and feasibility in a small group of volunteers who do not have the disease or patients with symptoms.

Phase II trial

A clinical trial to measure efficacy, that is, the effect of a treatment under ideal conditions, in patients with the disease.

Phase III trial

Large randomised controlled trial or multi-centre study to measure effectiveness in the community, that is, the effect of a treatment in general clinical practice.

Phase IV surveillance

Post-marketing survey to measure rare adverse events.

Positive predictive value

Proportion of test-positive people who have the disease.

Prevalence

The total number of people in a population with a condition at a given point in time.

r value

Pearson's correlation coefficient that measures the strength of a linear relationship between two continuous normally distributed variables.

r^2

The coefficient of determination is equal to the squared correlation coefficient and provides an estimate of the per cent of variation in one variable that is explained by the other variable.

Random selection

Sample taken from a population in which all people have an equal chance of being selected.

Randomised controlled trial

A study which is conducted to measure whether a new treatment is superior or equivalent to no treatment or an existing treatment and in which participants are randomly allocated to the study groups.

Relative risk

Ratio of the probability of the outcome occurring in the exposed group divided by the probability of the outcome occurring in the non-exposed group.

Residuals

Distance between an observed value and its predicted value, in this case the value predicted by the regression line.

Risk

The probability of an event or outcome occurring, such as the risk of an infection, death or cure.

Screening test

Test used for early identification of disease in a population without symptoms.

Sensitivity

Proportion of disease-positive people who are test-positive.

Specificity

Proportion of disease-negative people who are test-negative.

Standard deviation (SD)

A measure of variability that describes how far the data spreads on either side of the central mean value. The standard deviation is the square root of the variance and therefore is in the same units as the data values.

Standard error (SE)

A measure of the precision with which the mean value has been measured.

Treatment received analysis

Participants are re-grouped according to the treatment they actually received irrespective of the treatment to which they were allocated. Using this method, there is no control of confounders.

***t* value**

A t value, which is calculated by dividing a mean value by its standard error, gives a number from which the probability of the event occurring is estimated from a *t*-distribution. A *t*-distribution is closely related to a normal distribution but depends on the number of cases in the sample.

Type I error

A difference between groups is statistically significant although a clinically important difference does not exist. In this case, the null hypothesis is incorrectly rejected. That is, a difference between groups is statistically significant although a clinically important difference does not exist.

Type II error

A difference between groups is not statistically significant although a clinically important difference exists. In this case, the null hypothesis is incorrectly accepted.

Unpaired *z*-test

Test used to compare the mean values of two independent samples using a normal distribution. This test is only used when the sample size is very large or the mean and standard deviation of the population are known.

Variance

A squared term that describes the total variation in the sample.

Index